KW-249-930

Midwifery

R. G. LAW, MD, FRCOG

Consultant Obstetrician and Gynaecologist, Whittington Hospital, London;
Consultant Gynaecologist, Hornsey Central Hospital, London;
Lecturer in Obstetrics and Gynaecology, Hornsey Central Hospital, London;
Examiner to The Central Midwives Board

M. FRIEDMAN, PhD, MD, MRCP, FRCPE

Consultant Paediatrician, Whittington Hospital; Honorary Consultant Paediatrician,
University College Hospital, London; Lecturer in Paediatrics, University College Hospital
Medical School, London

Staples Press   London

Granada Publishing Limited
First published 1972 by Staples Press
3 Upper James Street London W1R 4BP

Copyright © 1972 by R. G. Law and M. Friedman

All rights reserved. No part of this publication
may be reproduced, stored in a retrieval system,
or transmitted, in any form or by any means,
electronic, mechanical, photocopying, recording
or otherwise, without the prior permission of
the publishers.

ISBN 0 286 62753 1 (board)
ISBN 0 286 11013 X (paper)

Printed in Great Britain
by Richard Clay (The Chaucer Press), Ltd,
Bungay, Suffolk

Physiotherapy Dept.

Duberies Centre.

Midwifery

Foreword

This book has been written with the needs of the student of midwifery very much in mind. The basic principles outlined provide a good foundation of theoretical knowledge to which practical experience can be added.

The authors have always shown great interest in midwifery and obstetric nurse training; and Mr Law, as an examiner of the Central Midwives Board is well aware of the Board's requirements.

The student of midwifery should find this a useful textbook when preparing for examinations.

M. E. Turner, D.N.(Lond), SRN, SCM, MID
Formerly Superintendent Midwife,
Whittington Hospital, London

Acknowledgments

No textbook can ever be written without the help and coopera-
tion of many different people. For this reason it is impossible
for me to acknowledge all those who, in their various ways,
have contributed towards the production of this book. To some,
however, my particular recognition is due. Firstly, to Miss
M. E. Turner and to Miss M. Box, for their invaluable and painstaking comments and criticism of the original draft. Secondly,
to Dr W. G. G. Loyn, for producing so willingly and promptly
the important section on obstetric analgesia and anaesthesia.
Next, to Mr Peter Janson-Smith and Mr Robert Coates for their
help over the many problems inseparable from publication.
Lastly, but very far from least, I would like to thank the many
classes of Pupil Midwives who, over the years, by being kind
enough to listen to my lectures, have really provided the impetus
necessary for starting what has turned out to be a demanding,
time-consuming but completely absorbing work. To these
pupils, past, present and future, this book is gratefully dedicated.

R. G. LAW

Contents

List of Figures

Preface

The Pupil Midwife, on starting her six months' training, is often faced with what appears to be a most confusing situation. The subject she is about to study is one which is to a great extent new to her, involving new concepts, new ideas and a new terminology. In addition, while having to attend lectures, demonstrations and classes, she is also expected to work in the delivery suites, the clinics and the post-natal wards of what is usually an unfamiliar hospital with unfamiliar staff. Over and above this, and due to a large extent to the nature of the obstetric course itself, it is usually impossible for her to start at the beginning of her new subject and work through it systematically. Pregnancy, labour and the puerperium, both normal and abnormal, are hopelessly intermingled and as a result it is often hard for her to see the wood for the trees and to understand the basic objects of obstetrics because of the innumerable problems and difficulties with which she is faced.

All this is to be regretted, the more so since, of all medical specialties, obstetrics is the most logical and the one where a solid grasp of first principles enables almost any problem to be understood and at least partially solved without extensive and detailed knowledge.

It is with this in mind that this book has been written. Its object is to offer the pupil midwife what we believe to be a simpler approach to obstetrics than is provided by more elaborate text-books on the subject. It is not intended to replace these but merely, by serving as an introduction, to make them more understandable and hence more valuable to the pupil as she first approaches this fascinating subject.

PART ONE

Normal Pregnancy

CHAPTER ONE

Introduction

The Objects of Obstetrics

To be logical and straightforward, the approach to obstetrics must start by considering the objects of this branch of medicine, since until these are understood it will be impossible to appreciate our reasons for pursuing the subject at all. Fortunately these objects are few in number and clear by nature. They are as follows:

1 To produce a healthy, undamaged baby, capable of independent existence

It is not enough for the baby merely to be born alive, although this is clearly necessary and was, in fact, accepted as a partial success in the not too distant past. Nowadays, however, the stress of life is so great that anyone who is in any way handicapped is at a severe disadvantage. For this reason it is therefore necessary to emphasise *morbidity* – the possession of abnormalities attributable to the obstetric background – as well as *mortality* – life or death itself.

2 To conclude the process of childbirth with a healthy mother, capable both physically and mentally of having further successful pregnancies

This object will be clear if it is realised that it is uneconomical from the point of view of the survival of the species for a mother to have only one child. A woman who is unable to have further pregnancies, whether she wishes to or not, is a failure of obstetric management. Similarly, a mother who is seriously damaged by her experiences during childbirth, either in mind or in body, must also be regarded as a failure of obstetric care, since her ability to enjoy and profit from life has been to some extent reduced.

3   To improve, if necessary, the general health of the mother
This is not such an important object, and indeed in those cases where the patient is already in good health it need not be considered. At times, however, the physical or mental state of the patient leaves much to be desired and in such cases considerable improvements are often possible during the months they are under ante-natal supervision.

In order to achieve these three objects, the following four basic problems must be solved:

1   That of assuring normal intra-uterine development of the foetus and the continued health of the patient during pregnancy. This can be achieved only by continuous and painstaking obstetric care in order to detect, as early as possible, the development of any abnormality affecting the safety of the foetus or of the mother and, having detected it, to deal with it both speedily and effectively.

2   That of assuring a safe delivery, since it is clearly absurd to supervise the development of the foetus during pregnancy merely to allow it to perish during labour.

This second problem may be subdivided into three parts:

a   In the first place, the question arises whether the foetus will be able to pass safely through the maternal pelvis. This is really the fundamental problem of obstetrics, since if a vaginal delivery is liable to prove fatal to the foetus all previous efforts at maintaining its health have obviously been futile.

b If the answer to the above question is 'Yes', it then becomes necessary to consider the method of delivery which offers the greatest safety to the foetus and to the mother. If, on the other hand, the answer is 'No', delivery by Caesarean section is the only acceptable alternative.

c Lastly, it must be decided where ante-natal care should be given, where the delivery should take place and under whose immediate supervision labour should be conducted.

Although a decision on these three points may not always be possible until the patient is at or near term, in general they should be answered, if only provisionally, during early pregnancy. The reason for this is that such a course is clearly in the patient's best interests as it avoids the worry and indecision which otherwise will almost inevitably arise. It is also far more convenient from an administrative point of view for such issues to be decided as soon as possible.

3 The third problem to which a solution must be found is that of assuring a safe return of the mother to her everyday life and of supervising the progress of her baby.

4 Lastly, no midwife, whatever her personal feelings, can consider that she has done everything possible for her patient until she has made certain that the mother has been offered, at the end of the puerperium, adequate and acceptable contraceptive advice.

Ovulation

Pregnancy is a state in which a fertilised ovum is embedded and growing in the maternal tissues. This rather cumbersome definition is designed to cover *all* pregnancies, both those which are situated *within* the uterus – intra-uterine – as well as those in which the foetus is growing *outside* the uterus – extra-uterine or ectopic. In the vast majority of instances and, of course, in all normal pregnancies, the fertilised ovum is embedded in the uterine cavity and grows there until delivery.

Ovulation

For pregnancy to take place, an ovum must first be produced and then fertilised. Other than actually seeing the ovum, a procedure which is rarely if ever possible in human beings, there are no *absolute* signs of ovulation, although of course a pregnancy is proof positive that this must have occurred. With certain exceptions, the best outward sign that the genital tract as a whole is functioning normally, and that ovulation is occurring at definite and regular intervals, is menstruation. There are also other less straightforward presumptive signs of ovulation, such as a sudden and copious discharge of clear mucus from the vagina about a fortnight after the start of a period, or a slight rise in body temperature, but as a rule menstruation is the most obvious and the most usually accepted indication that ova are being produced.

Ovulation is thought to occur about fourteen days after the start of a period. As the average time between periods is twenty-eight days, an ovum is produced almost exactly half-way between one period and the next, that is at Mid-Cycle.

Each ovary at birth contains a large number – about 100,000 – of what are called primordial follicles. These are small clusters of cells, each one of which contains a special cell capable of developing into a mature ovum. As the number of periods a woman may expect in the course of her life will not amount to more than between 350 and 400, it follows that of all the primordial follicles present in the ovaries at birth only a few will actually produce ova and that only a very small proportion of these ova will ever be fertilised.

The process whereby the ovum reaches maturity is, in outline, as follows:

Under the influence of one of the hormones of the anterior pituitary – Follicle Stimulating Hormone or F.S.H. – one of the primordial follicles starts to increase in size and grows from a solid cluster of cells into a small, cystic cavity containing a clear fluid. Attached by a small stalk to the side-wall of this cavity is an unusually large cell which is to become the mature ovum. By continued growth this small cyst becomes much larger, and projects above the surface of the ovary. At this stage it is known as a Graafian follicle. About the fourteenth day of the menstrual cycle, calculated from the first day of the last period, the Graafian follicle bursts, the ovum breaks away from its stalk and passes into the outer end of the Fallopian tube, which is specially designed to receive it. Once in the tube, the ovum passes slowly towards the uterus.

At the same time the lining of the uterus – the endometrium – has been prepared for the arrival of the ovum by the action of hormones produced both by the Graafian follicle and by the

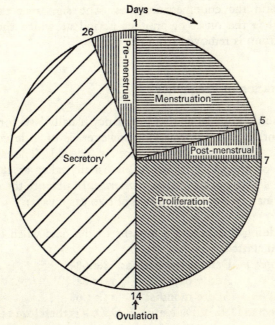

Fig. 1   Pie diagram of the menstrual cycle

structure into which it develops after ovulation – the corpus luteum. These hormones – oestrogens and progesterone – alter the structure of the endometrium in such a way that it will allow the ovum, if fertilised, to embed in it and start to grow into a foetus. The ovum itself, again only if fertilised, produces yet another hormone – Human Chorionic Gonadotrophin or H.C.G. – which has the effect of prolonging the activity of the corpus luteum in the ovary. Thus kept alive, the corpus luteum will continue to produce the oestrogens and progesterone necessary to maintain the pregnancy for about the first ten weeks, after which time the ovum itself starts to produce its own hormones and, in effect, to look after itself.

If, on the other hand, the ovum is not fertilised, no H.C.G. is produced, the normally short life of the corpus luteum is not prolonged and it starts to degenerate some eight to ten days after ovulation. With degeneration its production of hormones fails, the support these provide for the endometrium is withdrawn, and the endometrium dies. The sign that this has happened is the onset of another period at which the dead endometrium is removed from the uterus.

The Duration of Pregnancy

It is common knowledge that pregnancy usually lasts for about nine months. Such information, however, is of little value in obstetrics where greater accuracy is needed. The average duration of pregnancy, therefore, is usually taken as 280 days from the *first* day of the *last normal period*. In practice the date of delivery may be calculated in one of two easy ways:

1   By adding 7 days and 9 months to the date when the last period started.
    Example 1   Date of last period: 8.2.68
                  Add 7 days: 15.2.68
                  Add 9 months: 15.11.68
The Expected Date of Delivery – E.D.D. – is therefore 15.11.68.

2   At times it may be more convenient to add 7 days and *subtract* 3 months from the date when the last period started.
    Example 2   Date of last period: 6.5.68
                  Add 7 days: 13.5.68
                  Subtract 3 months: 13.2.69
Here the expected date of delivery is 13.2.69.

In carrying out these calculations it is necessary to be careful about two points:

a Always to be certain, where applicable, to add a year – Example 2.

b Equally, and more importantly, to be certain that, where necessary, a month is added. This point is made clear in Example 3.

> *Example 3* Date of last period: 27.4.68
> Add 7 days: 4.5.68 *Not* 4.4.68
> Subtract 3 months: 4.2.69 *Not* 4.2.68

In this example the expected date of delivery is not 4.1.69, as it would have seemed to be if the addition of the necessary month had been overlooked. The significance of this is that if this point is forgotten, a woman may be thought to be due a month before this is really the case, an error which may have serious consequences for her or for the foetus.

These methods of calculation, which are based on a knowledge of the first day of the last menstrual period, include the days elapsing between this event and the actual start of pregnancy, which probably occurs soon after ovulation. They are therefore of use only where there is reason to believe from the past menstrual history that the woman's periods have been regular and that there is no indication that they would not have continued to be so. Difficulties arise when the periods have previously been irregular, especially when they have been occurring at widely-spaced intervals, such as every two to three months, since it is then by no means certain that ovulation occurred only fourteen days after the start of the last period. For this reason, any method of calculating the probable date of delivery which is based solely upon past menstrual history will be bound to be inaccurate in such women.

In circumstances of this sort it would obviously be helpful to know the precise date of fertilisation, but this is never available. Of less value is the date of ovulation, but this can be estimated only approximately and then only if special signs are noted. Lastly, although the date of the coitus responsible for the pregnancy may sometimes be known, there is never any way of knowing the exact time which elapsed between intercourse and conception.

For these reasons, where the menstrual history is unreliable, or when the patient has forgotten when her last period occurred, other means must be sought of estimating the duration of pregnancy and the probable date of delivery. Here the size of the uterus as estimated by vaginal examination in early pregnancy, preferably before the fourteenth week, is of the greatest importance. From such an examination, which is carried out only by a doctor, it is possible to gauge the duration of pregnancy to within one or two weeks. This procedure gives more reliable results than those obtained by calculating the length of gestation from the date on which the patient first felt foetal movements, since this varies within very wide limits.

Even where the menstrual dates are apparently reliable, vaginal estimation of the size of the uterus should always be carried out in early pregnancy to make sure that the duration of pregnancy it suggests corresponds to that calculated from the patient's dates. While these two methods usually provide a good measure of agreement, there are occasions where this is not so. In such cases two very different situations may be encountered:

1 *The uterus is larger than expected.* The main reasons for this are as follows:

a Wrong dates

b A multiple pregnancy

c A very large foetus

d A tumour of the uterus, with or without a co-existing pregnancy

e A hydatidiform mole, which is a rare cystic degeneration of the ovum

f A pelvic swelling which is not the uterus at all, such as an ovarian cyst or a distended bladder.

2 *The uterus is smaller than expected.* Here one of the following conditions is probably present:

a Wrong dates

b A foetus which is failing to grow properly

c A foetus which has died and has been retained in the uterus

d A patient who is not pregnant at all.

In all such cases the midwife should get in touch with a doctor without delay, since the management of the case is now his responsibility. It cannot be too strongly emphasised that the midwife's part in present-day obstetrics is to treat the normal and to recognise and refer for a medical opinion anything abnormal. There are few exceptions to this rule.

Summary

Objects of Obstetrics

Obstetrics has three main objects:

a To produce a healthy baby

b To produce a healthy mother

c To improve the health of the mother during pregnancy

To achieve these objects, four problems must be solved:

a That of assuring a normal intra-uterine development for the foetus.

b That of assuring a safe delivery:

   (i) By considering the best *place* for delivery
   (ii) By considering the best *method* of delivery

c That of assuring the speedy return of the mother to everyday life.

d That of offering the newly-delivered mother acceptable contraceptive advice.

Ovulation

Other than pregnancy, there are no absolute signs of ovulation as the ovum itself cannot be seen.

The best presumptive sign of ovulation is regular menstruation, others being a mid-cycle discharge and a slight rise in body temperature.

Ovulation usually takes place midway between the periods, provided that these are occurring at regular twenty-eight-day intervals.

An ovum develops in a primordial follicle which grows into a Graafian follicle. When this bursts the ovum passes into the Fallopian tube and from here into the uterus. The Graafian follicle then changes into the corpus luteum.

Under the influence of hormones from the Graafian follicle and the corpus luteum the endometrium is altered to receive the ovum.

If the ovum is fertilised, it embeds in the uterine cavity and starts to produce its own hormones. These first preserve the activity of the corpus luteum and later maintain the life of the ovum itself.

If the ovum is not fertilised the corpus luteum dies within a few days and another period starts.

Duration of Pregnancy

The average duration of pregnancy is 280 days.

The methods of calculating the expected date of delivery are straightforward provided that certain simple points are remembered. Otherwise serious mistakes may occur.

Where the menstrual history is unreliable, the duration of pregnancy is best estimated from the size of the uterus as judged by a vaginal examination. This method is more accurate than that based upon the date on which foetal movements were first felt.

If the uterus is larger than expected this may be due to:

a Wrong dates

b A multiple pregnancy

c A very large foetus

d A tumour of the uterus

e A hydatidiform mole

f A pelvic swelling other than the uterus.

Where the uterus is smaller than expected this may be due to:

a Wrong dates

b A poorly growing foetus

c A dead foetus

d No pregnancy.

In all such cases medical aid should be called.

CHAPTER TWO

The Diagnosis of Pregnancy

The Clinical Diagnosis of Early Pregnancy

It does not follow that because a woman thinks she is pregnant that this is really so. It is therefore sensible to confirm her suspicions in every case. It is perhaps surprising to learn that an absolute diagnosis of pregnancy cannot be made until the foetus can either be heard, felt or seen by means of X-rays. In early pregnancy, therefore, the diagnosis has to be based upon a number of presumptive symptoms and signs of which the following are the more common:

1 Amenorrhoea

Although the great majority of healthy women with normally regular periods who suddenly cease to menstruate are pregnant, this is not always so. In certain cases irregular vaginal bleeding may occur in early pregnancy, either from the cavity of the uterus or from some abnormality of the lower genital tract (pages 85–86). Although such bleeding is often thought to be a period, this is not so, the various changes in the endometrium which allow true menstruation being suspended during pregnancy.

On other occasions there may be amenorrhoea without pregnancy. The causes of this are varied; hormone imbalance, systemic diseases and psychological disturbances all playing their part. When such cases are encountered by the midwife, medical aid should, of course, be asked for without delay.

2 Morning Sickness
A feeling of nausea, sometimes culminating in vomiting, is said to be a reliable symptom of early pregnancy. However, such nausea is by no means invariably present, being seen in rather less than 50 per cent of cases. Typically, nausea is noticed on waking, but it may occur at other times, its main feature being that it occurs about the same time every day. Unless vomiting is persistent and accompanied by specific changes in the urine, morning sickness need not be regarded as pathological and requires no medical treatment.

3 The Breasts
In early pregnancy, many women complain that their breasts feel heavy and uncomfortable. In some cases such discomfort may amount to pain and tenderness. These symptoms are more marked in women who experience premenstrual symptoms of a similar but milder nature. While such breast changes are of value in the diagnosis of pregnancy, their absence in no way excludes this possibility.

4 Vaginal Discharges
An increased vaginal discharge, which may be white or colourless, mucoid or thick, is experienced by many women in early pregnancy. However, since the amount of such discharge varies widely, and since it may frequently be present for other reasons, this again is not a definite symptom of pregnancy but merely one which, if encountered along with several others, helps to support the diagnosis.

5 Other Symptoms
Other symptoms often complained of in the early weeks of pregnancy are:

a   Discomfort from varicose veins and haemorrhoids

b   Frequency of micturition, especially at night

c Abnormally persistent and otherwise inexplicable lassitude. This last, often most distressing to the patient, is frequently encountered and may be a valuable additional diagnostic feature, especially in a multipara who has experienced it in previous pregnancies.

Physical Signs

Pregnancy should never be diagnosed solely on a variety of symptoms, no matter how convincing these may be. It is necessary to examine every patient, since otherwise mistakes will inevitably arise which may prove embarrassing and even dangerous.

In examining a patient who believes herself to be pregnant, it is best to keep to a definite routine so that no point may be overlooked. As the details of this routine naturally vary according to a midwife's training and personal preference, the following is intended to provide only a general guide in this matter.

1 Breast Changes

It is obviously impossible to tell if the breasts, when seen for the first time, are larger than normal, though the patient may herself volunteer this information. Moreover, if the duration of amenorrhoea is only six to eight weeks it is pointless to look for the classical changes of areolar pigmentation, Montgomery's tubercles or enlargement of the nipples, since these are evident only later. What must be sought is the presence of multiple superficial veins, running around the border of the areola and crossing the midline from one breast to the other. These veins present an altogether typical appearance difficult to describe but easily recognised with practice and although not diagnostic of pregnancy, are highly suggestive of this state. Although the breast changes of pregnancy regress after delivery and lactation, they never completely disappear and for this reason their presence is of greater diagnostic value in a primigravida than in a multipara, especially one whose last child is still very young.

2 Skin Pigmentation

The gradual development of pigmentation on certain parts of the body is another sign of pregnancy often emphasised in text-books. It is, however, of less importance in practical obstetrics. The reason for this is that in the first place pigmentation in its fully-developed form is seen only in dark-skinned women such as Asians, Africans, West Indians and European brunettes and is less marked in blondes and red-heads, in some of whom it may be altogether absent. Secondly, it tends to develop relatively late in pregnancy, by which time the diagnosis has as a rule already been established.

When pigmentation does occur, it is usually seen in the following places:

a In the mid-line of the abdomen, where it creates a narrow band, the Linea Nigra or black line, extending from the pubis to the umbilicus and sometimes reaching upwards towards the xiphisternum

b On the areolae and nipples where, in very dark-skinned people, it may spread outwards to form a secondary areola beyond the true areola itself

c Over the perineum

d On the cheeks and forehead. Here it takes on a 'butterfly patch' distribution and is known as Chloasma or the Mask of Pregnancy. This disfiguring sort of pigmentation is fortunately rarely present in anything but a mild form and almost always disappears soon after childbirth.

3 Changes in the Uterus

In the final analysis, a clinical diagnosis of pregnancy depends on detecting certain typical changes in the uterus. Due to the fact that in early pregnancy this organ is entirely contained within the pelvis, it cannot be felt abdominally until after the twelfth week. Abdominal examination before this time will therefore reveal no palpable mass unless some abnormality is present, either in the form of an extra-uterine tumour – ovarian, intestinal, renal or hepatic – or of a uterus larger than the duration of amenorrhoea would suggest (page 10). Normally, therefore, the size, shape and consistency of the uterus can be determined, during the early weeks of pregnancy, only by vaginal examination, a procedure which, as already pointed out, is carried out only by a doctor. It might be imagined that this could present some risks to the patient in the sense that it might provoke an abortion, but in practice this is not so, although when there has been bleeding during early pregnancy, this method of examination may possibly present such a danger. When all is straightforward no such risk exists and in these circumstances a vaginal examination is a safe as well as a necessary diagnostic measure.

The particular features which a doctor would look for at vaginal examination are as follows:

a The cervix becomes softer than normal. This sign is not well marked in early pregnancy but becomes better developed later

b The uterus is enlarged, its precise size depending upon the duration of pregnancy

c The uterus alters its shape. In the non-pregnant state it is usually pear-shaped; during pregnancy it becomes globular

d The uterus becomes softer, so much so that it may be taken for an ovarian cyst

e *Hegar's Sign*. This particular sign, said to be present at the eighth week, depends on the fact that at this time the uterus is filled by the ovum only in its upper half, the lower part still being empty. As a result, if the softened cervix is trapped between a hand on the lower abdomen and two fingers in the anterior vaginal fornix, the impression is gained that the fingers of both hands almost meet between the cervix below and the uterine body above. The value of this sign has, however, been overrated. It is difficult to elicit, unreliable, possibly dangerous and almost always unnecessary, and thus has little to commend it.

Following the bimanual examination a speculum is usually passed. This may reveal a moderate amount of vaginal discharge, already referred to, and also a bluish discoloration of the vaginal walls and of the cervix. This blueing, considered by some to be of great diagnostic value, does, however, occur in other conditions. It is merely due to an increased blood flow through the lower genital tract, the blue colour being that of the reduced haemoglobin in the blood showing through the thin and transparent vaginal and cervical epithelium.

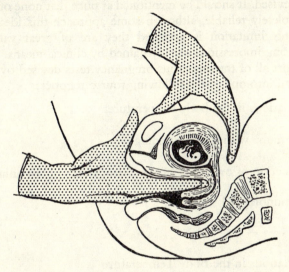

Fig. 2   Hegar's sign

Only after enquiring into the various symptoms mentioned above and carrying out the necessary examinations can a firm but still not absolute diagnosis of pregnancy be reached. In the great majority of patients this is all that is needed, since time itself will dispel any remaining doubts. It must, however, be stressed that while it is rarely necessary to proceed further in establishing a diagnosis of pregnancy, to do less than what has been suggested above cannot pass as good obstetrics. At this important time in her life a woman has a right to expect a diagnosis based not on a vague probability but on a carefully taken history and a thorough clinical examination.

B

Pregnancy Tests

Although, as already pointed out, a careful history and clinical examination will allow an acceptably reliable diagnosis of pregnancy to be reached in most instances, there are occasions where, for one reason or another, further diagnostic methods are needed. It is because of this that various pregnancy tests have been devised. It should be mentioned at once that none of these is completely reliable, although some approach this ideal, but once this limitation is accepted they are of great value in supporting impressions already gained by clinical means.

Almost all of the numerous pregnancy tests devised over the years fall into one of the following four categories:

1   Variations in the body temperature

2   Hormone withdrawal bleeding

3   Induction of ovulation or spermatogenesis in test animals

4   Immunological reactions.

1   Variations in the Body Temperature
If taken on waking, the morning temperature usually shows a small but definite rise once ovulation has taken place. This rise usually disappears at the start of the next period, but if pregnancy supervenes this fall will not occur and the temperature will remain at its higher level. A test of this sort is obviously impossible unless the patient has kept a careful and continuous temperature record for several months. For practical purposes, therefore, its use is restricted to a few highly motivated women, usually with a long history of sub-fertility, who are anxious to become pregnant and who wish to know of this at the earliest opportunity.

2   Hormone Withdrawal Bleeding
If, in women who develop amenorrhoea for reasons other than pregnancy, oestrogens and progesterone are given for a few

days and then stopped, the endometrium built up by these hormones as in the normal menstrual cycle will die and bleeding will occur. This is the basis for one type of pregnancy test. Hormone-containing tablets, usually either Orasecron – one tablet five times a day for two days – or Primodos – one tablet daily for two days – are taken by mouth. Within a few days vaginal bleeding will start if the woman is not pregnant. If she *is* pregnant nothing will happen and her amenorrhoea will continue. A positive test – bleeding – is therefore a sign that the patient is *not pregnant*. Women often imagine that by taking these pills they will abort but this is not so and where they are, in fact, pregnant, no harm will be done to the foetus by this test.

3   Induction of Ovulation and Spermatogenesis in Test Animals
On page 7 it was said that the ovum starts to produce its own hormones soon after fertilisation. In early pregnancy the most important of these are Human Chorionic Gonadotrophins – H.C.G. – the value of which seems to lie in preserving the corpus luteum until its functions can be taken over by the placenta. An important side-effect of these gonadotrophins, which are excreted in large quantities in the urine, is that they can cause growth or maturation of the gonads or sex-glands – ovaries or testes – resulting in either ovulation or spermatogenesis. Thus if urine from a pregnant woman is injected into an animal, the contained gonadotrophins will cause either ova or sperm to be produced, according to its sex. It would normally be hard to make sure that this event was due to the injected gonadotrophins as the animal might be producing germ cells on its own. However, if an immature animal is used for this test, this possibility can be excluded and if ova or spermatozoa are found they must have been produced by the action of the gonadotrophins in the injected urine. In such an event the woman who provided the specimen must be pregnant.

In the past several varieties of test animal have been used, such as mice, rats and rabbits, all of which were female. At present, where employed at all, the test is carried out on male toads. These, within two hours of being injected with urine from a pregnant woman, produce spermatozoa which are easily recognised under the microscope. If, on the other hand, the woman is not pregnant, no spermatozoa will be seen. This test is cheap, rapid, easy and reliable but for various reasons it has now been largely replaced by immunological reactions.

4 Immunological Reactions

These depend upon what are called Antigen–Antibody Reactions and once again involve H.C.G. Since H.C.G. contains proteins it can cause antibody formation if injected into another animal. Several tests of pregnancy have been devised which make use of this principle. In the simplest of these, the Gravindex Test, urine from the woman to be investigated is mixed with serum containing antibodies prepared against H.C.G. If the woman is pregnant her urine will contain H.C.G. and this will combine with the antibodies in the serum. If to this mixture of urine and serum is now added a suspension of Latex particles coated with H.C.G., there will be no antibodies for this added H.C.G. to react with, since these will already have been used up when they combined with the H.C.G. in the patient's urine. In these circumstances the Latex particles stay in suspension and the mixture remains clear. If, on the other hand, the woman is not pregnant, her urine contains no H.C.G., the antibodies in the serum will have nothing with which to combine and will thus still be present to react later with the H.C.G. which is added on the Latex particles. This reaction makes the urine cloudy as the particles clump together. Such a *positive reaction* shows that the patient is *not pregnant*, while a *negative reaction* – no clumping of the particles – shows that she *is*.

In practice this test is quick and easy to carry out. It is also cheap, needs little in the way of apparatus and does not involve the use of a live animal. Its main drawback lies in its extreme sensitivity. This is because the antibodies in the serum cannot distinguish between H.C.G. produced by the ovum and very similar gonadotrophins which come from the pituitary gland in amounts which, at times, may be abnormally high. A very accurate test, unlike the animal tests which are rather less sensitive, may therefore produce what are called False Positive results. The times in a woman's life when these false positives may arise are as follows:

a Puberty
b The menopause
c Post-partum and during lactation
d Between episodes of metropathic uterine bleeding.

With the possible exception of the last, these are times when few women would welcome a pregnancy and as a result false positive tests, when they occur, are liable to cause a great deal of concern. It is therefore as well to be on one's guard and to be sure that the pathologist is told when the urine to be tested is from a pubertal girl, a menopausal woman or a lactating mother. In such circumstances false positive results can be avoided by using a specimen of urine diluted with water.

Diagnosis in Late Pregnancy

As a rule it is not hard to diagnose pregnancy after the twentieth week, although at times difficulties may arise, particularly where any possibility of pregnancy is emphatically denied by the patient. While it might be imagined that in such circumstances a pregnancy test would answer the question, this is not necessarily the case. Due to the fact that the production of H.C.G. decreases after the tenth or twelfth week, most of the usual tests become negative after this time. Other means must therefore be sought of reaching a correct diagnosis.

Of the various symptoms associated with the second half of pregnancy, the chief one is still amenorrhoea. It may, in fact, be the only one, morning sickness, subjective breast changes and frequency of micturition having usually subsided by this time. Foetal movements may have been felt by the patient – they are usually noticed around twenty weeks in a primigravida and somewhat earlier in a multipara – but these may be misinterpreted, the patient maintaining that she has never felt them when she wishes to deny that she is pregnant, or falsely claiming that they are present if she is abnormally anxious to have a child. When they first occur, these movements cannot usually be felt by an observer, although this is possible later in pregnancy when they provide a valuable proof of the presence of a living foetus in the uterus.

It is therefore necessary in these perplexing cases to look for certain physical signs on which a diagnosis may be based. Of these the size of the uterus is the most important, since not only will this help in reaching a diagnosis of pregnancy but will also allow a more or less accurate estimation to be made of its duration.

1 The Size of the Uterus
The size of the uterus is usually estimated by measuring, on abdominal palpation, the height of the fundus. As a rule this reaches the level of the symphysis pubis at twelve weeks, and the upper border of the umbilicus at twenty-four weeks. It will thus be one-third of the distance between these two points at sixteen weeks and two-thirds at twenty weeks. After this the relation of the fundus to the duration of pregnancy becomes variable, since it is influenced by many different factors. As a general rule, however, it may be expected to reach half way between the upper border of the umbilicus and the xiphisternum at thirty weeks and to the xiphisternum itself at thirty-six weeks. In the last month of pregnancy the fundal height sinks down a little, more commonly in a primigravida than in a multipara.

As has been said, these later levels are most inconsistent and vary according to the parity of the patient, the size of the foetus and the amount of liquor present in the uterus, quite apart from depending to some extent upon the way in which the foetus is lying in the uterus. For these reasons, too great a reliance should not be placed on the height of the fundus in estimating the duration of pregnancy after the twenty-eighth week.

2 Uterine Contractions
Another sign to be looked for is that of intermittent uterine contractions. These are felt as periodic hardening of the uterus and appear either spontaneously or after stimulation by rubbing or firm palpation. As no other abdominal organ behaves in this way, these contractions are a diagnostic sign of great value.

3   Palpating the Foetus

Palpable foetal parts provide one of the definite signs of pregnancy. At about the twenty-second to twenty-fourth week they may best be made out by what is called 'ballottement'. This depends on the fact that at this time there is a relatively large

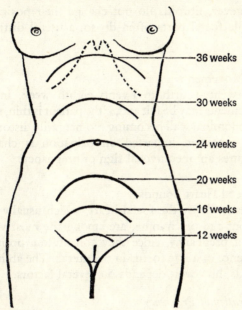

36 weeks

30 weeks

24 weeks

20 weeks

16 weeks

12 weeks

Fig. 3   Height of the fundus at different times in pregnancy

amount of liquor amnii and that in consequence the foetus can often be persuaded to change its position in the uterus. Some firm part, such as the head or the breech, can therefore sometimes be felt to move away from the side of the uterus by tapping it gently with the fingers. This is called 'External Ballottement' and gives a very characteristic sensation. Alternatively, a doctor can, by vaginal examination, often make the head or the breech float upwards by tapping it with his fingers and, a moment later, feel it fall back on them again. The impression given by this sign, which is known as 'Internal Ballottement', is again unmistakable.

Later in pregnancy, palpation of the uterus allows individual foetal parts to be felt, since they are now larger. The rounded head and breech can usually be made out after the twenty-fourth week, although it is often hard to distinguish between one or the other. Limbs can also be felt, though it is generally impossible to say precisely what they are. It should perhaps be mentioned that foetal parts are sometimes mistaken for fibroids and vice versa. However, fibroids do not change their position in the uterus, while foetal parts often do so, a useful distinguishing feature.

4   Foetal Movements

After the twenty-fourth to twenty-eighth week, intermittent foetal movements may be felt and, if the patient is thin, sometimes seen, the abdominal wall becoming momentarily distorted. Once again, the sensation imparted on palpation is characteristic and constitutes an unequivocal sign of pregnancy.

5   The Foetal Heart Sounds

The sounds made by the foetal heart, which usually beats at a rate of about 140 per minute, are among the most valuable of the signs of pregnancy, since they constitute a positive proof of the presence of a live foetus in the uterus. The ability to hear these sounds, however, depends on several factors.

a   *The Duration of Pregnancy*

Although the heart starts beating at a very early date, it is literally too small to be heard without the aid of special equipment until the foetus has reached a certain size and age – usually between 18 and 20 weeks. After this time, depending upon the various factors described below, the heart beat becomes progressively easier to perceive, although it is never possible to be certain of hearing it, no matter how advanced the pregnancy.

b   *The State of the Patient's Abdominal Wall*

Fat is a poor conductor of sound. The thicker the patient's abdominal wall, the more difficult will it be to hear the foetal heart and the more advanced must pregnancy become before success is achieved.

c   The Position of the Foetal Stethoscope
If the foetal heart is to be heard, the mouth of the foetal stethoscope must be placed more or less directly above it, the actual
point depending upon the way in which the foetus is lying in the
uterus. If this is already known it is relatively easy to position
the stethoscope correctly, but if not, a search will have to be made
over the anterior surface of the uterus. Until this has been done
it is wrong to say, in cases of doubt, that the foetal heart cannot
be heard, since this implies intra-uterine death.

d   The Experience of the Midwife
The more the foetal heart is listened to, the easier does it become
to hear. The ability to detect the foetal heart sounds under a
variety of conditions therefore comes only with practice. For
this reason the midwife should not be discouraged by early
difficulties or failures. Even when it is thought that the foetal
heart can be heard, there are certain points which must be checked
in order to be certain that no mistake has been made.

i   The blood flowing through the larger uterine vessels often
    makes a noise similar to that of the foetal heart. As this
    'Uterine Souffle' comes from the maternal blood vessels,
    it will be in time with the patient's pulse and not at a
    different rate, as is the case with the foetal heart. In order to
    exclude this particular error, the patient's pulse should
    always be taken when listening to the foetal heart.

ii Sometimes, instead of the usual sound of the foetal heart,
    a rapid, blowing noise is heard, at a different rate and usually
    considerably faster than the patient's pulse. This noise is
    made by blood flowing through the umbilical cord of the
    foetus, which at that moment is trapped under the stetho-
    scope. From a diagnostic point of view this Funic Souffle, as
    it is called, is as valuable a sign as hearing the foetal heart
    itself.

6   The Breasts
The superficial veins running just under the skin of the breasts
and around the areolae, already mentioned on page 16, in-

crease in size as pregnancy progresses and become even more obvious. In addition the areolae and nipples enlarge and become more prominent while their colour darkens. Lastly, a further sign of breast activity is the production of a clear, watery secretion which, with practice, may be expressed from the nipples after about the twenty-sixth week, although the precise time when this is possible varies greatly from case to case.

7 X-ray Evidence of Pregnancy

Although the dangers to the foetus of irradiation have probably been over-emphasised, it is not usual to attempt to diagnose pregnancy by X-ray examination unless this is absolutely necessary. While there are few occasions when this is the case, it may be important to differentiate a normal pregnancy from the condition known as Hydatidiform Mole (page 86). Here, X-ray evidence of foetal bones is valuable in proving the presence of an intra-uterine pregnancy. At other times the patient may deny pregnancy so vehemently that actual visualisation of the foetus becomes a sheer necessity. Fortunately, such cases are seldom encountered.

Where, for one reason or another, an X-ray of the uterus in early pregnancy is under consideration, it is worth remembering that although foetal bones are present from a very early date, these are so small that they will not at first show up on a film, the more so since they lie in front of the dense maternal sacrum. For this reason, such X-rays are unlikely to be of much value in the diagnosis of pregnancy before the sixteenth or eighteenth week.

Summary

Clinical Diagnosis of Early Pregnancy

Since absolute proof of pregnancy rests upon hearing, feeling or seeing the foetus in the uterus in early pregnancy, the diagnosis can be based only on a number of presumptive symptoms and signs.

The symptoms of early pregnancy are as follows:

a   Amenorrhoea

b   Morning sickness

c   Subjective breast changes

d   Increased vaginal discharge

e   Frequency of micturition – especially nocturia.

Pregnancy should never be diagnosed on these symptoms alone; physical signs must be looked for in every case. Of these the following are the more important:

a   *The Breasts* may show the presence of distended veins over their surfaces, especially around the areolae and across the midline.

b   *Skin Pigmentation* may be seen in the midline of the abdomen, on the nipples and areolae, on the perineum and sometimes on the face.

c   *The Uterus* is enlarged, soft and globular. Since it is not large enough to be felt abdominally before the twelfth week, in earlier pregnancy this finding can be determined only on vaginal examination carried out by a doctor.

d   The vaginal and cervical epithelium take on a blue colour.

A firm but not absolute diagnosis of pregnancy can usually be reached if all these points are considered in every case. To do less than this is bad obstetrics.

Pregnancy Tests

At times it may be necessary to resort to special tests in order to establish a diagnosis of pregnancy. These tests fall into four groups:

a   Variations in body temperature

b   Hormone withdrawal bleeding

c Induction of ovulation or spermatogenesis in certain animals

d Immunological reactions.

Variations in Body Temperature

If the normal post-ovulatory rise in body temperature is maintained beyond the expected time of the next period, pregnancy is possible. This test is seldom practicable.

Hormone Withdrawal Bleeding

By injecting certain hormones the endometrium can be built up. On stopping these hormones the endometrium will die and bleeding will result. This will not happen if the woman is pregnant.

Induction of Ovulation or Spermatogenesis

Urine from a pregnant woman contains H.C.G. which will cause immature animals to ovulate or to produce sperm. A variety of animals has been used for this type of test, the latest being the common toad. This test has, however, been superseded by immunological reactions.

Immunological Reactions

The H.C.G. in a pregnant woman's urine will react with a serum prepared against it. This reaction is then checked by using Latex particles as an indicator. Tests of this sort, of which the Gravindex is the simplest, are much in use at present.

False positive results to immunological tests may arise in puberty, at the menopause and during lactation. Special precautions are necessary when carrying out these tests at such times.

Diagnosis in Late Pregnancy

Since pregnancy tests are usually negative during the second half of pregnancy, other means are needed for diagnosing this condition at that time.

The only *symptom* which may still be present is amenorrhoea; morning sickness, subjective breast changes and frequency of micturition having often disappeared after the first weeks, while foetal movements are liable to misinterpretation.

Physical signs, therefore, are of greater value. Of these the following are the more important:

a *The Height of the Fundus* – also of use in estimating the duration of pregnancy.

b *Uterine Contractions*

c *Palpation of the Foetus* – either by external or internal ballottement or by actually feeling foetal parts.

d *Foetal Movements* – usually felt but occasionally seen.

e *Hearing the Foetal Heart* – this depends upon the duration of pregnancy, the thickness of the patient's abdominal wall, the position of the foetal stethoscope and the experience of the midwife.

f *Superficial Veins on the Breasts* – may be more prominent.

g *Pigmentation of the Areolae and Nipples* – is more evident.

h *Watery Secretion* – may be expressed from the nipples.

i *X-ray Visualisation of the Foetal Bones* – although very rarely needed for diagnosis may be of help after the sixteenth to eighteenth week.

CHAPTER THREE

The Management of Pregnancy

The Place of Delivery and of Ante-natal Care

Within the National Health Service a woman may be delivered in one of three places. These are:

1 A Maternity Hospital or Maternity Unit of a General Hospital

2 A General Practitioner Maternity Home

3 The Patient's Own Home.

1 Maternity Hospitals and Maternity Units of General Hospitals

These establishments are under the overall charge of one or more consultant obstetricians. Adequately staffed at all levels from a medical as well as from a nursing point of view, they are equipped with modern labour wards, operating theatres, ante-natal and post-natal wards and special care cots. They thus provide facilities for dealing with every type of obstetric abnormality.

2 General Practitioner Maternity Homes

These usually possess a simply-equipped Labour Ward but have no operating theatres or any other special departments.

They are staffed by midwives and by non-resident general practitioner obstetricians. Although sometimes attached to the maternity unit of a general hospital, in which case they enjoy some of the advantages of such an establishment, they normally lack facilities for managing abnormal labours.

3   The Patient's Own Home
Although obviously subject to variation, the patient's own home must always be considered, whatever her economic status, as possessing minimal obstetric facilities and as suitable only for a normal confinement.

In view of these wide differences, it is necessary to bear two main points in mind when selecting the most suitable place of confinement for a patient.

1   The wishes of the patient herself

2   The probable nature and outcome of the labour.

Wherever possible, the patient should be allowed to choose her place of confinement. This choice, however, must never take precedence over the needs for her safety. Thus, should she want to be delivered at home, this can be agreed to only if she belongs to a category of patient in whom a normal delivery may confidently be expected. On the other hand, if there is no reason to suppose that labour will be difficult or abnormal, but should she still wish to be delivered in hospital, this wish must, if possible, be granted. In no circumstances should the midwife try to persuade such a patient to alter her views and agree to a home delivery unless the number of hospital beds available is severely limited. Where any difference of opinion exists, the views of a doctor should be sought without delay.

Where the patient is willing to leave the choice of the place of confinement to the midwife, the following cases are suitable for delivery either at home or in a general practitioner maternity home:

1   *Primigravidae* over eighteen and under thirty years of age, provided that the patient herself is healthy, that pregnancy pro-

gresses normally and that there is no reason to anticipate an abnormal labour or the delivery of an affected infant.

2 *Multiparae* under the age of thirty-five having their second, third or fourth child, subject to the same provisions regarding pregnancy and labour, provided that the past obstetric history has been normal.

Any patient *not* included in one or the other of the above two categories should be delivered in hospital. Such cases would include:

Primigravidae

1 Where the patient is under eighteen and over thirty years of age

2 Where pregnancy has been abnormal

3 Where there is any abnormal medical or surgical condition, such as cardiac, pulmonary, renal or hepatic disease

4 Where there is any reason to suspect that labour will be abnormal

5 Where labour starts prematurely – before the thirty-seventh week (page 276)

6 Where it is thought that the baby will be 'Small-for Dates' (page 116)

7 Where the baby is liable to be adversely affected in some way.

Multiparae

1 Where the patient is over thirty-five years of age

2 Where she has already had four children, or, more precisely,

four previous pregnancies of over twenty-eight weeks'
duration

3   Where there is a bad past obstetric history, especially involving some abnormality liable to recur or to lead to difficulties at delivery

4   Where there is a history of a previous perinatal death – a
still-birth or a first-week death

5   Where pregnancy has been abnormal

6   Where there is any abnormal medical or surgical condition

7   Where it is possible that labour will be abnormal or the baby
adversely affected in some way.

At first sight this list suggests that almost every pregnant
woman would qualify for a hospital delivery. In fact, pregnancy
is essentially a straightforward affair, the vast majority of patients,
by virtue of their relative youth, being unlikely to have anything seriously wrong with them. A very large proportion of
cases will therefore be eligible for a domiciliary confinement.
On the other hand, in a number of instances social reasons may
render such an arrangement unsuitable. In such cases, a hospital
booking will be necessary on social rather than on medical
grounds. It is here that the opinion, advice and assistance of the
Local Authority or the Medical Social Worker are invaluable,
and the latter should always be consulted regarding the social
background of the patient.

The Duration of Stay in Hospital

A patient booked for a hospital confinement may either stay
there for between eight and ten days, or return home within
forty-eight hours of delivery. In the latter event she would need
to be looked after by a domiciliary midwife for the remainder
of the first fortnight of the puerperium. The third variant,

namely allowing a mother home within five or six days, has nothing to recommend it since it lacks the advantages of either of the other two procedures while possessing none of its own.

A '48-Hour Discharge' appeals to many patients, especially multiparae with small children, since it allows them to get back to their homes with the least delay while at the same time offering them the advantages of a hospital confinement. However, before agreeing to such a course, the midwife must satisfy herself on the following points:

1 Is the case suitable for such management?

2 Are the home conditions satisfactory?

3 Will the mother be able to rest once she is home?

Assuming that the answer to the last two of these questions is 'Yes', it remains to consider the obstetric grounds for a 48-hour discharge. These are that labour should have been normal and that the baby should be healthy and likely to progress satisfactorily. Many patients booked for a hospital confinement because of the possible development of some abnormality of labour have, in fact, uneventful confinements and therefore may safely be allowed home within 48 hours. However, since it is never possible to say in advance that labour will not be complicated, no one should be *promised* a 48-hour discharge since neither the obstetrician nor the midwife is in a position to give such an undertaking. If this point is not made clear when booking arrangements are discussed, misunderstandings and disappointments are bound to arise.

Bearing these points in mind, the two main indications for a 48-hour discharge are as follows:

1 Where the parity or age of the patient is such that a hospital delivery is indicated

2 Where there is a history of some past abnormality of labour involving either the patient or the baby.

Always provided that labour is normal and the baby making good progress.

Lastly, where such a booking is contemplated, the Local Authority must be asked to arrange a visit to the patient's home to ensure that conditions there are satisfactory.

The Place of Ante-natal Care

Just as one of a number of places may be selected for the patient's delivery, so may a wide choice be exercised in the matter of the place or places of ante-natal care. For example, this may be conducted in a hospital ante-natal clinic, in a Local Authority clinic, by a general practitioner obstetrician in his surgery or by a domiciliary midwife in the patient's home. To add variety to these four basic possibilities, supervision may be, and very often is, shared between two or more of these places and persons.

The Hospital Ante-natal Clinic

In general, the hospital ante-natal clinic should be attended by the following categories of patients:

1 Those, booked for a hospital confinement, who have a special reason for attending there throughout pregnancy. Such patients are those with a bad past history, either obstetric or medical, those with medical or surgical conditions, and those in whom pregnancy is in some way abnormal.

2 Certain social cases, either women who are doctors, midwives or nurses, or those who for some reason find the hospital clinic particularly convenient to attend.

3 Women who lack confidence and feel safer if seen throughout pregnancy in a hospital clinic, among doctors and midwives whom they have come to know and trust.

The very great majority of patients attending the average hospital ante-natal clinic can be placed in the first of these three groups. By their very nature, they need careful consideration at every visit and for this reason are liable to take up a good deal of time. It is therefore desirable to keep down the numbers in the other two categories, in order to avoid overcrowding the clinic and defeating its main object of allowing a proper amount of attention to be given to each patient.

Other Places of Ante-natal Care

Where attendance at a hospital ante-natal clinic is not considered necessary ante-natal care may either be carried out in the nearest Local Authority clinic or be provided by a general practitioner obstetrician in his surgery or by a midwife in the patient's home. In such cases, arrangements will usually have been made for the delivery to take place either at home or in a General Practitioner Maternity Home. These particular patients, therefore, need not be seen in a hospital ante-natal clinic during pregnancy save for a particular reason. This may be either because of the development of some abnormality or because it seems that the place of confinement originally selected may be unsuitable.

Shared Ante-natal Care

Unfortunately, not all patients booked for delivery in hospital can be seen there throughout pregnancy, since facilities are lacking for dealing with the large numbers this would involve. In many instances, therefore, ante-natal supervision must be shared between two or more of the places and people mentioned above, the patient being seen for some of the time either at the Local Authority clinic or in the general practitioner obstetrician's surgery. Where this arrangement is in force it is usual for her to attend the hospital ante-natal clinic at the following times:

1 At booking

2 At the thirty-sixth week of pregnancy

3 At term.

In addition, a patient should be given an appointment to a hospital ante-natal clinic at any other time that the Local Authority or the general practitioner obstetrician may wish and such an appointment must be arranged without any unnecessary delay.

It will be readily appreciated that once ante-natal care is shared between two or more authorities, difficulties are liable to arise. These difficulties may assume the following forms:

1 The patient may fail to attend either because she simply does not wish to do so, is prevented from doing so by illness or some social commitment, or because she does not realise that she is expected to do so. This lapse may not be immediately evident if she is believed to be attending different clinics on different dates.

2 A failure to communicate important information about the patient may arise between the various people concerned with her ante-natal supervision.

3 Valuable time may be wasted in obtaining a consultation appointment at the local hospital clinic.

4 Patients may not always be properly examined or certain special investigations may be omitted on the assumption that these will be carried out elsewhere.

These difficulties can to a large extent be avoided if the midwife adopts the following procedure *in all cases*.

1 Make sure that the patient knows *where* to attend for her next visit and *when* this is to be. Stress the importance of this and tell her to let the clinic concerned know if she cannot get there so that alternative arrangements may be made.

2   See that the clinic she is to attend at her next visit knows of this so that the staff there can get in touch with the patient should she fail to appear.

3   See that the patient's personal ante-natal card is properly completed at the end of each visit so that the clinic she next attends will have the necessary information about her.

4   In arranging a hospital consultation, stress the need for urgency and be prepared to be insistent about this. Should this course fail, as may from time to time happen, do not hesitate to ask a doctor for help in this matter.

Provided that these rules are obeyed, the system of ante-natal care outlined above, although cumbersome, time-consuming, unwieldy and uneconomical, will work reasonably well. For this to happen, however, three more factors must be present:

1   There must be a close liaison and a good understanding between the various authorities concerned.

2   Hospitals *must*, whatever their state of over-crowding, agree to accept all cases referred to them with the least possible delay.

3   Hospitals must also provide ante-natal care for those patients for whom such a course is medically or socially necessary.

The Management of Normal Pregnancy: I

The objects of ante-natal care may be summarised as follows:

1   To bring to term or near to term a healthy foetus capable of surviving.

2   To safeguard the health of the patient both with regard to pregnancy itself as well as in respect of any general diseases from which she may be suffering or which she may develop.

3 To determine the safest method of delivery for the patient as well as for the foetus.

4 To provide acceptable ante-natal education for the patient and for her husband.

These objects may be achieved by acting in accordance with the following principles:

1 The patient's first attendance at the ante-natal clinic should take place as early as possible in pregnancy, certainly not later than the twelfth week. This will allow sufficient time for adequate obstetric care and for the treatment of any abnormalities or deficiencies which may already be present or which may arise during pregnancy.

2 The patient should be seen at regular intervals during pregnancy in order to be sure that all is progressing normally and, if not, to make certain that any abnormality which has arisen is detected as soon as possible.

3 At every visit enough time should be given to each patient to allow for careful and thorough examination and for discussing any questions she may wish to raise.

4 Any abnormalities discovered should be reported at once to a doctor.

Failure to conform to any of these general principles means that ante-natal care has been in some way deficient and that any accidents arising from this must be looked upon as avoidable.

It should perhaps be mentioned here that although the various methods of examination during the ante-natal period may sound involved and complicated, few, in fact, actually are so, the great majority being extremely straightforward. This, in effect, means that in almost all women safe and satisfactory ante-natal care can be provided by any competent and conscientious midwife provided that she keeps to the basic principles set out below and never fails to carry out the few simple procedures which are necessary.

The First Visit

The patient's first attendance at the ante-natal clinic is perhaps the most important of all since upon it depends to a very large extent her subsequent management and progress throughout pregnancy as well as during labour. At this first visit the following points should be considered:

1   The diagnosis of pregnancy should, if possible, be established beyond all reasonable doubt.

2   An estimate of the patient's state of health and of the normality of the pregnancy should be made.

3   The place of ante-natal care and of confinement should, at least provisionally, be decided upon.

These three features are a *doctor's* rather than a *midwife's* responsibility.

4   Advice regarding morning sickness, diet, work, exercise, rest and hygiene during pregnancy should be given.

5   Advice on maternity benefits must be made available.

6   The patient should be told of the Ante-Natal Education Classes available to her.

7   The date, time and place of the patient's next attendance must be made clear to her and entered upon her personal ante-natal card.

These aspects of ante-natal care lie primarily within the *midwife's* province.

1   Establishing the Diagnosis of Pregnancy
The way in which this may be done has already been considered on page 14. It should be remembered that although the great majority of women who visit an ante-natal clinic for the first

time are obviously right in believing themselves to be pregnant, this is not necessarily true in every case and as a result pregnancy should always be confirmed through the patient's history and by a full medical examination. Failure to do this will sooner or later end in a woman who is not pregnant being booked for ante-natal care and delivery, a mistake which is both distressing to the patient and embarrassing to the doctor concerned.

2   The State of the Patient's General Health and of the Pregnancy

An accurate assessment of the patient's general state of health and of the normality of the pregnancy can be reached only by means of a detailed history and a proper physical examination.

a   The Menstrual and Obstetric History

Although the examination of the patient is a doctor's responsibility, a midwife is often asked to take the history. In such an event information should first be sought about the menstrual pattern and in particular about the date of the last menstrual period. The expected date of delivery may then be calculated (page 8). If, for some reason, this cannot be done, a note to this effect should be made and a doctor informed.

The patient should also be asked whether she has had any vaginal discharge or bleeding since her last normal period. It might be imagined that such obviously abnormal symptoms as these would be reported as a matter of course, but in practice this is frequently not the case. On the other hand, once questioned about them, patients usually reply truthfully. Naturally, where such a history is obtained the clinic doctor must be told without delay, since urgent hospital admission for observation and treatment may be necessary (see pages 85 and 118).

The patient should also be questioned about her past pregnancies, both with regard to their number and the years in which they occurred, and their outcome in terms of the weight and fate of the babies must be recorded. It is also useful to know whether past pregnancies and labours were normal or abnormal, and if abnormal, in what respect. While many patients are unable to provide these details – indeed some appear utterly indifferent to the reasons for past interference – in other cases much useful information comes to light. The reason for asking questions of this sort is that what has happened in the past often influences the present, either because certain abnormalities are liable to recur or because they predispose to some other defect which itself might complicate pregnancy or labour.

b Medical and Surgical History

It is necessary to know whether the patient has, in the past, suffered from any serious medical diseases or has had any surgical operations, particularly abdominal, since these might affect her in a manner liable to cause trouble during pregnancy or labour. In particular, she should be asked whether she has ever had rheumatic fever, diphtheria, scarlet fever or recurrent tonsillitis – because of the effect these illnesses sometimes have upon the heart – tuberculosis, especially pulmonary tuberculosis, jaundice – possibly indicating permanent damage to liver function – and a urinary tract infection, either cystitis or pyelonephritis. These last may result in renal function being permanently impaired, and even if this is not the case, they are particularly liable to recur during pregnancy, thus often needing special investigations and treatment (page 92).

Next, the patient should be asked whether she has ever had German measles – rubella – in view of the effect this outwardly trivial illness may have upon the early development of the foetus. She should also be assured that if she has had this particular illness in the past she will never get it again, no matter how close a contact she may be to an active case.

It is also useful to ask about a history of twins in the patient's family since in some cases this may indicate a familial trait, liable to be repeated in her own pregnancy (page 284). She should also be asked whether she has ever had a blood transfusion, since here the possibility exists that this was of blood of an incompatible Rhesus group, in which case her baby might be affected at birth (page 140). In present-day medicine, however, much care is taken to ensure that any blood given is accurately crossmatched in this respect and this particular risk, therefore, belongs more to the past than to the present. Lastly, before the patient is examined, it is usual for the midwife to weigh her, to test her urine for albumen, sugar and ketone bodies and to arrange for a

Mid-Stream Specimen of Urine – M.S.U. – to be sent to the Pathology Laboratory for culture and microscopy. Both these procedures are discussed in greater detail in the following section.

c The Clinical Examination of the Patient
Since the clinical examination of the patient at her first visit is always carried out by a doctor, it need not be described in great detail. Essentially, this procedure consists of recording the blood pressure, auscultating the heart and lungs and inspecting the legs to exclude the presence of varicose veins. The breasts are examined to determine the state of the nipples and to exclude the presence of any abnormal masses and the abdomen is palpated to check the height of the fundus, should pregnancy be sufficiently advanced for this to be palpable. Finally a vaginal examination is carried out. Here the points of particular importance, other than those already considered on page 18, are the position of the uterus – it should be flexed anteriorly and not posteriorly – and its size, which should correspond to the duration of amenorrhoea. Vaginal examination will also help to exclude the presence of pelvic tumours such as ovarian cysts and fibroids, both of which may cause trouble during pregnancy or in labour and thus may require medical or surgical treatment.

d Special Examinations
i *The Blood*   A specimen of the patient's blood should be taken at the booking clinic and sent to the pathology laboratory for ABO and Rhesus grouping and Haemoglobin estimation as well as for the determination of the Wassermann Reaction – W.R. – for Syphilis and of the Gonococcal Complement Fixation Test – G.C.F.T. – for past gonorrhoeal infection. Should the Rhesus grouping show that the patient is Rhesus negative – Rh. negative – it will be necessary to check that she does not develop antibodies to the foetus' blood group. This can only be done by testing her blood at intervals during pregnancy (page 142).
ii *X-ray Examination of the Chest.* An X-ray of the patient's chest is usually taken during early pregnancy to exclude a tuberculous lesion or other pulmonary abnormality. Owing to the high irradiation dosage offered to the foetus, mass radiog-

raphy is unsuitable at this time and a standard film is therefore needed.

iii *The Examination of the Teeth.* It is usually wise to refer a pregnant woman for a dental opinion as early in pregnancy as possible, especially if superficial examination of the teeth suggests that they are in need of attention. Most hospitals nowadays have a Dental Department to which such patients may be sent with the least possible trouble and delay.

3 The Place of Ante-natal Care and of Confinement
This question has been considered on page 32.

4 Advice on Morning Sickness, Diet, Work, Exercise, Rest and Hygiene

Following her physical examination and after she has discussed with the doctor the place of ante-natal care and of confinement, it is usual for the midwife to advise the patient on such matters as morning sickness – when complained of – diet, work, exercise, rest and what is rather vaguely called 'The Hygiene of Pregnancy'. Although, in general, text-books devote a good deal of space to this aspect of ante-natal care, this probably represents, to a large degree, misdirected effort and wasted time, since women as a rule have well-established notions of what they want and what they need. It is therefore difficult if not impossible to persuade them to alter these views. Moreover, unless they have developed unusually unsatisfactory habits, it is probably best to allow them to continue as they wish rather than to try to influence their way of life, since this generally succeeds merely in worrying them to no good effect. For these reasons, only an outline of what is usually recommended is given here.

a Morning Sickness
As already stated on page 15, unless vomiting is persistent and accompanied by the excretion of ketone bodies in the urine it need not be regarded as pathological and requires no medical treatment. On the other hand, even mild morning sickness can prove distressing to the patient who is thus anxious to obtain advice about its correct management.

While no hard and fast rules can be laid down on this matter, a good general plan is to advocate a break with routine regarding eating and drinking. A cup of tea and a biscuit before getting up in the morning, preferably brought to the bedside by the husband, frequent small meals rather than a few heavy ones and fluids taken between rather than with food may all be of benefit. Above all, a sympathetic and confident attitude on the part of the midwife, together with reassurance that the condition is purely temporary and will soon pass, is of the utmost value in limiting the distress and annoyance that morning sickness can bring to the sufferer.

b   Diet in Pregnancy

Broadly speaking, a person's diet depends in part on habit and in part on economic necessity. It is therefore doubly hard to alter it, especially at a time when the need for money is apt to increase rather sharply. However, as a general rule, to be good a diet should be mixed and contain as much first-class protein such as meat, fish, eggs and cheese, and as little carbohydrate – potatoes, bread, cake, biscuits, sweets and chocolate – as possible. The amount of fat taken as butter, cream and margarine should not be excessive. Fresh foods, although often more expensive and less easily obtained than the tinned variety, are on the whole to be preferred and the day's meals should always include as much as can reasonably be afforded of fresh fruit and green vegetables. It is usual to recommend offal in the form of liver, kidneys or sweetbreads two or three times a week, but this particular advice is usually ignored by the average patient who appears to find such foods distasteful and will go to some lengths to avoid them. Although the tendency these days is to eat a preponderance of carbohydrates mainly because foods containing these substances are cheaper and more filling, this should be discouraged during pregnancy owing to the liability of such a diet to cause obesity.

Lastly, the patient should be reminded of the availability of cheap milk (page 50) and be encouraged to use in her cooking or drink one pint every day. It should also be made certain that she has been supplied with Iron and Vitamins such as Pregnavite Forte, one tablet three times a day, to be taken throughout pregnancy.

c Work
Nowadays most women work in their homes looking after their families or have some outside employment. The former cannot be given up during pregnancy while to discontinue the latter too soon may cause unnecessary financial hardship. Provided that the patient remains fit and well and that her work is not unduly demanding from the viewpoint of physical effort, she should be encouraged to continue in it until the twenty-eighth week. If, on discussing this matter with her, it is felt that her present duties are too demanding, it may be possible to persuade her employers to offer her some alternative work of a less arduous nature. When her duties lie solely in the home she should be told to reduce all heavy work to a minimum, if possible persuading her husband to take over certain chores, certainly for the time being and preferably on a more permanent basis.

Women often worry about the possibility of returning to work after childbirth, fearing that they will not be able to do so. While much depends upon the individual circumstances of each case, the midwife should never be depressing on this score and as a rule it will be best to reassure the patient that she will be ready to resume her occupation, should she still wish to do so, some six to eight weeks after her child has been born.

d Exercise
Women vary widely in the amount of exercise they take and for this reason no hard and fast rules can be laid down as to what constitutes an ideal arrangement during pregnancy. In general, the best advice is that whatever exercise is usually taken should continue during pregnancy, provided that this progresses normally, but that exertion to the point of physical exhaustion should not be allowed to happen. There is therefore no need to urge drastic reduction of physical exercise in a patient accustomed to this any more than to demand increased efforts of one who is of essentially sedentary habits.

e Rest
Here again, people vary widely in the amount of rest and sleep they seem to require. As a rule, however, the lassitude which is so often a feature of early pregnancy means that more sleep will be needed and should therefore be taken at this time. As a

general guide, it is best to advise eight hours a night, if possible even more than this, while, if facilities exist, a short rest in the middle of the day has much to commend it. In later pregnancy, especially after the thirty-second week, it is best to insist on a period during the afternoon of at least two hours' rest, taken in or on a bed rather than merely sitting in a chair, while the time spent in bed at night should be increased. If the patient finds it hard to get to sleep, or wakes up for long periods during the night, she should be advised to ask her doctor for a hypnotic drug, of great help in such cases. She must, however, be warned not to get into the way of relying too greatly on such an aid to sleep and she should certainly be discouraged from taking any such substance once pregnancy is over, for fear of starting a habit which may prove very difficult to break.

f Smoking and Drinking
If the patient feels able to give up cigarettes during pregnancy she should be strongly advised to do so, since among its more adverse effects, smoking appears to interfere with the rate of growth of the foetus. Where such a sacrifice is beyond her powers she should, if possible, reduce her cigarette consumption to fewer than ten a day, since the less smoking is indulged in the smaller will be its effects on the patient and the foetus. So far as alcoholic drinks are concerned, provided that these are not consumed to excess, and this is very rarely the case, they seem to harm neither the patient nor the foetus and there is thus no need to forbid them during pregnancy.

g Sexual Intercourse
It is said that humans are the only members of the animal kingdom to practise intercourse during pregnancy and that this is probably fundamental to their basic psychological make-up. This being so, it is pointless to forbid or to discourage this activity and unless there is evidence of some abnormality of pregnancy, especially vaginal bleeding, there is no need to recommend that intercourse be given up. It is customary to dissuade a woman from coitus during the last six weeks of pregnancy, but the reasons for this are obscure and it is doubtful whether any of those offered this particular advice actually avail themselves of it.

5 Maternity Benefits*
The maternity benefits available in this country may be considered under two headings, financial and nutritional:

a Financial
A pregnant woman is entitled:

i To a Maternity Grant of £22, payable after the twenty-eighth week against the signature of a doctor or a midwife.

ii If working and in possession of the required number of National Insurance stamps, she may also claim a Maternity Allowance of £4·50, paid weekly, usually for eleven weeks before and for seven weeks after delivery.

Details of these payments are given in Leaflet N.I.17A, obtainable from the Local Pensions and National Insurance Office.

b Nutritional
i All pregnant women are entitled to claim one pint of milk per day at a reduced price. This is available throughout pregnancy and is transferred to the baby after delivery.

ii Supplements such as vitamin tablets, orange juice and cod liver oil are available either free or at nominal prices.

iii All iron supplements are provided free of charge.

6 The Date and Time of the Next Visit
Either the midwife or the clinic doctor will have already discussed with the patient the place or places of further antenatal care, taking into account her history and the findings on examination. She should also have been told when to attend again and a note to this effect entered in her case records. It is a midwife's responsibility to see that her patient, before leaving the clinic, understands these arrangements and fully appreciates the need to return on the arranged date and at the correct time. It is also necessary to be certain that she realises that should she be unable to attend she must tell the clinic concerned.

Lastly, the patient should be reminded to bring up to the

* Since writing this these benefits have been extensively altered.

clinic at her next attendance a specimen of her urine in a small, clean bottle.

The Management of Normal Pregnancy: II

The previous section was mainly concerned with the patient's first visit to the ante-natal clinic and with the procedures carried out at that time. It now remains to discuss the ante-natal care needed during the remainder of pregnancy. This may most easily be considered under the following headings:

1   The intervals between clinic attendances

2   Routine obstetric examinations and investigations

3   Special examinations.

1   The Intervals between Clinic Attendances
Since the liability to develop an abnormality of pregnancy increases as term approaches, the patient should be seen more often in late than in early pregnancy. For this reason attendances at the ante-natal clinic should take place as follows:

a   Four-weekly until the twenty-eighth week

b   Fortnightly until the thirty-sixth week

c   Weekly until term.

At this stage the patient must be referred to the clinic doctor who will decide whether to allow pregnancy to continue or whether, on the other hand, labour should be induced without further delay, since naturally this is not a matter for which a midwife can assume responsibility.

It should be stressed that the above times of attendance represent those suitable for cases where pregnancy is proceeding normally and that they are the least that can safely be recommended. Should pregnancy become abnormal, or if it is thought that an abnormality is likely to arise, it will be better to see the patient more frequently. Here again, however, the advice of a doctor will be needed before any decision is taken.

c

2 Routine Examinations and Investigations

The following simple examinations must be carried out every time a woman is seen at the ante-natal clinic:

a Urinalysis must be carried out

b The blood pressure must be taken

c The weight must be recorded

d The patient must be examined for the presence of oedema

e The breasts and legs must be examined

f The abdomen must be palpated.

With the exception of the last of these, none is in the least difficult or time-consuming, yet, if correctly and conscientiously carried out, they make all the difference between a well-managed pregnancy in which any abnormality which arises is detected and hence treated early and effectively, and a mismanaged pregnancy in which an abnormality remains undiagnosed and hence untreated until it assumes dangerous proportions.

a The Analysis of the Urine

As instructed, the patient will bring up to the clinic a sample of her urine. This should be tested for albumen, sugar and ketone bodies. The result of this investigation must then be entered on an appropriate form and handed to the patient to show to the doctor or midwife who is to examine her. Should the urine be found to contain albumen, a mid-stream specimen must be obtained and tested. The reason for this is that in an ordinary clean specimen, albumen may merely represent contamination from a vaginal discharge, which, in a properly collected mid-stream specimen will not be the case, the albumen, if still present, coming from some part of the urinary tract. In such an event, or if either sugar or ketone bodies are found to be present, or if the patient complains of symptoms such as frequency, urgency or dysuria, a doctor must be informed at once, since any of these findings may indicate a serious abnormality of pregnancy.

Where any of these urinary abnormalities are discovered it is usual to send a further mid-stream specimen in a sterile container to the Pathology Laboratory for culture and microscopy.

If for some reason this sample cannot be sent off at once, it must not be allowed to stand at room temperature, since this would allow the bacteria present in small numbers in nearly every specimen of urine to grow and thus to interfere with the laboratory findings. Instead, it should be kept for the time being in the clinic refrigerator at a temperature of 4°C. This will prevent further bacterial growth while allowing the survival of those organisms already present, thus providing the laboratory staff with an uncontaminated specimen on which to carry out the necessary investigations.

b   The Blood Pressure

If possible, the blood pressure should not be taken before the patient is in the examination room; usually it is recorded in the course of her physical examination, sometimes before this starts. She should be lying down on the couch at rest and if she has had to hurry to the clinic she should be allowed a few minutes in which to settle down and relax. Failure to observe these simple rules may result in unduly high readings being obtained.

The level of the systolic and diastolic pressures must be carefully noted and entered on the patient's case records. If the pressure is above 130/90 mm Hg or if it shows a rise of over 10 mm Hg, either systolic or diastolic, above the level noted at her previous visit to the clinic, the doctor should be told.

In a normal pregnancy the blood pressure rarely rises above 120/80 mm Hg and as a rule shows what is called the Mid-Trimester Drop, the pressure being lowered during the middle third of pregnancy, sometimes to a marked degree. Provided that the woman feels well and can carry out her daily routine without physical distress, there is no need to worry if what seems to be an extremely low pressure is recorded, such as 85/40 mm Hg or even less. This apparently severe hypotension may in part be due to the fact that when lying down the return of blood to the heart is delayed by the pressure exerted on the vena cava by the heavy, pregnant uterus. This at times may result in transient faintness when the patient is lying on her back, easily remedied by turning her on to her side. As a rule, however, as already mentioned, the only manifestation seems to be an occasional abnormally low blood pressure.

c The Patient's Weight

The patient should be weighed before she is examined and the result entered in her case notes. Ideally she should be unclothed for this procedure, since otherwise marked fluctuations may occur, depending upon what she happens to be wearing at the time. In practice this particular source of error is ignored, shoes and outdoor clothes only being removed. Although at first sight this arrangement may seem to be unscientific, in practice it combines an acceptable degree of accuracy with the greatest amount of convenience and saving of time to all concerned.

The amount of weight gained during a normal pregnancy depends on a number of different factors and thus tends to vary rather widely around an average of 13·0 kg. Of considerably greater importance than the total weight gain is the increase to be expected at various times in pregnancy. These increases are as follows:

By the 10th week: 500 grammes
By the 20th week: 4·0 kg
By the 30th week: 9·5 kg
By the 40th week: 13·0 kg.

Two points of special importance in relation to weight gain in pregnancy are:

1 The increase between the twentieth and the thirtieth week should not exceed 4·5 kg. If it does, there is a possibility that the patient may later develop pre-eclampsia (page 97).

2 For the same reason, from the thirtieth week onwards, the amount of weight gained during any one week should not be more than 1 kg.

Sometimes a slight drop in weight, amounting at the most to about 1 kg, occurs just before the onset of labour. This is taken by some as an indication that the patient is 'due'. While this sign is admittedly of some value, it must not be relied upon too much, if only because weight fluctuations of this magnitude are fairly common in the non-pregnant as well as in the pregnant.

d The General Appearance of the Patient

Although appearances are misleading, it is unusual for normal healthy women to look ill during pregnancy. The midwife should therefore pay careful attention to her patient's appearance, noting in particular her colour and the state of her hair, her skin and her teeth. Pallor, a poor complexion and lustreless hair are all, at times, manifestations of ill-health and as such should be reported to a doctor.

Oedema

The development of oedema, especially where this involves the fingers, may be a sign that the condition known as pre-eclampsia is either already present or is liable to develop in the near future. In consequence, oedema should be looked for at every visit. This is usually done by pressing the skin over some firm, unyielding structure, such as a bony point. If such pressure is kept up for a few seconds, the oedema fluid in the tissues is displaced outwards resulting in pitting of the skin which may be both seen and felt. The parts of the body most easily tested in this way are the ankles – over the medial malleoli – the shins, the fingers – where the pressure of rings produces a characteristic groove – and the abdomen – where the pressure from a foetal stethoscope soon causes a circular depression to form. It is often said that puffiness of the face is also noted in these cases, but unless the patient is particularly well-known to the midwife, or the swelling abnormally pronounced, it is usually impossible to be certain that such an appearance is not normal. Sacral oedema, although sometimes present when the patient has been in bed for some time, is rarely detected in the ante-natal clinic.

e The Breasts

At the patient's first visit to the ante-natal clinic her breasts will have been examined by a doctor. Although it is not necessary for this examination to be repeated at every subsequent visit, it is usually wise to exclude the presence of abnormal masses in the breasts at the twenty-eighth and thirty-sixth weeks. In addition, it is usual to check the size and shape of the nipples and whether they can easily be made to protrude, since these features are of importance should the patient wish to breast-feed her baby.

Varicose Veins

At each visit the patient's legs should be inspected for the presence of varicose veins, which often arise in the course of pregnancy and can cause considerable discomfort and annoyance. Where there is evidence that such varicosities have either developed or are increasing in size, a doctor should be informed, since it may be necessary to prescribe supportive stockings, which can be ordered only on medical advice. Once these have been supplied, the midwife should see that they are a good fit and that they provide adequate control of the veins when the patient is standing up.

f The Abdomen

Even if it is not thought likely that the uterus will be palpable, the abdomen should be examined at every visit, since part at least of the value of this procedure is to exclude the presence of any abnormal masses and to make sure that the uterus is not larger than the period of amenorrhoea would warrant.

To derive the maximum accuracy from this examination the height of the fundus should be determined and recorded in the patient's notes *before* checking on the duration of amenorrhoea, instead of *first* finding out how long pregnancy has lasted and *then* seeing whether the size of the uterus corresponds more or less to this time. This latter method is both slovenly and inaccurate and leads to endless difficulties in those cases, by no means rare, where the uterus is either larger or smaller than expected.

As suggested above, these problems may be avoided by *first* estimating the height of the fundus in terms of weeks of pregnancy and *then* seeing from the notes whether this corresponds to what would be expected. If there is any gross discrepancy between the uterine size and the patient's dates, the matter must be discussed with the clinic doctor.

Having assessed the height of the fundus, it is next necessary to make sure, so far as is practicable, that there is only one foetus present. This can sometimes be difficult, but if not borne in mind as a possibility, the diagnosis of a multiple pregnancy will be even less frequently made than is at present the case. This point is further considered on page 286; here it need only be said that a uterus larger than the period of amenorrhoea would warrant, a multiplicity of foetal parts, or unexpected difficulty in outlining the foetus, should all lead a midwife to suspect a multiple pregnancy and to ask for a doctor's advice on the matter.

The lie of the foetus should next be determined. This is said to be *longitudinal* if the foetal back is more or less parallel to the patient's. If the foetal back is at right angles to the mother's the lie is *transverse*. Since the foetus is constantly altering its position in the uterus during early pregnancy, it is not necessary to attach much importance to the lie until the thirtieth week, by which time it normally has become longitudinal.

The Foetal Head

It is now necessary to discover the whereabouts in the uterus of the foetal head; whether this is in the fundus or, as is usually the case, in the lower part or *lower pole* of the uterus. Although the foetal head is usually felt easily and convincingly, difficulties can always be encountered and in certain circumstances it may well be mistaken for the breech. Here practice is of the greatest value, while it is also useful to remember that nothing in obstetrics should ever be taken for granted. Although for reasons already mentioned, the lie, and hence the situation of the head, is of little importance before the thirtieth week, if at or after this time the midwife suspects that it is *not* in the lower pole of the uterus but somewhere else, such as in the fundus or one or other of the flanks, medical aid should be sought since this is a clear indication of an abnormal presentation.

The Engagement of the Foetal Head

The examination of the uterus to make out the lie of the foetus and the situation of the foetal head will also serve to determine the *presentation* of the foetus. This may be either by the head – Cephalic – or by the breech – Podalic. Of the two the former is by far the more common. If the head presents it is necessary to find out if it is *engaged*, that is, whether it has passed through the brim into the cavity of the pelvis. This does not usually occur much before the thirty-sixth week of pregnancy, indeed in a multipara engagement may not take place until after the onset of labour, although this is not as common as is often taught. It is not easy to describe the exact way in which to test for engagement, although practice will soon teach this. Basically, if on abdominal palpation more than half of the foetal head can be felt above the pelvis or if the impression is gained that the fingers can get below the widest part of the head, it is *not engaged*. This point will be considered in greater detail on page 167, in which Normal Labour is described. At this stage it is only necessary to say that the importance of engagement lies in the fact that it indicates that since the foetal head has managed to reach the cavity of the pelvis it will as a general rule be able to negotiate the outlet with safety. Moreover, if the head of the foetus can pass through the pelvis the body will do so as well. Engagement therefore means that unless something unexpected is amiss either with the patient's pelvis or with the foetus, there will be enough room for a safe delivery.

The Thirty-sixth-Week Examination

The examination of the patient at the thirty-sixth week should always be carried out by a doctor, since it is important at this time to decide whether labour is likely to be straightforward or whether complications are liable to arise which require special management.

In the main, such a decision centres around the engagement of the foetal head, which, as just mentioned, should now have taken place. If the head is still above the brim it may be necessary to see whether it can be made to engage artificially. To do this the patient should be on her back with her head slightly raised and her knees moderately flexed, in order to relax the abdominal muscles. Firm pressure applied to the head in a downward and backward direction will usually make it enter the pelvis. Although this test is carried out by a doctor at the thirty-sixth week, at the patient's subsequent visits the midwife may wish to repeat it in order to confirm the previous findings. In this connection it should be mentioned that at times the Head Fitting Test, as it is often called, is not easy to perform and that considerable practice is needed to interpret it accurately. For this reason, even when the midwife is confident about her ability in this respect, she should still request a medical opinion on any woman, primigravida or multipara, in whom the foetal head is not engaged after the thirty-sixth week of pregnancy.

It may be of help at this stage to summarise the times in pregnancy at which the various points mentioned above should be checked with particular care.

At twenty-eight weeks:	Exclude the possibility of a multiple pregnancy
At thirty weeks:	Discover whether the lie is longitudinal or transverse
At thirty-two weeks:	Determine the presentation – head or breech
At thirty-six weeks:	See if the foetal head is engaged and if not whether it can be made to enter the pelvis.

3 Special Examinations

The Blood

Although a full examination of the blood is carried out only at the patient's first attendance at the ante-natal clinic, some of the investigations performed at this time should be repeated at intervals during pregnancy.

a The Haemoglobin Level

Unless the haemoglobin level is under 70 per cent – 10 G per cent – when first estimated, it need not be checked again until the thirty-second week. This will allow sufficient time before delivery for Iron therapy, should this be indicated. Ideally, a further haemoglobin estimation should be made at the thirty-sixth week to exclude the development of an anaemia late in pregnancy.

b   Rhesus Antibodies

In all Rhesus negative women, particularly those who have had a child, the presence of antibodies should be looked for at the first clinic attendance. If these are absent, further checks should be made at the twenty-eighth, thirty-second and thirty-sixth weeks. If, on the other hand, antibodies are present from early pregnancy, their concentration or *titre* must be estimated more frequently (page 142).

c   Vaginal Discharges

Where a patient complains of a vaginal discharge, particularly if it is profuse or irritating, a high vaginal swab should be taken for culture and microscopy. For this purpose a clean speculum and a sterile swab are needed. The swab, together with the appropriate request form, must then be sent without delay to the pathology laboratory, either in a glass test-tube or in a suitable transport medium.

Miscellaneous Points

At the end of each visit, the following points should be checked with the patient:

a   Has she any questions she would like answered or any worries she wishes to discuss? These may concern her pregnancy or some other feature of her life, either business, social or family, which is in some way affected by the pregnancy. However fanciful or odd some of these questions and worries may appear, it must be remembered that to the woman concerned they are of importance and need careful and sympathetic handling. For that reason, enough time must be found at each visit to allow the patient an opportunity to discuss any matters which may be uppermost in her mind.

This is one of the most important of the various aspects of normal ante-natal care and is one which the midwife, by her training, is particularly well-equipped to deal with, often in collaboration with the Medical Social Worker, whose advice should always be asked for if this seems at all necessary. The help and encouragement which can be given to the patient in this way can easily make the difference between a straight-forward and enjoyable pregnancy and one which, although physically normal, is beset throughout by a succession of doubts, fears and worries.

b Has she enough supplies of Iron and Vitamin tablets to last until the next visit?

c Does she know where and at what time to come for her next visit?

It will be realised from this review of the management of normal pregnancy that all must ultimately depend upon liaison and teamwork involving many different authorities, depart-ments and individuals – medical, nursing and administrative. The present-day complexity of clinic work has made any com-pletely individual system of ante-natal care virtually impossible. While such co-operation has undoubtedly produced great benefits and has much to commend it, it is important to bear in mind the value to the patient of a more personal approach and to arrange so far as possible that she sees the same midwife or doctor at each of her clinic visits. If this can be done it will add greatly to the value of the ante-natal care provided while the amount of work involved, far from being increased, will be considerably reduced, owing to the simplicity of seeing the same patients each time. An arrangement of this nature repre-sents the best possible solution to the problem of providing efficient yet personal supervision, and, by encouraging an individual approach within the wider concept of co-operation between numerous different people, allows the greatest benefit to be brought to the greatest number of pregnant women at the least cost in man-power and materials.

The Uterus and Its Contents at Term

In order to understand how certain of the abnormalities of pregnancy arise as well as the way in which the uterus acts during labour, it is necessary to have some knowledge of the anatomy of the uterus, the placenta and the foetus.

The Uterus

The non-pregnant uterus is a small, pear-shaped organ, about 7·5 cm long, 5 cm wide and 2·5 cm thick situated in the pelvis between the bladder and the rectum. It is divided into four parts which are, from above down, the fundus, the body, the isthmus and the cervix. The uterine cavity, which is lined with endometrium, is a flat triangular space, communicating above and laterally with the Fallopian tubes and below with the cervical canal, at the lower end of which is the external os, opening into the upper part of the vagina.

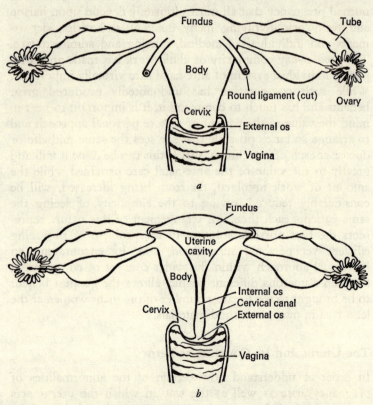

Fig. 4   The non-pregnant uterus
(a) general appearance (b) coronal section

Outer Coverings

Both the front and the back of the uterus are covered by peritoneum, the upper part of which encloses the two Fallopian tubes. This peritoneal covering is continued laterally on to the side-walls of the pelvis to form the Broad ligament. Anteriorly, at the level of the isthmus, the peritoneum is reflected on to the upper surface of the bladder, posteriorly it dips into the hollow of the Pouch of Douglas between the vagina and the rectum. The peritoneum is firmly attached to the underlying uterine muscle – the myometrium – save in the region of the Broad ligament laterally and the isthmus anteriorly. Here it is loosely applied to allow for upward distension of the bladder.

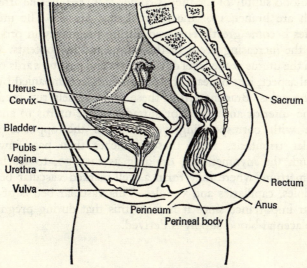

Fig. 5   Lateral view of non-pregnant uterus

The Myometrium

The myometrium consists of three layers:

1   An outer longitudinal layer
2   An inner circular layer
3   An intermediate layer

Of these, only the intermediate layer is of obstetric importance. This consists of a mass of interlacing muscle fibres, running in all directions. It makes up the bulk of the uterus and during labour provides the necessary force for the descent and delivery of the foetus. The myometrium varies in depth, this being greatest in the fundus and upper part of the body. It is less thick in the region of the isthmus. The cervix is composed mainly of fibrous and connective tissue, lined internally with endothelium.

Blood Supply

The blood supply of the uterus comes from the uterine arteries, which are branches of the internal iliac vessels. The uterine arteries become greatly enlarged during pregnancy in order to meet the increasing needs of the uterus and its contents. They reach the uterus at the level of the cervix and pass upwards on its lateral aspect, just beneath the peritoneum, accompanied by the uterine veins. Branches from these main vessels run medially on the anterior and posterior surfaces of the uterus to anastomose with corresponding vessels from the opposite side. Smaller tributaries from these branches then pass inwards through the myometrium, dividing as they go, to reach the endometrium where they form a well-marked vascular bed of arterioles, capillaries and venules. This vascular bed is of particular importance since it is from this that during pregnancy the placental blood supply is derived.

The Uterus at Term

The uterus at term is ovoid in shape and is enlarged to 30 cm in length, 25 cm in width and 20 cm in depth. Owing, however, to the fact that the fertilised ovum usually implants in the upper part of the body, the rate of growth of this part of the uterus is greater at first than that of the lower half. This, although eventually sharing in the general increase in size, does so both at a later date and to a lesser extent, that portion immediately above the cervix – the isthmus – developing into the lower uterine segment only during the last weeks of pregnancy. The cervix itself undergoes no appreciable enlargement.

Uterine growth is due in part to an increase both in the number and in the size of the myometrial fibres and in part to distension by the developing ovum. As a result, the thickness of

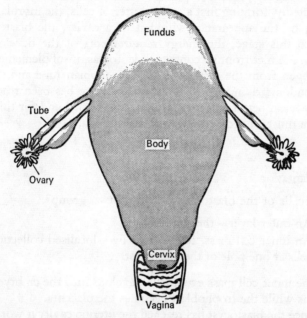

Fig. 6 The uterus at term

its walls increases only during early pregnancy, after the third month these actually become thinner, so that at term they are barely 1 cm thick at the fundus and considerably less in the region of the lower segment.

The cavity of the uterus contains the foetus, the placenta, the foetal membranes and the liquor amnii. It is lined by a modified type of endometrium known as Decidua.

The Placenta

To understand the anatomy of the placenta the early development of the fertilised ovum must be briefly reviewed.

At ovulation the ovum is the largest cell in the body, its size being due to the presence within it of yolk or deutoplasm. Fertilisation takes place in the outer part of the Fallopian tube. Following this, during its passage to the uterus, the ovum divides repeatedly, forming first a solid cluster of cells, the morula, and later, by the appearance within it of a cavity, the blastocyst. Up to this stage, the energy requirements of the developing ovum are met from its contained deutoplasm, supplemented by glycogen from the secretions of the Fallopian tube and, later, the endometrium. After the blastocyst stage has been reached, however, a better means of nutrition is needed and for this the ovum must embed or *implant* in the decidua.

Implantation

The cells of the blastocyst consist of two groups.

1 An outer layer – the trophoblast
2 An inner cell mass, represented by a localised collection of cells at one pole of the blastocyst.

The inner cell mass eventually develops into the embryo and foetus while the trophoblast becomes the placenta.

Once the blastocyst has reached the uterine cavity it works its way into the decidua, eventually becoming completely covered over by this layer. This process of implantation is made possible by the specialised trophoblastic cells. These now send out small projections into the surrounding decidua, dissolving its cells and opening up minute capillaries. In this way small pools of maternal blood form around the embedded ovum which can now derive its oxygen and nutrition from this source. In addition, wedges of trophoblast burrow into the deeper layers of the decidua to anchor the ovum to its site of implantation and to secure a firm base for its future development.

Further growth of the trophoblast results in the formation of numerous finger-like villous processes, some of which are attached, as were their predecessors, to the deeper layer of the decidua – the anchoring villi – while others lie with their ends free in the pools of maternal blood, now known as the inter-villous space. These chorionic villi, which are made up of two sorts of cells, the syncytium and the cytotrophoblast, are originally formed over the whole surface of the ovum, but as this grows it projects more and more into the uterine cavity, stretching its decidual and villous coverings, impeding their blood supply and eventually causing their death. This does not, of course, happen to those villi situated more centrally between the ovum and the uterine wall, which continue to grow and to subdivide at an enormous pace, eventually forming the placenta.

The Placenta at Term

The placenta at term is a plate-like structure, about 23 cm in diameter and 2·5 cm thick. It weighs about 550 grammes. It is usually situated in the upper part of the uterine cavity, either

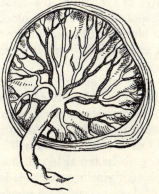

Fig. 7   Foetal surface of the placenta

anteriorly or posteriorly, secured there by its anchoring villi. Its smooth foetal surface is directed inwards and is covered by the amnion. Below the amnion a mass of veins and arteries, tributaries of the umbilical vessels, run over the surface of the placenta, dividing as they pass outwards. Branches from these vessels turn at right angles into the substance of the placenta, dividing as they go and eventually reaching the chorionic villi.

The bulk of the placenta is composed of vast numbers of these chorionic villi, each one of which contains an arteriole, a venule and a small capillary plexus, covered by endothelium and a thin

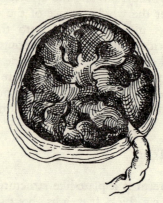

Fig. 8   Maternal surface of the placenta

and incomplete layer of syncytium, the cytotrophoblast having by now largely disappeared. The foetal blood is thus separated from the maternal blood in the intervillous space for the most part only by the endothelial lining of these small chorionic vessels.

The chorionic villi are grouped together somewhat hap-hazardly into twelve to sixteen Cotyledons, separated one from the other by well-defined septa, which represent the original wedges of trophoblast that first grew out into the decidua from the margins of the early ovum. The intervillous space, as already explained, is filled with maternal blood, derived from the de-cidual vessels which originally ran towards the implantation site. The mouths of these vessels open directly into the base of the intervillous space, and blood from them slowly circulates around the villi, draining back into the mother's vascular system through multiple short, wide-mouthed veins. In addition, maternal blood from the periphery of the placenta is collected into a thin-walled channel, the Marginal Sinus, which forms an incomplete circle around the edge of the placenta.

The Functions of the Placenta

The placenta has four main functions:

1 *Respiratory.* Due to the close relation of the blood in the intervillous space to that in the chorionic villi, oxygen can readily pass from the mother to the foetus while carbon dioxide from the foetus can as easily be returned to the maternal circulation.

2 *Nutritional.* In the same way, nutrients from the mother's blood cross into the foetal circulation either directly or after modification by the syncytial cells.

3 *Excretory.* The break-down products of foetal metabolism can be removed only by being passed across the villi into the intervillous space for excretion by the mother.

4 *Endocrine.* The placenta is a complex endocrine gland, numerous hormones, principally gonadotrophins, progesterone and oestrogens, being formed by the cells lining the chorionic villi. These hormones have several functions:

a The gonadotrophins suppress ovulation and probably maintain the corpus luteum until its functions can be taken over by the placenta.

b The oestrogens and progesterone are responsible for the growth of the uterus, the changes in the uterus, cervix and vagina necessary for labour and the growth and secretory activity of the breasts. Progesterone can also relax smooth muscle, and while this is useful in reducing uterine irritability and ensuring that its contents are not too readily expelled, it has the unfortunate side-effect of predisposing to constipation, urinary stasis, varicose veins and haemorrhoids.

The Placental Barrier

It is usually taught that the placenta acts as a barrier in preventing certain substances from reaching the foetus from the mother. Recent work, however, has cast some doubt on this view and it seems that while considerable variation exists in the rate in which substances reach the foetus, all will eventually do so.

Ageing of the Placenta

Since the placenta is an organ with a very limited life-span, it is not surprising that towards the end of pregnancy it should show signs of age and of impaired function. It is generally thought that this ageing is due to the formation of placental infarcts – greyish-white areas of villous occlusion and thrombosis – together with calcification of the villi and deposition of fibrin plaques in the intervillous space, all of which would tend to reduce the efficiency of the placenta. Such macroscopic evidence of ageing is, however, by no means always present, and even if seen is not necessarily related to the actual performance of the placenta. It is therefore possible that less well-defined but equally sinister microscopic changes occur towards term, the effect of which is to place the foetus at risk by interfering with normal placental function and causing placental insufficiency (page 99).

The Foetus

As already said, the foetus develops from the inner cell mass of the blastocyst. This collection of cells soon becomes separated from the trophoblast surrounding it, being connected to it only by the body stalk, the forerunner of the umbilical cord. Further growth of the inner cell mass results in the formation of a flat embryonic plate, from which the primitive embryo develops with early differentiation of such essential structures as the brain, the gut, the heart and the main vessels. These last send out branches into the body stalk to join the arteries and veins of the chorionic villi and establish the rudiments of a foetal circulation.

At an early stage a membrane grows around the embryo,

which up to this point has been lying in the cavity of the blastocyst. This membrane, the amnion, soon comes to enclose the foetus and obliterates the cavity of the blastocyst, reaching the inner aspects of the trophoblast – the chorion – and of the early

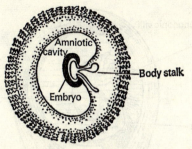

Fig. 9   Later ovum showing foetal membranes

placenta. The amnion is filled with a clear fluid, the liquor amnii, which protects the foetus from injury, allows it room for movement and growth and prevents the formation of adhesions between it and the uterine wall. As the ovum increases in size, it comes to occupy progressively more space, completely filling the cavity of the uterus by the twelfth week. After this time, the inner surface of the uterus is, with the exception of the area covered by the placenta, entirely lined by amnion, under which is a thin layer of chorion while deep to both lie the compressed remnants of the decidua.

The Umbilical Cord

This structure, derived from the body stalk of the early ovum, connects the foetus to the placenta. Covered by a layer of amnion, it is composed of a translucent, gelatinous material called Wharton's Jelly, and is about 2 cm in diameter. Its length varies greatly, being normally between 25 and 75 cm. It contains the umbilical vessels, usually one vein and two arteries, which run from the placenta to the foetus. On rare occasions an abnormal number of vessels is present in the cord. Since this is often associated with other foetal abnormalities, it is important always to check this point at delivery. False Knots (bulbous outgrowths of Wharton's Jelly) are frequently seen along the length of the cord. They are of no clinical significance. True knots, on the other hand, which are rare, are of great importance since,

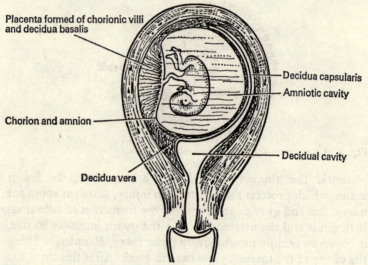

Placenta formed of chorionic villi
and decidua basalis

Decidua capsularis

Amniotic cavity

Chorion and amnion

Decidual cavity

Decidua vera

Fig. 10 Ovum filling uterus cavity

if pulled tight, they may cause the death of the foetus by interfering with its blood supply. More commonly, the same accident may result from the cord, which during pregnancy often becomes wound around the neck of the foetus, being stretched and compressed during labour as the head descends into the pelvis.

The Foetus at Term

At term the foetus normally weighs between 3·0 and 3·5 kg and measures about 40 cm from crown to rump. For reasons of space it is folded up upon itself within the uterus and, since the flexor muscle groups are usually stronger than the extensor at this stage of life, it commonly adopts an attitude of flexion, the back being gently curved, the head bent forwards at the neck, the arms folded across the chest and the legs flexed and crossed on one another. In this attitude the shape of the foetus is an ovoid, the larger pole of which is formed by the breech and legs while the smaller consists of the well-flexed head. Since the uterine cavity is also ovoid in shape, its greater pole being uppermost, it follows that the foetus will fit the uterus best with its head lowest while its larger breech and flexed legs occupy the more capacious fundus. It is unlikely that any reason more complicated than this determines the normal lie, attitude and presentation of the foetus at term.

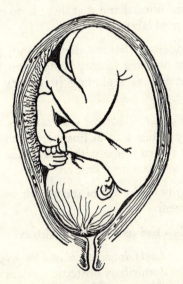

Fig. 11   The foetus at term showing flexed attitude

Summary

The Place and Delivery of Ante-natal Care

A patient may be confined in one of three places:

a   A Maternity Hospital or Maternity Unit of a General Hospital
This is an establishment equipped to deal with any obstetric abnormality.

b A General Practitioner Maternity Home
Here facilities are lacking for the safe management of abnormal labours.

c Her Own Home
Only if the delivery is normal should it be conducted here.

The following types of case are suitable for delivery either at home or in a general practitioner maternity home:

a Primigravidae over 18 and under 30, provided that pregnancy has been normal and that there is no reason to anticipate an abnormal labour

b Multiparae under 35, having their second, third or fourth baby, the past obstetric history being normal and subject to the same restrictions regarding pregnancy and labour as primigravidae.

All other patients should be delivered in hospital.
A mother may either stay in hospital for eight to ten days after delivery or return home within 48 hours. The two main indications for a 48-hour discharge are:

a Where the parity or the age of the patient was the reason for hospital confinement.

b Where there is a bad past obstetric history.

Provided always that labour is uneventful and the baby normal.
In such cases the domiciliary obstetric services must be willing to accept the subsequent care of the mother and the baby.

The place of ante-natal care may be a hospital, a Local Authority clinic or a general practitioner obstetrician's surgery. Care is frequently shared between two or more of these places and people.

Patients attending a hospital ante-natal clinic throughout pregnancy are usually those booked for a hospital confinement.

Where a patient is booked for delivery in a general practitioner maternity home or in her own home, ante-natal care is usually provided either by the Local Authority clinic or by a general practitioner obstetrician. Should any such case need a hospital consultation, this must be arranged without loss of time.

Most patients booked for a hospital delivery need to be seen at the hospital ante-natal clinic only at booking, at the thirty-sixth week and at term. The bulk of the ante-natal care is provided either by the Local Authority or by a general practitioner obstetrician.

Where ante-natal care is divided between two or more places, difficulties may arise. These may be avoided by maintaining a close liaison between the various authorities concerned, by ensuring that every patient knows the time and place of her next visit and by making sure that her personal ante-natal card is properly completed at the end of each visit.

The Management of Normal Pregnancy: I

The three basic objects of ante-natal care are:

a To bring to term a healthy foetus

b To safeguard the health of the mother during pregnancy

c To determine the safest method of delivery.

To achieve these objects the following principles must be observed:

a The patient must attend the clinic for the first time in early pregnancy, if possible before the twelfth week

b She must be seen regularly and frequently during pregnancy

c Enough time must be devoted to her at each visit

d Any abnormalities discovered must be reported to a doctor.

The First Visit
The following points must be considered at the first visit:

a The diagnosis of pregnancy must be established

b The patient's health and the state of her pregnancy must be checked. This involves:
i Consideration of the menstrual and past obstetric history.
ii Consideration of the past medical and surgical history with

special reference to cardiac, renal, pulmonary and liver diseases, rubella and blood transfusions.

iii A full clinical examination, conducted by a doctor.

iv Analysis of a sample of urine, including a mid-stream specimen.

v A full haematological examination.

vi An X-ray of the chest.

vii If necessary, a visit to a dentist.

c The place of ante-natal care and of confinement must then be agreed.

d Advice on the following points should then be given:
i Morning sickness
ii Diet, including milk and iron and vitamin tablets
iii Work – whether at home or at paid employment
iv Exercise
v Rest – both at night and in the day-time
vi Smoking and drinking
vii Sexual intercourse
viii Maternity benefits

e The date and time of the next visit must then be arranged, particular emphasis being laid upon the importance of keeping this appointment.

The Management of Normal Pregnancy: II

A patient's subsequent ante-natal care may be considered under three headings:

a The intervals between clinic attendances

b Routine obstetric examinations and investigations

c Special examinations.

The intervals between clinic attendances should normally be as follows:

Every four weeks until the twenty-eighth week
Every fortnight until the thirty-sixth week
Every week until term.

These represent the minimum number desirable and must be increased should any abnormality develop.

The following routine examinations and investigations are necessary during normal pregnancy:

a   *The urine* should be tested at every visit for the presence of albumen, sugar and ketone bodies. If any abnormality is discovered a doctor should be informed and a mid-stream specimen of urine sent to the laboratory for further investigation.

b   *The blood pressure* should be recorded at every visit and a doctor informed if it is over 130/90 mm Hg or if there is a rise of over 10 mm Hg – systolic or diastolic over the last recorded level.

c   *The patient should be weighed* at every visit, attention being paid to:
Total weight gained: The average for pregnancy is 13·0 kg.
Weight gained between twenty and thirty weeks: Not to exceed 4·5 kg.
Weekly gain after thirty weeks: Not to exceed 1 kg.

d   *The general appearance of the patient* and in particular the state of skin, hair and teeth should be noted.

e   At every visit *Oedema* must be looked for over the ankles and on the fingers and the abdominal wall.

f   *The breasts* must be examined for abnormal masses at the twenty-eighth and thirty-sixth weeks. The state of the nipples should be checked at these times.

g   The legs should be inspected for the presence of *varicose veins*, elastic stockings being ordered if necessary.

h   *Abdominal palpation.* Attention must be paid to the height of the fundus, the number of foetuses present, the lie of the foetus and the position in the uterus of the foetal head. From this information the presentation of the foetus may be determined.

i *Engagement of the head.* If the head is presenting it must be seen whether it is engaged or can be made to engage. If any doubt exists on this point after thirty-six weeks, medical aid must be sought.

j The times in pregnancy when these various points should be checked are:
At twenty-eight weeks: Exclude a multiple pregnancy
At thirty weeks: Determine the lie of the foetus
At thirty-two weeks: Determine the presentation of the foetus
At thirty-six weeks: Determine whether the head is engaged or will engage.

Special Examinations

a *The Blood.* The haemoglobin level should be estimated at thirty-two and thirty-six weeks. Rhesus antibodies should be looked for at twenty-eight, thirty-two and thirty-six weeks

b *Vaginal Discharges.* If a vaginal discharge is present a high vaginal swab should be sent for culture and microscopy.

Miscellaneous Points
Before leaving the clinic the patient should always be asked:

a Whether there are any particular points she wishes to discuss

b Whether she has enough iron and vitamin tablets

c Whether she knows where and when to come for her next visit.

The Uterus and its Contents at Term

The non-pregnant uterus, which measures $7 \cdot 5 \times 5 \times 2 \cdot 5$ cm, is divided into a fundus, a body, an isthmus and a cervix. Its triangular cavity communicates with the Fallopian tubes above and with the vagina below.

The peritoneal covering of the uterus is reflected on to the bladder anteriorly and the rectum posteriorly. Laterally it extends to the side-walls of the pelvis as the broad ligament which encloses the Fallopian tubes in its upper fold.

The muscle of the uterus – myometrium – consists mainly of a thick intermediate layer of interlacing fibres. It is greatest at the fundus, thinner in the lower part of the body and absent in the cervix.

The blood supply of the uterus is derived from the uterine arteries, which run upwards on its lateral aspect, sending branches through the myometrium to form a vascular plexus in the endometrium.

The uterus at term measures 30 × 25 × 20 cm, the increase in size involving its upper half more than its lower. It contains the foetus, placenta, membranes and liquor amnii and is lined by the decidua, a modified endometrium.

The placenta develops from the chorionic villi which are trophoblastic outgrowths appearing after implantation. Some of the villi anchor the ovum to the decidua while others lie free in the intervillous space. With continued growth of the ovum the villi, which at first cover its entire surface, become restricted to a central area destined to become the placenta.

The placenta at term measures 23 cm in diameter and is 2·5 cm deep. It weighs about 560 grammes. Its foetal surface is covered with vessels which subdivide in its substance and eventually reach the chorionic villi. The maternal blood supply to the placenta is developed from those decidual vessels which originally ran to the site of implantation. In addition, blood from its periphery collects into a thin-walled marginal sinus.

The functions of the placenta are respiratory, nutritional, excretory and endocrine. The chief hormones produced are gonadotrophins, oestrogens and progesterone.

Ageing of the placenta, which takes the form either of infarcts or of microscopic changes in the villi themselves, may, if pronounced, reduce its efficiency and predispose to foetal anoxia.

The foetus develops from the inner cell mass of the blastocyst. It is connected to the trophoblast by the body stalk, forerunner of the umbilical cord. The foetus soon develops the rudiments of a brain, a gut and a cardio-vascular system which, by uniting with the chorionic vessels, establishes the foetal circulation.

The foetus is enclosed in the amniotic membrane, filled with liquor amnii. This protects it from trauma and allows it room for growth and movement.

The umbilical cord is between 25 and 75 cm in length and about 1·5 cm thick. It is composed of Wharton's Jelly and usually contains a vein and two arteries. An additional vein is sometimes present and this may be associated with a congenital malformation of the foetus. Although false knots are of no significance, true knots, which are occasionally seen, may lead to foetal asphyxia. This may also occur if the cord happens to have become twisted around the foetal neck.

The foetus at term weighs between 3 and $3\frac{1}{2}$ kg, and measures 40 cm from crown to rump. It is in an attitude of flexion with the head lowermost. The probable reason for this is that it is best accommodated to the cavity of the uterus when in this position.

PART TWO

Abnormal Pregnancy

CHAPTER FOUR

Abnormalities of Early Pregnancy

Introduction

To the midwife, the importance of the various abnormalities which may arise in the course of pregnancy lies primarily in their diagnosis and only secondarily in either their aetiology or their management. The reason for this is that while a midwife is often the person who first recognises an abnormality, once it has been discovered its subsequent treatment is usually the responsibility of a doctor, the duties of a midwife in the actual management of such a case being nursing rather than medical. In this subdivision of obstetrics, therefore, a midwife is concerned more with clinical symptoms and signs rather than with therapeutic measures.

This point has been stressed because, in the description of the abnormalities of pregnancy and of labour, where, to a large extent, the same division of responsibility exists, emphasis will be laid more upon symptomatology and diagnosis than upon treatment, which will be considered less fully.

It is customary to separate the abnormalities of pregnancy into two main subdivisions, according to whether they arise before or after the twenty-eighth week. The reason for selecting this particular moment is that it represents the time when the foetus

D

becomes legally viable and when, in theory if not in fact, it is capable of survival if delivered.

The types of abnormality that may be encountered in pregnancy can be classified as follows:

Bleeding from the Genital Tract. This may occur either during early or in late pregnancy. In the former event it is simply called bleeding in early pregnancy, in the latter it is referred to as antepartum haemorrhage.

Hypertensive States. These, of which the most common are pre-eclampsia, eclampsia and essential hypertension, usually complicate late pregnancy but may sometimes arise during the first twenty-eight weeks.

Vomiting. This generally occurs during the early weeks of pregnancy when, as mentioned on page 15, it is sometimes of value as a diagnostic point. During late pregnancy it is less frequently encountered, but it may at times be a symptom of some underlying abnormality such as a urinary infection, severe pre-eclampsia or a hiatus hernia.

Urinary Infections. Although these may be met with in any period of pregnancy, they are typically regarded as complications of its middle third.

Maternal Diseases and Pathological States. These are conditions which although not caused by pregnancy nevertheless complicate it in some way. They include:

a   Anaemias

b   Cardiac and pulmonary diseases

c   Diabetes mellitus

d   Fibroids and ovarian cysts.

Malpresentations. Although occurring in pregnancy, particularly during the last weeks, malpresentations seldom influence its progress although they naturally have a profound bearing upon the course and outcome of labour.

Multiple Pregnancies. These affect both pregnancy and labour from the point of view of the foetus as well as that of the mother.

In the sections which follow, the chief abnormalities of early pregnancy, namely bleeding, vomiting and urinary infections will first be considered. Next, the complications of late pregnancy such as pre-eclampsia, eclampsia, essential hypertension and ante-partum haemorrhage will be discussed. Lastly, some space will be devoted to subjects such as the Small-For-Dates Foetus and Rhesus Isoimmunisation. Multiple pregnancy and malpresentations, however, will be considered in the section devoted to abnormal labour. In view of their purely medical nature, no description will be given of the various maternal diseases and pathological states which may complicate pregnancy.

Bleeding in Early Pregnancy

Bleeding from the genital tract during early pregnancy should be assumed to be from the placental site unless proved otherwise. It must therefore always be taken seriously and investigations and treatment started without delay.

Bleeding in early pregnancy may be due to a variety of causes, of which the following are the more common:

1 Bleeding in Association with an Otherwise Normal Pregnancy

a Bleeding from the Uterine Cavity

i *Implantation Bleeding*

Here the ovum, when implanting in the decidua, erodes a small vessel. The resultant haemorrhage is as a rule too slight to disturb the pregnancy. Owing to the time that elapses before its appearance at the vulva, the blood is brown in colour rather than red. As the uterus is not irritated into contracting there is no pain. Bleeding of this sort often occurs about the time of the first missed period, which it is sometimes mistakenly thought to represent.

ii *Bleeding from a Larger Vessel*

Here the trophoblast opens up a larger vessel and haemorrhage is more severe, often disrupting and killing the ovum. Pain is felt, due in part to distension of the uterus with blood and in part to uterine contractions. These contractions may either expel the ovum whole – a *complete abortion* – or merely part of it – *an incomplete abortion*. Where the bleeding is less heavy and damage less extensive the ovum may survive – a *threatened abortion* – but the function of the trophoblast may be permanently impaired. This may later result in placental insufficiency and a small-for-dates baby (page 116). Finally, although the ovum may die, the uterine contractions may not be strong enough to expel it. It is then retained within the uterus and is known as a *missed abortion*.

b   Bleeding from the Lower Genital Tract
Cervical polyps and erosions and, very rarely, carcinoma, may cause vaginal bleeding during pregnancy. As a rule this is both slight and painless. Trauma, either accidental or deliberately inflicted in an attempt to procure an abortion, may also give rise to bleeding which may then be thought to be coming from the placental site.

2   Bleeding in Association with an Abnormal Pregnancy

a   Bleeding from the Uterus: Hydatidiform Mole
In this condition there is no foetus and the development of the placenta is grossly abnormal, the villi being swollen and resembling clusters of small grapes. Characteristically, bleeding is recurrent, often severe and frequently accompanied by painful uterine contractions. Occasionally pale, grape-like vesicles are passed per vaginam – a valuable diagnostic point.

b   Bleeding from an Extra-uterine or Ectopic Pregnancy
An ectopic pregnancy is one which is situated outside the cavity of the uterus, usually in the Fallopian tube, less commonly in the ovary or the peritoneal cavity. These structures produce only a scanty decidua which cannot prevent the trophoblast invading the underlying blood vessels. Bleeding results which eventually disrupts the ovum and distends the tube with blood, causing a variable amount of pain and shock. Uterine bleeding is usually slight and is due to hormone withdrawal following the death of the ovum rather than to leakage of blood through the tube. For this reason, the loss tends to *follow* the pain, the reverse of what is usually seen in an intra-uterine abortion.

The Diagnosis of the Cause of the Bleeding
This must be based upon the case history and the physical findings, the midwife as a rule being concerned only with the

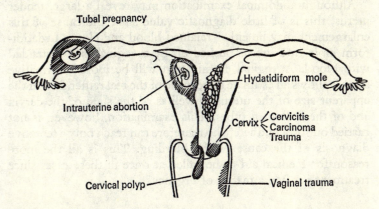

Fig. 12   Sources of bleeding in early pregnancy

former. To reach a provisional diagnosis of the cause of the bleeding the following questions should be asked:

1   *Has there been any recent amenorrhoea and if so, for how long? Did the patient know that she was pregnant?* This is usually the case save in certain very early ectopic pregnancies, although naturally the patient may deny the possibility.

2   *Did the bleeding follow any interference or trauma?* Although this would not necessarily rule out an intra-uterine abortion, since the trauma might have been successful, it does raise the possibility of local damage to the vagina or cervix.

3   *Was the bleeding excessive and/or accompanied by the passage of clots?* Such a history suggests an intra-uterine abortion rather than an ectopic gestation.

4   *Was there any pain, and if so, did it precede or follow the bleeding?* This will further help to differentiate between an intra-uterine and an extra-uterine pregnancy.

5   *Had the pregnancy previously been apparently normal or had there been excessive vomiting, malaise, headache or hypertension?* The latter conditions strongly suggest a hydatidiform mole.

Although abdominal examination may reveal a large, tender uterus, this is of little diagnostic value since the cause of this enlargement may be either retained blood and clot, a hydatidiform mole or a uterus pushed up by a vagina itself distended with blood. A vaginal examination will be more informative since it allows an estimate to be made of the real rather than of the apparent size of the uterus as well as of the state of the cervix and of the Fallopian tubes. This examination, however, is not carried out by a midwife who therefore can reach only a tentative diagnosis of the cause of the bleeding. This is all the more reason for medical aid to be called at once in these cases since treatment is often a matter of urgency.

Treatment

As these patients are usually admitted to a gynaecological ward, a midwife is seldom directly concerned with their subsequent care. This needs therefore only to be briefly summarised.

1   Threatened Abortion
Treatment here consists of bed-rest, sedation and possibly hormone replacement, using a progesterone derivative. If bleeding stops and pain disappears, the patient may be allowed up within three to four days and sent home in a week. In view of the late danger of placental insufficiency, a hospital confinement should be arranged.

2   Missed Abortion
These cases are often difficult to diagnose and are usually admitted to hospital for further observation. Once a diagnosis has been made and if the bleeding settles, the patient may be allowed home. There is no need to evacuate the uterus, the more so since the diagnosis might be at fault and the pregnancy still intact.

3   Incomplete Abortion

Here it is useless to attempt to preserve the pregnancy as the ovum is dead. Resuscitation of the patient, evacuation of the uterus and a return home within two to three days is the usual sequence of events.

4   Complete Abortion

It is often difficult to be sure of this diagnosis. Bleeding, however, will soon settle if the uterus is empty and there will therefore be no need for its evacuation. The patient may be allowed home in about three days.

5   Hydatidiform Mole

Here the uterus *must* be emptied, either vaginally or by abdominal hysterotomy. A most careful follow-up is necessary owing to the possibility of later malignancy – chorioncarcinoma.

6   Ectopic Gestation

Where the diagnosis is in doubt, as is often the case in these patients, careful supervision in hospital is imperative. A doctor must be called if pain recurs, particularly if this is severe. Once a diagnosis has been reached, laparotomy is carried out and the pregnancy removed. Failure to do this may result in serious internal haemorrhage.

7   Cervical Polyps and Erosions

Once a carcinoma has been excluded, only out-patient treatment is needed in these cases.

8   Traumatic Bleeding

If trauma is slight, no treatment will as a rule be needed. If it is serious, suturing after preliminary resuscitation is usually indicated. The scarring from certain chemical abortifacients such as potassium permanganate can be exceedingly severe and cause permanent damage to the lower genital tract.

Hyperemesis Gravidarum

Excessive vomiting in early pregnancy is known as Hyperemesis Gravidarum. It is usually regarded as a pathological development of the morning sickness experienced in some form or another by about 40 per cent of pregnant women. In hyperemesis, however, certain abnormal developments occur, involving in particular the urine, which, from an early stage contains ketone bodies.

Basic Pathology

No cause has ever been discovered for this disease, although factors such as nutritional imbalance, vitamin deficiency, toxins, hormonal changes and psychological upsets have all at various times been incriminated. Whatever the *cause*, the *course* is that of any uncontrolled vomiting. Since the body cannot store either water or carbohydrates, prolonged or excessive vomiting soon leads to their depletion, energy requirements then being met from fats and proteins. The ketones which are excreted in the urine provide a sign of this disturbed metabolism, while these and other abnormal by-products have a toxic effect upon the liver, the kidneys, the heart and the central nervous system, predisposing to further vomiting. In addition to this, dehydration, by restricting the elimination of these by-products, adds still further to the difficulties of the situation. A vicious circle is thus set up.

Diagnosis

Diagnosis is based upon a history of vomiting, starting several days or weeks previously and gradually increasing in severity to a stage at which no solids or fluids can be retained. The urine is reduced in volume, highly concentrated and contains ketone bodies. Hyperemesis must always be distinguished from vomiting due to conditions such as a duodenal ulcer, cholecystitis or some other abdominal emergency; toxins, drugs, infections –

particularly renal – or cerebral tumours. This, however, is a matter for a doctor rather than a midwife and rests upon the results of further clinical evaluation of the patient.

Clinical Course

Since it is rare nowadays for hyperemesis to remain untreated, its natural course is never seen. It is said, however, that the excessive vomiting ultimately leads to changes in the organs mentioned above, shown by the development of jaundice, albuminuria, tachycardia and hypotension, low-grade pyrexia and neurological signs such as paralyses and mental disturbance.

Management

All but mild cases of hyperemesis must be admitted to hospital for treatment, the nature of which depends upon the severity of the disease and its response to an altered environment. Basic-ally, the management of this condition consists in replacing water, carbohydrates and vitamins, either orally or intravenously, and in giving anti-emetic drugs such as Cyclizine or Fentazin.

Investigations necessary include keeping accurate blood press-ure, pulse, temperature and fluid balance charts, and testing all urine passed for ketones and albumen.

As improvement occurs, oral feeding is gradually started and once established on a full diet, the patient is allowed home. Although relapses are common, once the sixteenth week has been reached improvement is usually permanent. It should be em-phasised that in addition to the medical measures outlined above, good nursing care is of the utmost value in this condition. This applies in particular to the sympathetic and tactful handling which these patients so often need.

Where the condition is mild enough to allow treatment to be carried out in the home, too great reliance should not be placed upon anti-emetic drugs; and simpler measures such as those outlined on page 47 should first be tried. Sugar, in the form of boiled sweets or barley sugar is also valuable and unless taken in excess will not cause undue weight gain. Above all, the patient should be reassured that the condition, although distressing, is not in itself dangerous and that it will settle down within a short space of time.

Should such simple measures fail to bring about a rapid improvement, or should the midwife feel that more specific treatment is needed, she must seek medical advice.

Urinary Infections in Pregnancy

Although urinary infections most commonly occur between the twentieth and the twenty-fourth weeks, they may be encountered at any time during pregnancy and, in addition, frequently complicate the early puerperium.

Cause

In many instances a pre-existing latent urinary infection, acquired either in childhood or in adult life, may be re-activated in pregnancy. On other occasions the infection apparently arises for the first time during the present pregnancy. The basic cause seems to be a combination of urinary stasis in either the bladder, the ureters or the renal pelvis, and infection, either introduced by a catheter or by upward spread along the urethra. At other times the infection reaches the urinary tract by way of the blood stream or the lymphatics. Of particular significance in pregnancy is ureteric reflux, urine being forced up the dilated ureters into the renal pelvis during micturition. This constitutes an important route for the spread of infection should the urine in the bladder contain bacteria.

Diagnosis

The classical signs and symptoms of a urinary infection, namely pyrexia, tachycardia, headache and backache, together with pain and tenderness in one or both renal angles, frequency, urgency and dysuria and a cloudy offensive urine, render the diagnosis clear. These manifestations, however, rarely appear in such a clear-cut form and as a rule the symptoms, both general and local, are less obvious. Thus pyrexia may be mild or absent and the general constitutional disturbance minimal. There is usually, however, a certain amount of pain and tenderness in one or both loins and a history of recent frequency of micturition, together with some discomfort or burning on passing water. The urine, however, in such cases is not necessarily offensive and unless the infection is very severe it will not contain obvious pus or blood.

Investigations and Treatment

The main danger of a urinary infection is that it may become chronic, when it may easily cause severe long-term damage to the urinary tract. It cannot therefore be too strongly emphasised that in every suspected case a doctor should be informed and arrangements made for a mid-stream specimen of urine to be sent for culture and microscopy.

Treatment consists in giving a suitable antibiotic or sulphonamide for seven to ten days, after which a further specimen of urine is sent for examination. If this is found to be sterile, maintenance therapy, usually of a sulphonamide, should be started and kept up until some weeks after delivery.

In severe cases hospital admission is necessary. Here, in addition to the measures outlined above, general medical and nursing care, in the form of free fluids, a light diet, analgesics, and antipyretics, together with a hypnotic at night, can be provided.

Bacilluria

The routine testing of the urine of all pregnant women for the presence of bacteria is now carried out in most ante-natal clinics at the patient's first attendance and has much to commend it. Although a urine which contains a significant number of bacteria – over 100,000 per ml – but gives rise to no symptoms, is passed by only about five per cent of women, nearly all clinical urinary infections in pregnancy are derived from this small group of patients. Where evidence of such bacilluria is obtained, treatment must be given. This usually takes the form of long-term maintenance sulphonamide or antibiotic therapy. As with clinical infections, such therapy, to be of lasting benefit, must be continued at least until term and preferably for several weeks after delivery.

Summary

Bleeding in Early Pregnancy

Bleeding from the genital tract in early pregnancy must be assumed to be from the placental site unless proved otherwise.
   The most common causes of such bleeding are:

a *Implantation Bleeding.* Occasionally mistaken for a scanty period.

b *Bleeding from a Large Decidual Vessel.* Often resulting in the death of the ovum. This may then either be retained in utero; missed abortion; expelled entire: complete abortion, or only partly: incomplete abortion. If the ovum survives: threatened abortion, placental function may be impaired.

c *Bleeding from the Lower Genital Tract.* Polyps, Erosions or Trauma.

d *Bleeding from a Hydatidiform Mole.* The loss here being often severe and accompanied by the passage of vesicles on occasion.

Bleeding from an Ectopic Gestation. Bleeding here being often slight and usually preceded by cramp-like pains. Rupture of a large vessel causes shock and internal haemorrhage.

   Diagnosis is based upon history and physical examination, of which only the former is as a rule available to the midwife. Points of importance are:

a The duration of amenorrhoea

b A history of trauma or interference

c The amount and type of bleeding

d The presence or absence of pain.

To reach a firm diagnosis, however, a vaginal examination should be carried out by a doctor.

Treatment depends upon the cause of the bleeding and may either be conservative or operative. Since these patients are almost always admitted to a gynaecological ward, their subsequent care is rarely within the province of the midwife.

Hyperemesis Gravidarum

Excessive vomiting in early pregnancy is known as hyperemesis gravidarum.

Basically, the vomiting results in depletion of the body stores of carbohydrates, water and vitamins and in the production of ketones which are excreted in the urine. The abnormal metabolites which are formed in this condition have a direct effect upon the liver, the kidneys, the heart and the central nervous system. The accompanying dehydration serves to aggravate the situation.

Diagnosis depends upon a history of persistent vomiting and ketonuria, the latter being a most important sign.

Management depends upon restoring water, carbohydrates and vitamins, either orally or intravenously, together with the use of anti-emetic drugs. The importance of good nursing care in this condition cannot be overemphasised.

Relapses after apparently successful treatment are frequent, but once the sixteenth week is reached, improvement is usually permanent.

In mild cases, simple measures coupled with reassurance are generally preferable to more specific measures.

Urinary Infections in Pregnancy

Urinary infections may occur at any time during pregnancy, most commonly between the twentieth and twenty-fourth weeks.

In many cases the underlying pathology is a latent infection acquired during childhood or early adult life.

The infecting organisms are either introduced from below – often by catheter – or reach the urinary tract by the bloodstream or lymphatics.

Urinary stasis and ureteric reflux are important factors in determining whether an infection will take root.

In general, the constitutional upset and local signs of infection are slight, the classical symptoms being only occasionally encountered.

In all suspected cases a mid-stream specimen of urine must be sent for full laboratory investigation.

Treatment consists of general medical and nursing care and of the administration of an antibiotic or sulphonamide. This should be maintained for several months if relapses are to be avoided.

Bacilluria, present in about five per cent of pregnant women, must be treated since it is from this small group of cases that nearly all urinary infections are derived.

CHAPTER FIVE

Major Abnormalities of Late Pregnancy

Pre-eclampsia

Pre-eclampsia is the most important as well as the most common abnormality of late pregnancy. It is characterised by a rise in blood pressure accompanied by oedema, albuminuria, or both. It must at once be stressed that, for a diagnosis to be made, all three of these cardinal signs need not be present and that, in fact, when albuminuria is detected the pre-eclampsia has already reached a severe stage.

The disease owes its particular importance to three features:

1 Its high incidence

2 The dangers it presents to the patient and to the foetus

3 The fact that in all but its most advanced form it is symptom-free.

Incidence

Since pre-eclampsia is not a notifiable disease and since no general agreement exists as to the precise criteria for diagnosis, it is impossible to determine its exact incidence. It appears, however, to complicate about ten per cent of all pregnancies, assuming a mild form in the great majority of instances. Severe pre-eclampsia is not common and is seen in less than one per cent of gestations.

Pre-eclampsia is particularly liable to arise in association with the following types:

1 Women who are over 35 years of age, particularly primigravidae

2 Women who are overweight

3 Women with a past history of pre-eclampsia

4 Women with essential hypertension and renal disease

5 Women with multiple pregnancies.

Dangers

The dangers of pre-eclampsia are largely related to its severity. They are comparatively slight if it assumes a mild form, as is usually the case in the early stages of the disease, but increase greatly if treatment is withheld or is inadequate. As with other abnormalities of late pregnancy, these dangers may be considered under two headings: maternal and foetal.

Maternal Dangers

The most important maternal danger is Eclampsia. This condition resembles severe pre-eclampsia with the addition of fits and carries a high maternal and foetal mortality (page 106). Other unusual complications are cerebral haemorrhage and cortical necrosis of the kidneys. Accidental ante-partum haemorrhage (page 126), often regarded as a serious complication of pre-eclampsia, is not, in fact, especially common in these cases, while renal damage, other than cortical necrosis, does not occur. In the same way, pre-eclampsia will not cause a permanently raised blood pressure, although, as said earlier, it is more likely to arise in people whose blood pressure is already high.

Foetal Dangers

These are largely related to the fact that in pre-eclampsia the placenta is often small and unable adequately to maintain the foetus. This condition of placental insufficiency leads to retarded growth, the foetus being small-for-dates and having an increased liability to die either in utero or during the neo-natal period. Further foetal dangers stem from these risks in that, in attempting to avoid them, delivery is often effected long before term, thus subjecting the baby to the hazards of prematurity.

Physical Signs

Pre-eclampsia is unusual in that in all but its severe form it is a disease without symptoms, the patient generally feeling perfectly well. It can thus be diagnosed only upon the physical signs it presents, which themselves can be discovered only by clinical examination. This explains the need for regular ante-natal supervision, especially in those women who are liable to develop the disease.

The three cardinal signs of pre-eclampsia, namely hypertension, oedema and albuminuria, must now be considered more fully.

a Hypertension

It is usually agreed that a blood pressure of over 130/90 mm Hg, accompanied by either oedema or albuminuria, justifies a diagnosis or pre-eclampsia. Of greater importance, however, is a *rising* blood pressure, that is to say, one which is higher by 10 mm Hg or more than that recorded at the patient's previous attendance.

b Oedema

In late pregnancy a certain amount of oedema of the feet is accepted as normal. When, however, this extends to the shins, the fingers or the abdominal wall, or when the face becomes unnaturally puffy, it must be regarded as pathological.

c Albuminuria

It has already been said that albuminuria need not be present for a diagnosis of pre-eclampsia to be made and that in fact its presence usually means that the condition has reached a severe stage, the foetal hazards in particular rising steeply in such cases. The albumen must, of course, be present in a mid-stream specimen of urine and a urinary tract infection must be excluded.

Symptoms

Where symptoms as well as signs are present, pre-eclampsia has usually reached a very severe stage and eclampsia itself may be imminent. These symptoms, which are of considerable clinical importance, are as follows:

1 Headache

2 Vomiting

3 Epigastric Pain

4 Visual Disturbances – blurring of vision, dimness of vision, flashes of light before the eyes but *not* spots before the eyes.

5 Oliguria.

It need scarcely be emphasised that if a midwife notices the development of any of the signs or symptoms of pre-eclampsia, whether in the ante-natal clinic or in the ward, she must inform a doctor immediately. Even where the disease seems to be present in a very mild form, it is most unwise either to disregard it or to delay treatment.

Types of Pre-eclampsia

Pre-eclampsia may be subdivided into three main types:

1 *Mild Pre-eclampsia* is characterised by a blood pressure of under 140/90 mm Hg, together with oedema. Albuminuria is absent and there are no symptoms. This is the commonest type seen and presents minimal maternal or foetal risks.

2 *Moderate Pre-eclampsia* is characterised by a blood pressure of between 140/90 and 160/100 mm Hg, with oedema but no albuminuria and no symptoms. Here the foetal risks are increased, especially if the condition has persisted for several weeks, as placental insufficiency is then liable to develop, often insidiously. The maternal risks are still small.

3 *Severe Pre-eclampsia* is characterised by a blood pressure of over 160/110 mm Hg together with oedema, which may be extensive. It is usually a late manifestation of the disease. Pre-eclampsia is also severe if, regardless of the level of the blood pressure, there is albuminuria or if symptoms develop.

Management

The management of pre-eclampsia is founded upon the principle that pregnancy should be allowed to continue for as long as this is safe both for the patient and for the foetus but that delivery should be effected as soon as the maternal or foetal risks start to rise. For this principle to be safely applied, it must be remembered that pre-eclampsia is never cured so long as the patient remains undelivered and that the best that can be hoped for is to bring it under control. It must also be realised that such control, even when apparently satisfactory, may not necessarily be maintained and that relapses can occur at any time with little warning. Lastly, it must be borne in mind that mild pre-eclampsia is more easily controlled than severe pre-eclampsia. It follows that:

1 The earlier pre-eclampsia is diagnosed, the milder it will usually be and the greater the chance of effective control

2   The control of pre-eclampsia presents two aspects: that of the treatment needed to achieve it and that of the supervision needed to ensure that it is being maintained

3   The signs and symptoms suggestive of imminent eclampsia and of increased maternal and foetal dangers must be fully appreciated.

1   Diagnosis
It should by now be clear that the early diagnosis of pre-eclampsia is based upon a slight rise in blood pressure together with the presence of some degree of oedema and that the development of albuminuria must never be awaited. Where any doubt exists, a medical opinion must always be sought since the responsibility for the safety of the patient rests with the doctor rather than with the midwife.

2   Control of the Pre-eclampsia
It is in this particular aspect of management that the midwife has the largest part to play. As already said, this control presents two aspects: that of treatment and that of supervision, the details of which depend upon the place of treatment. This may be either the patient's home or a hospital.

a   Management in the Home
This should be contemplated only in cases of mild pre-eclampsia where the patient is able and willing to accept whatever supervision and treatment are necessary to prevent deterioration.

i   Treatment
Three principles govern the treatment of pre-eclampsia, namely rest, sedation and diet, of which the first two are the more important.

Rest

The patient should go to bed early, at 7 or 8 p.m. and get up late, at 9 or 10 a.m. She should also rest in bed from 2 to 4 p.m. every afternoon. While up, all but the lightest domestic duties must be avoided.

Sedation

While the choice of sedative naturally depends upon the doctor in charge of the case, as a general rule, a barbiturate such as Phenobarbitone – 30 to 60 mg – twice or three times daily is combined with a night sedative such as Soneryl – 100 to 200 mg.

Diet

A high protein, low carbohydrate diet should be given. Although it is usually taught that the amount of salt taken should be drastically reduced, this does not really seem to be necessary and therfore need not be insisted upon.

ii *Supervision*

It is necessary to supervise all pre-eclamptics, however mild, both in order to gauge the extent to which treatment is controlling their condition as well as to ensure that such control is being properly maintained. Naturally, when the patient is being nursed at home such supervision is necessarily less strict than in hospital, but even at home it must consist of daily or twice daily blood pressure recordings and daily examination of the urine for albumen.

b *Management in Hospital*

Although the principles of the hospital management of pre-eclampsia are the same as those obtaining in the home, since cases admitted to hospital are often of a more severe type, the amount of rest taken must, initially at least, be greater, confinement to bed being usually necessary until adequate control has been established. Similarly, heavy sedation such as Sodium

Amytal – 100 to 200 mg 3 to 6 hourly – is often required during the first few days. As control is gained the degree of sedation can usually be reduced and a change made to Phenobarbitone and Soneryl as given to patients treated at home.

Diet is subject to the restrictions already described, care being taken to ensure that no foods of high carbohydrate content are provided as supplements by well-intentioned but ill-advised friends and relatives.

In addition to the above measures, it is sometimes necessary to resort to drugs designed specifically to reduce the blood pressure. There are large numbers of these substances, which in general are of little use in pre-eclampsia. A trial of them is, however, sometimes made when severe pre-eclampsia develops at a time when immediate delivery would gravely impair the foetus' chances of survival. The actual choice and dosage of these drugs is a medical matter and need not be discussed. The same applies to the occasional use of diuretics in the treatment of severe oedema.

Supervision

As in the case of patients treated in their homes, supervision consists essentially of frequent blood pressure readings, initially four- or even two-hourly, later six- to twelve-hourly depending upon the severity of the condition. Daily urinalysis and quantitative estimation of albumen in the urine by Esbach's reagent is also necessary. In addition a fluid balance chart should be kept as this is a valuable index of the degree of fluid retention and hence of the amount of oedema.

3 Signs of Increasing Maternal and Foetal Dangers

These consist of a rising blood pressure, increasing oedema and, particularly, the development of albuminuria. This last sign is of especial significance and often necessitates immediate intervention. Other danger signals are the development of symptoms such as headache, abdominal pain and visual disturbances. A less dramatic but nevertheless serious clinical feature is failure of the foetus to increase in size. This suggests a diminishing placental function and may result in intra-uterine death unless steps are taken to deliver the patient without delay.

4 Later Management

The later management of pre-eclampsia, being of medical rather than of nursing interest, need only be summarised. The following probabilities may be encountered:

a The Pre-eclampsia improves with treatment, the foetus continuing to grow satisfactorily

If conditions are suitable, the patient may be allowed home, provided that the pre-eclampsia has been no more than mild at any time. However, if home treatment is impracticable, she must stay in hospital until delivered. Pregnancy must on no account be allowed to continue beyond the expected date of delivery owing to the possibility of placental insufficiency developing after term.

b The Pre-eclampsia improves initially but deteriorates later

If the thirty-sixth week has been reached the patient should be delivered. Otherwise a further effort may be made to regain control by means of stricter treatment, hypotensive drugs being sometimes used for this purpose. Should this fail, delivery will be necessary regardless of the risks to the foetus.

c The Pre-eclampsia deteriorates despite treatment

In such cases delivery must be carried out in a matter of days or hours.

d The condition of the patient improves but the foetus fails to grow

Here delivery offers the only chance to the foetus, despite its small size.

The Method of Delivery

In cases of pre-eclampsia, vaginal delivery is preferable to Caesarean section, as much for the sake of the foetus as for that of the patient. For this reason, operation is undertaken only if efforts at starting labour have failed or if deterioration has been so rapid that any further delay might risk the onset of eclampsia. In the majority of cases, therefore, induction of labour will be necessary, the actual procedure used depending upon the particular features of the case.

Post-partum Management

A rise in blood pressure immediately after delivery is often seen in cases of pre-eclampsia. Although this rise is usually slight, it may at times be severe enough to provoke post-partum eclampsia. There is some evidence that drugs such as Ergometrine, given to reduce the risk of a post-partum haemorrhage, may aggravate this blood pressure rise.

During the puerperium the blood pressure generally falls to its normal level within a few days, while albuminuria takes somewhat longer to disappear. Despite this excellent prognosis, it is still a good policy to persuade the patient to return to the post-natal clinic six weeks after delivery to allow a final check to be made upon the blood pressure and the urine.

Eclampsia

Nowadays eclampsia is a rare disease. The reason for this is that the great majority of cases arise from pre-eclampsia which has been allowed to progress unchecked. As this process usually takes several days, such a sequence of events is uncommon where good ante-natal care is available. Unlike pre-eclampsia, eclampsia is thus very largely preventable, its occasional rare occurrence being due to the fact that at times pre-eclampsia may deteriorate so rapidly that any form of control is impossible.

Eclampsia can arise before labour, during labour or after labour: ante-partum, intra-partum and post-partum eclampsia. In the past, the first of these possibilities was the most common, but, again owing to better ante-natal supervision, cases arising nowadays usually do so either during or soon after labour.

Symptomatology

The features of eclampsia are those of pre-eclampsia with the addition of one or more *fits*. As with pre-eclampsia, the severity of eclampsia varies greatly and a very high blood pressure or a gross degree of albuminuria, although usually observed, need not necessarily be present. It follows that any patient who has a fit during the second half of pregnancy must be managed as a case of eclampsia until proved otherwise.

The fit, which according to the severity of the condition may either be single or be repeated a number of times, presents the following characteristics:

1 *A Premonitory Stage* usually consisting of twitching of the small muscles of the face or hands.

2 *A Tonic Stage* in which the body is held rigid and respirations are suppressed, marked cyanosis therefore developing.

3 *A Clonic Stage* where violent, uncoordinated movements occur in which the tongue may be bitten and other injuries sustained.

Each of these three stages lasts for between one and two minutes, the patient remaining unconscious throughout.

4 *Coma* of varying depth and duration usually follows the clonic stage, being succeeded either by a further fit or by a gradual return to consciousness.

Dangers

Although modern treatment has reduced the dangers of eclampsia, these are still considerable. The *maternal risks*, which at times may even culminate in death, arise from the combined stresses of severe hypertension, repeated convulsions and prolonged unconsciousness. In order of frequency and of importance they are:

a Cerebral haemorrhage

b Cardiac failure

c Aspiration pneumonia

d Sepsis.

The *risks to the foetus* are those of:

a Placental insufficiency, from pre-existing pre-eclampsia

b Prematurity, from the need to deliver the patient before term

c Acute hypoxia, secondary to the maternal hypoxia common during fits.

The perinatal mortality from these combined hazards is about 25 per cent.

Prognosis

The outlook both for the patient and for the foetus depends upon the severity of the eclampsia, which in turn is related to the following signs:

a A rapid succession of fits

b Deep coma between fits

c A systolic blood pressure over 200 mm Hg

d A pulse rate over 120 per minute

e A temperature over 39·5°C

f Gross albuminuria and oliguria.

Management

This is essentially a medical matter and a doctor must therefore be called immediately the diagnosis of eclampsia is suspected.

His examination of the patient will take into account the following points:

a   The blood pressure and the pulse rate

b   The extent of the oedema

c   The lie and the presentation of the foetus

d   The foetal heart rate.

If it is suspected that labour has started, a vaginal examination will be carried out to assess progress and the outlook for delivery.

A picture of the type and severity of the eclampsia may thus be built up and management planned accordingly. This may be considered under the following headings:

a   Treatment designed to control the convulsions

b   Management of further convulsions

c   Observations required to assess progress.

a   *The Control of the Convulsions*

Here the two principles of treatment are to sedate the patient and to reduce her blood pressure. Within this context many different approaches have been suggested, all of which are mainly of medical interest. Sedation is usually achieved with drugs such as Morphia, Paraldehyde, Magnesium Sulphate, Avertin or Chlorpromazine or one of its derivatives. This in itself may bring about a fall in the blood pressure; usually, however, this is obtained by the use of certain hypotensive drugs of which Puroverine, Hydrallazine and Aldomet are the best examples.

Nursing Treatment

Since the nursing care of an eclamptic is essentially similar to that of any unconscious or semi-conscious patient with a liability to further convulsions, it need only be summarised.

i   The patient must be nursed in a single-bedded cubicle. All stimuli such as noise, light or movement must be kept to a minimum

ii. To reduce the chances of injury during a fit the bed should be placed alongside a wall

iii Similarly, all hard or sharp objects must be moved from the vicinity of the patient

iv Any dentures present must be removed

v If unconsciousness is prolonged, the patient's head must be kept low and turned to one side to allow secretions to drain away and to reduce the chance of their becoming aspirated during a fit

vi The patient should be nursed on her side, being turned at frequent intervals to avoid pulmonary congestion.

b Management during Convulsions
The essentials here are:

i To prevent damage to the tongue and consequent aspiration of blood and froth by the use of a gag and tongue clip. Failing these, a spoon bound with gauze may be inserted between the teeth. This must be done during the premonitory stage of a convulsion.

ii An airway must be maintained after the clonic stage by holding the chin forwards and pulling the tongue well out.

iii The severity of the fits themselves may sometimes be reduced by giving open chloroform. This, however, is not a midwife's responsibility.

c Observations Required to Assess Progress
The following observations must be carried out in all cases:

i Blood pressure: $\frac{1}{4}$–$\frac{1}{2}$ hourly record

ii Maternal pulse: $\frac{1}{2}$ hourly record

iii Foetal heart rate: $\frac{1}{2}$ hourly record

iv The urine must be tested four-hourly for albumen and Esbach's tubes set up on all specimens so tested. To facilitate this an in-dwelling catheter should be passed at the start of treatment.

v   A fluid balance chart must be kept.

Subsequent Management

When no further fits have occurred for between twelve and twenty-four hours, the patient should be delivered. As with pre-eclampsia, a vaginal delivery is to be preferred and induction of labour is therefore usually necessary. Caesarean section is reserved for women in whom induction has failed or who present some contra-indication to vaginal delivery.

While the above description applies to the management of a case of ante-partum eclampsia, cases occurring either during labour or after delivery may be managed along similar lines, although in intra-partum eclampsia delivery should be completed as soon as possible. In all cases sedation must be continued for several days, being slowly reduced when it becomes apparent that a recurrence of the eclampsia is improbable.

Essential Hypertension

Essential hypertension, a condition in which the blood pressure is raised for no obvious cause, differs from pre-eclampsia in that it is present *before* pregnancy. However, since women of child-bearing age are comparatively rarely examined in every-day life, their blood pressure is usually not known. Essential hypertension is therefore most commonly diagnosed in early pregnancy on the strength of a blood pressure of 140/90 mm Hg or more, discovered before the twentieth week, at a time when, for practical purposes, pre-eclampsia is never seen.

Like pre-eclampsia, essential hypertension presents no symptoms, its sole physical sign being that of a raised blood pressure. Oedema, other than slight swelling of the feet in late pregnancy, is not found, nor does the urine contain albumen.

Course in Pregnancy

During pregnancy essential hypertension may follow one of three main patterns:

1 The blood pressure, although raised, otherwise behaves normally, becoming somewhat lower in mid-pregnancy and rising again to its original level towards term. This pattern presents the least maternal and foetal dangers.

2 The blood pressure remains at a constant level throughout pregnancy. Here the risks to the patient and to the foetus are somewhat higher.

3 The blood pressure rises steadily throughout pregnancy, especially during the last few weeks. In addition, oedema and albuminuria develop. This indicates that pre-eclampsia has been *superadded* to the essential hypertension already present. This pattern, which is seen to a greater or lesser extent in about half of all cases, is associated with considerable maternal and foetal hazards.

Dangers

The dangers of essential hypertension are related in part to the level of the blood pressure and in part to the course the disease takes during pregnancy.

The *maternal hazards* are essentially those of pre-eclampsia, e.g., cerebral haemorrhage, eclampsia and renal failure. In addition, the blood pressure remains permanently raised in about one-third of all cases.

The main *foetal risks* are those of placental insufficiency, although prematurity may also prove to be a hazard, especially where delivery is necessary before the thirty-seventh week.

Management

The management of essential hypertension during pregnancy depends on the one hand upon the height of the blood pressure and on the other upon the severity of any superadded pre-eclampsia. It is therefore most easily considered in terms of its three subdivisions:

1 *Mild Cases*. Blood pressure under 150/100 mm Hg. No super-added pre-eclampsia.

Careful and frequent ante-natal supervision is needed in these patients to guard against deterioration, which may well be symptomless, and to ensure that the foetus continues to grow satisfactorily. Provided that all goes well in both these respects, these patients may remain at home, treatment being limited to mild sedation and increased rest. As in pre-eclampsia, pregnancy should never be allowed to go beyond term and delivery should always be carried out in a hospital.

2 *Severe Cases*. Blood pressure over 150/100 mm Hg. No super-added pre-eclampsia.

These patients are usually admitted to hospital in order to assess the degree of hypertension and its response to rest, sedation and, if necessary, hypotensive drugs such as Serpasil or Guanethidine. These are of considerably greater value here than in pre-eclampsia. Where the blood pressure can be controlled by rest and sedation alone, the patient may be allowed home under careful medical and nursing supervision, although readmission usually becomes necessary at or shortly after the end of the thirty-sixth week. Where the blood pressure cannot be easily controlled, the patient must remain in hospital. In all cases the time of delivery depends in part upon the response to treatment and in part upon the rate of growth of the foetus.

3 *Cases with Superadded Pre-eclampsia*. Since management here is in every way similar to that of severe pre-eclampsia (page 103), it needs no further comment.

The Time of Delivery

The following considerations must be taken into account in deciding the time of delivery:

1 However mild the hypertension, pregnancy must never be allowed to go beyond term.

2 Delivery before the fortieth week may be necessary if:
a The blood pressure rises despite hospital treatment
b Albuminuria appears and persists
c The foetus fails to grow.

Delivery

As in pre-eclampsia, vaginal delivery following induction of labour is the procedure of choice in patients with essential hypertension. Caesarean section should be reserved for those cases presenting specific indications for such an operation.

Albuminuria in Pregnancy

Although non-infective albuminuria in pregnancy is usually a complication of pre-eclampsia, eclampsia or essential hypertension with superadded pre-eclampsia, it sometimes appears to be unrelated to any of these conditions. In such circumstances it is usually assumed that chronic nephritis is present but this is unlikely for the following reasons:

1 In chronic nephritis there is an associated hypertension which is absent in pure albuminuria.

2 In chronic nephritis the albuminuria, being present before the start of pregnancy, is observed during the early weeks. Albuminuria of pregnancy on the other hand, tends to develop only during the latter weeks.

2   In chronic nephritis the urine contains casts while renal function tests are often abnormal. Such findings are not characteristic of albuminuria.

In the great majority of instances, therefore, the cause of the albuminuria is not known.

Dangers

Although, owing to the relative rarity of this condition, precise information on the maternal and, more particularly, the foetal dangers is lacking, it is generally agreed that these are considerable and that the high perinatal mortality is due to retarded foetal growth and a liability to intra-uterine death from placental insufficiency.

Management

Any case of albuminuria of pregnancy not attributable to a urinary infection must be admitted to hospital for investigation and treatment. In addition, unless the albuminuria disappears, a return home for further management cannot be allowed since careful supervision is necessary if the perinatal mortality is to be reduced.

Investigations

In addition to twice daily blood pressure recordings and a daily fluid balance chart, the following investigations are needed in these cases:

1   A mid-stream specimen of urine must be sent to the laboratory for culture and microscopy to exclude the presence of bacteria and casts

2   A urine concentration/dilution test must be carried out

E

3 A specimen of blood should be sent for estimation of the blood urea

4 Daily Esbach estimations must be set up.

Treatment

As in the case of pre-eclampsia and essential hypertension, the basis of treatment is rest and sedation. These measures alone may suffice to control the degree of albuminuria and may even, at times, lead to a satisfactory improvement.

a Provided that the patient's condition does not deteriorate and that foetal growth remains satisfactory, treatment should be continued until the end of the thirty-sixth or thirty-seventh week. The patient should then be delivered.

b If, despite treatment, the patient's condition worsens, as shown by increasing albuminuria and delayed foetal growth, delivery must, in the interests of both parties, be effected as soon as the risks of allowing pregnancy to continue outweigh those of prematurity.

The Small-for-Dates Baby

During the past few years increasing attention has been paid to the fact that the birth weight of some babies is considerably lower than might be expected from the duration of gestation. In view of their high perinatal mortality, such small-for-dates babies are of particular importance and deserve special consideration.

Definition

Although the definition of a small-for-dates baby is one whose birth weight is below the fifth percentile, this is a cumbrous and rather pedantic statement. For practical purposes it is best to regard as small-for-dates any baby weighing under $5\frac{1}{2}$ lb at term or one which if born before term is considerably smaller than would be expected.

Aetiology and Dangers

As mentioned in previous sections, pre-eclampsia, essential hypertension and albuminuria of pregnancy are all at times associated with small-for-dates babies, the cause of this being thought to be a failure of the placenta to supply enough nourishment for normal growth. Such placental insufficiency may also arise where there has been bleeding either in early or in late pregnancy or even where pregnancy has apparently been normal throughout, the reason for the placental failure in such cases being unknown.

Whatever its precise cause, the hazards of being small-for-dates concern only the foetus, being related to its small size and also to antecedent conditions such as congenital malformations, which themselves may be incompatible with life.

Where the foetus is otherwise normal, the associated placental insufficiency may result in intra-uterine death during the latter weeks of pregnancy, often with little or no clinical warning. In less severe cases, when the baby is born alive, it is particularly liable to nutritional and respiratory difficulties, death often resulting from hypoglycaemia or pulmonary haemorrhage.

Diagnosis

This rests upon the finding of a uterus which is considerably smaller than the period of amenorrhoea would suggest. In such cases it is often difficult to exclude a mistake in the patient's dates and here great assistance will be gained from information regarding the size of the uterus in early pregnancy (page 10). It might be thought that an X-ray of the foetus would decide its precise age but this is not so since when it is small-for-dates the appearance of the various ossification centres on which X-ray assessment is based is retarded.

Additional help may be afforded from estimations of the amount of hormones excreted by the patient in her urine, but these investigations need special laboratory facilities which are not generally available. In the majority of cases, therefore, diagnosis rests solely upon the clinical examination of the patient.

Management

This is dictated by the need to deliver the foetus as soon as it seems clear that its life is in danger from placental insufficiency, as shown by the finding that its rate of growth has practically ceased. Since it is always difficult to be sure of this point, mistakes are frequently made. However, it must be remembered that it is useless to allow pregnancy to continue in the hope that the foetus will once more start to grow and that it is better for it to be delivered too soon and alive than too late and dead.

Where the foetus, although small, is still growing, some advantage may be gained from admitting the patient to hospital for a prolonged period of rest, as there is reason to believe that this may allow the foetus' rate of growth to be maintained or even increased. Even where this occurs, however, delivery before term is almost always advisable and in no circumstances should pregnancy be allowed to go beyond the end of the fortieth week.

Ante-partum Haemorrhage

Ante-partum haemorrhage is defined as bleeding from the birth canal from the twenty-eighth week of pregnancy until the delivery of the foetus. It is one of the two main complications of pregnancy, pre-eclampsia being the other. Unlike pre-eclampsia, however, it is a symptom rather than a disease and is caused by a variety of factors. For this reason, any review of ante-partum haemorrhage must:

1 Provide an acceptable classification of the causes of the bleeding

2   Give a clinical account of the aetiology, signs, symptoms, dangers and management of these causes

3   Provide a means of differentiating between the various types of blood loss that may be encountered during late pregnancy.

The Classification of Ante-partum Haemorrhage

Ante-partum haemorrhage is best classified according to the origin of the bleeding:

1   *Bleeding of Foetal Origin*

2   *Bleeding of Maternal Origin*

a   From the placental site

b   From other structures

Bleeding from the placental site may come:

a   From a placenta situated in the lower part of the uterus – placenta praevia or unavoidable ante-partum haemorrhage

b   From the edge of a normally situated placenta – marginal sinus bleeding

c   From massive separation of a normally situated placenta – accidental ante-partum haemorrhage or abruptio placentae.

Bleeding from other structures may arise from lesions of the vulva, vagina, cervix or uterine body. It is sometimes known as Incidental Bleeding. In view of its medical as distinct from nursing interest, it need not be considered further.

1   *Bleeding of Foetal Origin*
The cause of bleeding of foetal origin is a torn vessel in the umbilical cord. Although normally the cord is attached directly to the placenta, at times its insertion is of the Velamentous type, in which the foetal vessels subdivide some distance from the

placenta. While this aberration is usually of no clinical significance, if the placenta is low-lying, these vessels may tear when the membranes rupture. Bleeding will then occur. Since the blood is of foetal origin, the patient will not be affected, but the loss may be severe enough to distress or even to kill the foetus. Diagnosis thus depends upon a relatively slight amount of bleeding, usually in relation to rupture of the membranes,

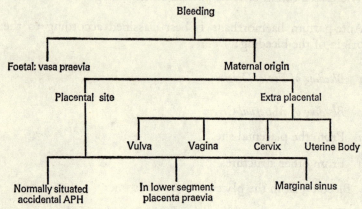

Fig. 13 Types of ante-partum haemorrhage

which is associated with marked foetal but no maternal upset. Treatment consists of immediate delivery provided that the foetus is still alive.

2   Bleeding from a placenta implanted in the lower part of the uterus – placenta praevia or unavoidable ante-partum haemorrhage

It has already been pointed out on page 64 that as pregnancy progresses and the ovum grows, the uterus provides the necessary room by stretching from above downwards, the last part to do this being the Isthmus, which develops into what is called the Lower Uterine Segment.

Normally this process takes place uneventfully, but if in early pregnancy the placenta has implanted in the region of the isthmus rather than in the body of the uterus, as the lower segment stretches, the placenta, being inelastic, will not follow suit and will be torn from its attachments to the uterine wall. This opens up blood vessels passing from the uterine artery to the placental site and bleeding results.

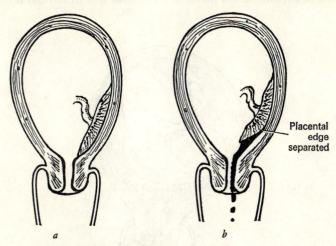

Fig. 14   Placenta praevia: mechanism of bleeding
(a) before bleeding (b) after bleeding starts

Signs and Symptoms

Since the stretching process described above continues as pregnancy advances, progressively more of the placenta may be detached and bleeding will therefore tend to be repeated. Typically the first loss is slight, the second moderate and the third severe. This must be remembered when considering treatment. Since the blood can escape from the cervical canal the uterus will not be distended by it and there will be no pain.

The cardinal signs of placenta praevia are thus painless, recurrent vaginal bleeding occurring for no apparent reason.

As the placenta is situated in the lower part of the uterus it tends to dislodge the foetus from its normal position. This results in an oblique or a transverse lie or in a presenting part which is displaced in a variety of ways depending on the position of the placenta – anterior, posterior or lateral. Since the amount of initial bleeding is usually small and the degree of placental separation slight, neither the patient nor the foetus is likely to be affected and the maternal pulse and blood pressure and the rate and rhythm of the foetal heart remain within normal limits.

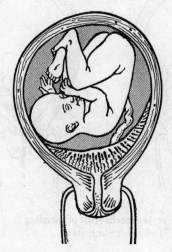

Fig. 15 Placenta praevia: oblique lie favoured

Types of Placental Praevia

It is usual to describe three types of placenta praevia:

1 *Lateral*. Here the placenta dips into the lower segment but does not reach as far as the cervical canal. Bleeding is usually slight.

2 *Marginal*. Here the placenta extends to the cervical canal. Bleeding is usually heavy.

3 *Central*. Here the placenta covers the opening of the cervical canal. Bleeding is variable, being at times slight or even absent.

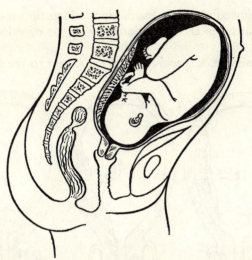

Fig. 16   Placenta praevia: forward displacement of head favoured

Diagnosis

Initially diagnosis is based upon the patient's history together with the findings on abdominal palpation. Due to the risk of causing further placental separation, vaginal examination is absolutely contra-indicated whenever a placenta praevia is suspected. In addition to these purely clinical measures, X-ray visualisation of the placental site is often possible and can be of great help in diagnosis.

Treatment

The basis of treatment is to prolong pregnancy until the foetus is mature, at the same time safeguarding the patient. This means that she must be admitted to hospital as soon as bleeding occurs and that she must stay there either until she has been delivered or until a placenta praevia can be excluded. Until this has been done no woman should ever be allowed home for fear of further and possibly heavy bleeding. Bed rest should be enforced for a week after all loss has ceased, following which the patient may be allowed up in the ward. Since a long time may have to be spent in hospital, occupational therapy is of value in these cases.

On admission, a specimen of blood is sent to the laboratory

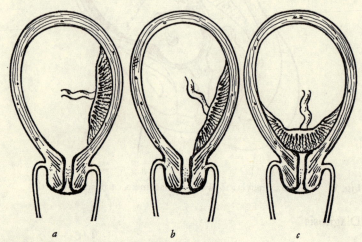

a   b   c

Fig. 17 Kinds of placenta praevia
(a) lateral (b) marginal (c) central

for grouping and for haemoglobin estimation, two pints of blood being available at all times in case of emergency. In view of the likelihood of further bleeding, any anaemia must be treated.

Further Management

a If no further loss occurs, the patient is usually examined under an anaesthetic in an operating theatre about the thirty-seventh or thirty-eighth week. All must be in readiness for a Caesarean section which may be carried out as an alternative to rupture of the membranes depending upon the position of the placenta. In either event the patient, on her return to the ward, must be carefully watched for further bleeding.

b Should haemorrhage recur before the thirty-seventh week, management depends upon its severity. In all cases a doctor must at once be called, the patient put back to bed, a half-hourly pulse and blood pressure record started and all pads saved so that the amount of blood loss may be estimated. If the bleeding settles, pregnancy may be allowed to continue, otherwise the patient must be examined in the operating theatre as soon as possible.

c If any bleeding, however slight, occurs after the thirty-seventh week, the patient should be delivered as there is no point at this stage in further prolonging pregnancy.

3   Bleeding from a normally situated placenta

a   Marginal Sinus Bleeding
It is sometimes taught that all bleeding from a normally situated placenta must be regarded as accidental ante-partum haemor-rhage, a condition characterised by extensive separation of the placenta and associated with considerable maternal and foetal risks. This view, however, is illogical, since in many instances bleeding during late pregnancy is merely due to rupture of a vessel on the placental margin, an altogether less urgent affair. Bleeding in these cases is characteristically slight and painless and is often repeated several times without becoming more profuse. In this it differs from bleeding from a placenta praevia, while the small amount of blood lost, together with the absence of other physical signs, distinguishes it from an accidental haemorrhage. The dangers of marginal sinus bleeding are usually slight, although at times some degree of anaemia may develop, while the irritant effect on the uterus of the extravasated blood is occasionally responsible for the onset of premature labour.

Management

No urgent treatment is needed in these cases. The tendency towards episodes of recurrent slight bleeding may be reduced by bed rest and sedation, which, however, may have to be con-tinued for a considerable time. Any tendency to anaemia must be treated. As labour may start prematurely the paediatric depart-ment should be warned that their help may be needed in caring for the baby after it has been delivered.

b Accidental Ante-partum Haemorrhage

Accidental Ante-partum Haemorrhage is one of the most serious and urgent complications of pregnancy as the associated maternal and foetal hazards are exceptionally high.

Aetiology

Essentially the condition is due to spasm and death of some of the decidual vessels, as a result of which bleeding occurs. This blood forms a haematoma beneath the placenta. This *retro-placental haematoma* has two effects, the nature of which depend upon its size and hence upon the extent of the original vascular spasm.

1 It separates the placenta from its attachments

2 It spreads into the uterine muscle.

The extravasated blood may either escape through the cervical canal into the vagina, more likely to occur when the placental implantation is low, or be retained, in which case the placental site is usually higher up in the uterus. In the former event the haemorrhage is known as *Revealed* and in the latter as *Concealed*. When part of the blood is retained and the rest escapes, bleeding is said to be of the *Mixed* type. It is probable that this is the most usual picture and that there is an element of both concealed and revealed bleeding in most cases of accidental haemorrhage.

Predisposing Factors

Classically, pre-eclampsia and essential hypertension are said to predispose to accidental haemorrhage, but this does not in fact seem to be the case. Certain types of anaemia, however, do appear to be associated with this condition which may thus be due to a vitamin deficiency of one sort or another. Certainly it is more common in women of poor social and nutritional standards who have borne a number of children in rapid succession.

Dangers

The *maternal dangers* of accidental haemorrhage are shock, renal failure and clotting defects. These, being directly related to retention of blood and clot behind the placenta are greatest when the bleeding is concealed and least when it is revealed. The blood which extravasates into the uterus and behind the

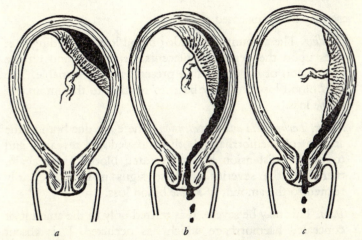

Fig. 18 Kinds of accidental ante-partum haemorrhage
(*a*) concealed (*b*) mixed (*c*) revealed

placenta disrupts and distends the tissues, producing pain and shock and predisposing to anuria from a reflex shut-down of renal function – Bilateral Cortical Necrosis. Simultaneously, the large haematoma tends to deplete the body's supply of fibrinogen a vital factor in the clotting of blood. A state of *Afibrinogenaemia* may thus arise, in which the blood will no longer clot and in which dangerous haemorrhage may, in consequence, occur.

The *foetal hazards*, on the other hand, are almost entirely due to placental separation. When this is extensive, as in large concealed haemorrhages, the foetus usually dies at once. In less severe instances it may survive initially but show signs of distress. The outcome will then depend upon the degree of this distress and the sort of treatment instituted. In very mild cases the foetus may be apparently unaffected. When born live, the baby may have to face the hazards of prematurity. The perinatal loss associated with accidental haemorrhage is therefore always high and in severe cases amounts almost to 100 per cent.

Physical Signs and Symptoms

These may be summarised as follows:

a   *Bleeding.* The amount of revealed blood loss, depending as it does upon the degree of placental separation and on the proportion of concealed loss present, is very variable. The *total* blood loss thus may bear no relation to the amount of *visible* loss.

b   *Shock, Tachycardia and Hypotension.* These are due both to the amount of haemorrhage, both concealed and revealed, and to uterine distension by extravasated blood. Once again, therefore, the severity of these signs is not necessarily related to the amount of *visible* blood loss.

c   *Pain.* This may be severe. It is related only to the amount of concealed haemorrhage which has occurred. It is absent when bleeding is entirely revealed.

d   *Uterine Enlargement and Tenderness.* The extravasated blood makes the uterus larger than normal, tender and hard. As a result, foetal parts are often felt only with difficulty if at all.

e   *The Foetal Heart Sounds.* Depending upon the degree of placental separation, the foetal heart sounds may be normal, rapid, irregular or absent.

Diagnosis

Although this is usually straightforward, the following possibilities should be remembered:

a   A purely *revealed* loss, being painless, may suggest a placenta praevia.

b An entirely *concealed* loss may be confused with a ruptured uterus or some general abdominal catastrophe.

Management

The objects of management are:

a To rupture the membranes and start labour as soon as possible

b To treat the shock

c To avoid complications such as clotting defects and renal failure.

The midwife, if confronted with a case of accidental haemorrhage must therefore act as follows:

a Call for medical aid at once

b Start a quarter-hourly record of the maternal pulse and blood pressure and of the foetal heart.

c Record all urinary output and test all specimens of urine passed for albumen and blood to determine whether renal function is being maintained

d Set up a trolley for artificial rupture of the membranes unless there is a possibility of a placenta praevia, when the patient must be examined in an operating theatre

e Prepare for saline, plasma or blood transfusion

f Prepare for blood to be taken for a clotting test.

Labour

Once labour has started, if the foetal heart is still present its rate must be checked quarter-hourly, as Caesarean section may have to be carried out as an emergency procedure should distress develop before the patient can safely be delivered vaginally.

In the majority of instances, once the membranes have been ruptured labour is rapid and easy. A severe post-partum haemorrhage is, however, likely unless any tendency to a clotting defect has been overcome in good time. Where this has been done, severe bleeding after the delivery of the placenta is usually more apparent than real and is mainly due to the passage of old retro-placental clots.

The Differential Diagnosis of Ante-partum Haemorrhages

The following summary may be of help in distinguishing between the various types of ante-partum haemorrhage:

1   Bleeding is slight and painless. The maternal and foetal states are satisfactory.

   The diagnosis here lies between:

a   *Incidental bleeding.* This may be excluded by a speculum examination

b   *Placenta praevia.* Abdominal and X-ray examination will point to the correct diagnosis

c   *Marginal sinus bleeding.* This may be diagnosed by excluding the other two possibilities.

2   Bleeding is slight and painless. The patient's condition is good. The foetus is distressed or dead.
Here the diagnosis is bleeding from Vasa Praevia. The blood is of foetal origin.

3   Bleeding is moderate or heavy. There may be some maternal tachycardia but no real shock. Moderate foetal distress may be present.

   Possiblities here are:

a   *Placenta praevia.* More likely to be present if the lie or presentation is abnormal or if the presenting part is abnormally high.

b   *Revealed accidental haemorrhage.* More probable if the lie and presentation are normal or if the presenting part is engaged.

Note. When haemorrhage is heavy, further investigations are usually pointless as immediate delivery is necessary. Examination under anaesthesia will therefore be carried out without delay.

4 Bleeding is slight or moderate. The mother is shocked and in pain. The foetus is distressed or dead.

The most likely diagnosis here is an accidental haemorrhage with a considerable degree of concealed loss and much placental separation. The alternative possibility, namely a ruptured uterus, is uncommon in pregnancy in the absence of any relevant past history.

Summary

Pre-eclampsia

Pre-eclampsia, a condition characterised by a rise in blood pressure together with the presence of oedema and/or albuminuria, owes its importance to its high incidence, the dangers it presents both to the patient and to the foetus, and to the fact that it is a disease of signs rather than of symptoms.

Pre-eclampsia complicates about ten per cent of all pregnancies, being particularly liable to occur in women over thirty-five, those who are overweight, those with pre-existing hypertension and renal disease and those with multiple pregnancies.

The chief maternal dangers of pre-eclampsia are eclampsia, cerebral haemorrhage and renal cortical necrosis. It is not, however, commonly associated with accidental ante-partum haemorrhage, neither does it cause permanent hypertension.

The foetal dangers are related in part to placental insufficiency and in part to prematurity.

The cardinal signs of pre-eclampsia are hypertension, oedema and albuminuria, the latter being absent from all save severe cases. Similarly, symptoms such as headache, vomiting, epigastric pain, visual disturbances and oliguria are usually seen only if eclampsia is imminent.

The basis of the management of pre-eclampsia is to prolong

pregnancy as long as this is safe for the patient and the foetus. For this it is necessary to diagnose the condition at an early and mild stage, to bring it under speedy and effective control and to ensure that this control is maintained. Within this context management may be either in the home or in hospital.

Management in the home is reserved solely for patients with mild pre-eclampsia who are willing to accept the necessary measures. Treatment consists of rest, sedation and some dietary restriction. The blood pressure must be taken once or twice daily and urine tested for albumen each day.

Hospital admission is necessary for patients with moderate or severe pre-eclampsia or where home treatment is impossible. The principles of treatment and supervision are similar to those used at home although stricter enforcement is usually necessary.

A rising blood pressure, increasing oedema and the development of albuminuria are signs that the maternal and foetal risks are increasing and that intervention may be necessary. A foetus which fails to grow is at special risk.

Later management depends upon the response to treatment. While pregnancy must never be allowed to go beyond term, on many occasions induction of labour before the expected date of delivery may be necessary for the sake of the foetus or of the patient.

A further rise in blood pressure after delivery is often seen. This may at times be high enough to precipitate eclampsia. It must be remembered that Ergometrine may aggravate this risk.

Eclampsia

Owing to improvements in the standard of ante-natal care, eclampsia is becoming a rare disease in this country.

Its symptomatology is that of severe pre-eclampsia with the addition of one or more fits. It may occur either before, during or after labour, the latter two types being the more common.

The convulsions themselves consist of three stages, Premonitory, Tonic and Clonic, each of which lasts for between one and two minutes. A period of coma of variable duration then ensues. Consciousness is lost throughout.

Eclampsia presents considerable maternal and foetal risks. The former consist of cerebral haemorrhage, cardiac failure, aspiration pneumonia and sepsis. The latter are those of placental insufficiency, prematurity and acute intra-uterine hypoxia.

Serious prognostic features are a rapid succession of fits, deep coma between fits, severe hypertension, tachycardia, hyperpyrexia and oliguria.

Management consists essentially in controlling the fits by means of sedatives and hypotensive drugs, the patient then being delivered regardless of the duration of pregnancy.

The following investigations are needed in a case of eclampsia:

Blood Pressure: $\frac{1}{4}$–$\frac{1}{2}$ hourly
Maternal Pulse: $\frac{1}{2}$ hourly
Foetal Heart: $\frac{1}{2}$ hourly
Fluid Balance Chart
Urinalysis for albumen and Esbach's Tubes.

Nursing care is that of any unconscious or semi-conscious patient liable to further fits. Points of particular importance are the maintenance of an adequate airway, the prevention of aspiration of blood and mucus and the avoidance of pulmonary congestion.

Vaginal delivery is preferable to Caesarean section in these patients. Labour is usually induced after the fits have been controlled for twelve to twenty-four hours. In cases of intra-partum eclampsia, however, delivery should be completed as soon as possible.

Essential Hypertension

Essential Hypertension differs from pre-eclampsia in that the blood pressure is raised before the start of pregnancy. It is, however, usually diagnosed by finding the pressure to be 140/90 mm Hg or more before the twentieth week.

Apart from the raised blood pressure, the condition presents neither signs nor symptoms.

During pregnancy essential hypertension may follow one of three courses:

a The blood pressure shows a mid-pregnancy drop

b The blood pressure remains at the same level throughout

c Pre-eclampsia is superadded to the existing essential hypertension.

The maternal hazards are those of pre-eclampsia. In addition, the blood pressure remains permanently raised in one third of cases.

The foetal risks are related to placental insufficiency and prematurity.

Management in pregnancy depends on the height of the blood pressure and the severity of any superadded pre-eclampsia. In mild cases treatment at home with rest and sedation is all that is required. In more severe cases hospital admission may be necessary for assessment of the degree of hypertension and for special treatment. In such cases hypotensive drugs are sometimes of value.

Due to the danger of placental insufficiency, in no case must pregnancy go past term. Delivery before the fortieth week may be needed if the blood pressure rises despite treatment, if albuminuria develops or if the foetus fails to grow.

Albuminuria

Non-infective albuminuria of pregnancy, although usually associated with pre-eclampsia, eclampsia or essential hypertension with superadded pre-eclampsia, occasionally arises in the absence of any of these conditions.

Although in such cases it is often assumed to be due to chronic nephritis, this is usually not the case.

The dangers of the condition are both maternal and foetal, the latter being due to placental insufficiency.

A case of albuminuria of pregnancy must be admitted to hospital for investigation of the urine and for renal function tests.

Treatment consists of rest and sedation, the patient being kept in hospital as long as the albuminuria persists.

Provided that the patient's condition remains good and that the foetus continues to grow, delivery may be postponed until the end of the thirty-sixth or thirty-seventh week. Otherwise it should be effected as soon as the risks of continuing the pregnancy outweigh those of prematurity.

Small-for-Dates Baby

A baby may be said to be small-for-dates when it weighs less than $5\frac{1}{2}$ lb at term or if, when born before term, it is considerably smaller than would be expected.

The condition of small-for-dates is associated with pre-eclampsia, essential hypertension, bleeding in early and late pregnancy and certain congenital malformations of the foetus. In some cases no obvious maternal or foetal causes can be found.

A small-for-dates foetus is particularly liable to die in utero before the onset of labour. Death from pulmonary haemorrhage or hypoglycaemia is likely to happen during the first week of life.

Diagnosis is usually reached solely on clinical grounds, it being important to exclude incorrect dates. X-ray examination of the foetus is of little value in determining its precise age. Hormone estimations, although useful, are not yet generally available.

Where its growth appears to have ceased, immediate delivery represents the best chance for the foetus. In other instances prolonged rest in hospital may be of some value in encouraging further foetal development. In no circumstances should pregnancy be allowed to go beyond term.

Ante-Partum Haemorrhage

Ante-partum haemorrhage is defined as bleeding from the birth canal from the twenty-eighth week of pregnancy until after the delivery of the foetus. A symptom rather than a disease, it is due to a variety of causes.

Bleeding of Foetal Origin. In cases of velamentous insertion of the cord a foetal vessel may be torn when the membranes rupture. Bleeding may be sufficient to kill the foetus. Treatment consists of immediate delivery if the foetus is still alive.

Bleeding from a Placenta Praevia. If the placenta is in the lower uterine segment its attachments are torn as the uterus stretches. Bleeding results. This is usually painless and recurrent. The low placental implantation also predisposes to a transverse or oblique lie and a presenting part which is often high or displaced laterally.

Diagnosis is based upon the history and abdominal findings, often helped by X-ray evidence. In no circumstances should a vaginal examination be carried out.

Treatment consists in prolonging pregnancy until the foetus is mature, provided that the patient's safety is not jeopardised. For this reason she must stay in hospital until delivered. If no further bleeding occurs, an examination under anaesthesia is done at thirty-seven to thirty-eight weeks, followed by rupture of the membranes or by Caesarean section. If further bleeding takes place before thirty-seven weeks, it is treated conservatively if slight, otherwise immediate delivery is indicated.

Marginal Sinus Bleeding. Here the placenta is normally situated; bleeding is from a vessel on its edge. The loss is slight and recurrent. Treatment consists of rest and sedation in hospital, any co-existing anaemia being corrected. The foetal risks of this condition are mainly those of prematurity.

Accidental Haemorrhage. Owing to spasm and death of some of the smaller decidual vessels, blood is extravasated behind the placenta, resulting in its separation. The blood may then either escape through the cervical canal or remain as a retroplacental clot in which case it also infiltrates the uterine muscle, producing pain and shock and predisposing to renal failure and clotting defects. Owing to placental separation, foetal distress and intra-uterine death often occur.

Management consists of immediate rupture of the membranes, treatment of maternal shock and prevention of renal or clotting complications.

Labour is usually rapid. A severe post-partum haemorrhage may occur unless a tendency to *afibrinogenaemia* has been overcome in good time.

CHAPTER SIX

Miscellaneous Abnormalities of Pregnancy

The Effect on the Foetus of Drugs Given During Pregnancy

Since the Thalidomide disaster, considerable concern has arisen over the possible effect on the developing foetus of drugs taken by the patient during pregnancy. While most of this worry is groundless, it nevertheless exists and for this reason many patients may ask for reassurance on this score.

When considering the possible effect of a drug upon the foetus, the following points should be borne in mind:

1　The drug, if extremely toxic, may kill the foetus outright.

2　If less toxic, it may affect it in some way short of death, either in a manner resembling its effect in the adult, as in drugs given for thyrotoxicosis or malignant disease, or differing markedly from this, as in the case of Thalidomide itself.

3　The earlier the pregnancy, the greater, in general, will be the effect of the drug upon the foetus.

4　The so-called Placental Barrier does not really exist. All drugs must therefore be regarded as able to pass to the foetus, although the rate and extent to which this happens varies greatly from drug to drug.

The Influence of Specific Drugs

1 Drugs Given for Malignant Disease

These highly toxic substances are, for obvious reasons, rarely prescribed during pregnancy. Little, therefore, is known of their effect upon the foetus. It is generally assumed that they are either lethal or that they cause severe congenital malformations. Recent work, however, suggests that their effect, save in very early pregnancy, may have been over-emphasised.

2 Hormones and Allied Substances

Certain progesterone-like substances, given in early pregnancy in cases of sub-fertility or threatened abortion, cause masculinisation of a female foetus. Modern drugs of this sort, however, such as Primolut Depot, do not have this effect.

Derivatives of Cortisone, sometimes used in the management of allergic or inflammatory conditions, may cause congenital malformations of the foetus, although the chances of this are remote. They are, however, likely to depress the foetal adrenal, an effect which must be corrected during the neo-natal period.

As stated earlier, drugs given in hyperthyroidism, itself rare in pregnancy, may depress the foetal thyroid, necessitating treatment after delivery.

3 Antibiotics and Sulphonamides

Antibiotics and sulphonamides are widely prescribed during pregnancy, being especially useful in the management of chronic urinary infections. Some of these drugs, notably long-acting sulphonamides such as Midicel, may damage the foetal liver, with resultant jaundice and kernicterus (page 399). Of the antibiotics, the Tetracyclines can sometimes cause developmental abnormalities of the teeth and interfere with normal epiphyseal growth of the long bones; while Streptomycin may, as in the adult, cause permanent lesions of the eighth cranial nerve with resultant deafness and vertigo.

4 Drugs Related Specifically to Liver Damage and Kernicterus
Certain drugs other than the sulphonamides may cause damage
to the foetal liver and hence predispose to kernicterus. These
drugs are:

a Salicylates – such as Aspirin.

b Synthetic Vitamin K – Konakion.

c Chlorpromazine – Largactil.

d Chlortetracycline – Aureomycin.

e Barbiturates.

Although the variety and number of drugs now believed to
have some adverse effect upon the foetus is considerable, in
assessing the hazards involved by their administration two important points should be borne in mind:

1 The number of foetuses actually *affected* by these drugs is
extremely small in relation to the number of women receiving
them.

2 The dangers presented to a foetus by any given drug must be
balanced against the benefits it offers to the patient. Expressed
differently, the dangers to a patient of withholding treatment
may be greater than those imposed on a foetus by giving it.

It is thus necessary to approach this question unemotionally
and to consider each case from the viewpoint of the patient's
future health as well as from that of the foetus. As a general rule,
therefore, where any drug is genuinely indicated for the treatment of a maternal complaint, it is probably best for it to be
given. On the other hand, where this is not so or where reasonable and, from the foetal point of view, safer alternatives exist,
they should always be preferred.

Rhesus Incompatibility

Recent interest in new measures to solve the problem of Rhesus incompatibility makes it necessary for the midwife to have some general knowledge of this problem. The following account has been written with this requirement in mind.

The Rhesus or Rh. Blood Groups

Although the A, B and O blood groups are those which are best known, many others exist, among which are the Rhesus or Rh. groups. These are three in number, designated by the letters C, D and E, but only group D is of clinical importance. For practical purposes, therefore, a person with blood group D may be regarded as Rhesus positive while one with the opposite group, shown as d, is Rhesus negative. The proportion of these two groups in the population is about 83 to 17.

Rhesus Sensitisation

If an Rh. negative woman becomes pregnant by a Rh. positive man, there is about a 70 per cent chance that the baby will also be Rh. positive. If this happens, there is a danger that some red blood cells from the foetus will pass across the placenta into her blood stream during pregnancy and stimulate her to produce antibodies. These antibodies will then pass back into the foetal circulation and affect its own Rh. positive cells, causing haemolytic disease.

This passage of foetal cells into the maternal circulation, which happens only in about twenty per cent of cases, does not usually take place to any great extent until labour. For this reason, any antibodies formed by the mother will have no effect upon the foetus responsible for them, since it will by now have been born. The antibodies, however, persist in the mother's blood stream long after delivery and may therefore affect a subsequent foetus, provided that it is Rh. positive. The chances of a first-born child developing haemolytic disease are thus virtually nil, while those of a second child are still only about ten per cent, this risk rising slowly in further pregnancies. It is therefore reasonable to re-assure a patient that the odds are *against* rather than *for* any of her children developing Rhesus incompatibility.

Types of Haemolytic Disease

Haemolytic disease may assume one of three forms:

1 *Hydrops Foetalis.* This is characterised by gross oedema and ascites of the foetus. It is invariably fatal, death occurring either during pregnancy or immediately after delivery.

2 *Icterus Gravis.* Here, jaundice and anaemia develop shortly after birth and may be severe. In such cases the jaundice often affects the brain and produces the condition known as Ker-nicterus, which is characterised by spasticity and mental and physical retardation. The originally high mortality of this variety of haemolytic disease has been much reduced by modern treatment.

3 *Anaemia of the New born.* This is the mildest type of haemo-lytic disease and the one which responds most readily to treatment.

Diagnosis

a During Pregnancy
This is done by detecting antibodies in the patient's blood by what is known as the Indirect Coombs Test. If antibodies are present and if their concentration or titre is rising, the foetus will probably be affected.

b After Delivery
Clinical examination of the baby immediately after delivery may suggest the diagnosis, confirmation being obtained by finding that the level of haemoglobin in the cord blood is low and that of

bilirubin is high. In addition, the presence of affected red cells will be shown by the Direct Coombs Test.

Management

There are two aspects of the management of Rhesus incompatibility, namely *treatment* and *prevention*, of which the latter is the more recent.

a   Treatment during Pregnancy

If treatment is to be successful, the presence of maternal antibodies must be discovered as early in pregnancy as possible. For this reason, the patient's blood should be tested at her first visit to the ante-natal clinic and checked again at the twenty-eighth, thirty-second and thirty-sixth weeks. If antibodies are discovered, a specimen of liquor amnii is withdrawn – Amniocentesis – in order that its bilirubin concentration may be estimated. This will provide a more accurate picture of the state of the foetus than that offered by the titre of maternal antibodies. If it seems probable that the foetus will be only mildly affected, labour is induced at or near term. In more severe cases it will be necessary to deliver the baby in a much more premature state. Where the foetus is likely to die of haemolytic disease if left in utero and of prematurity if delivered, intra-uterine transfusion offers it the best chance of survival. In this procedure Rh. negative blood is injected into its peritoneal cavity through a fine polythene cannula.

b   Treatment after Delivery

Treatment after delivery consists essentially of replacement transfusion, the baby's Rh. positive blood with its affected red cells and antibodies being replaced by Group O Rh. negative blood from a donor other than the mother. Such a transfusion, which is by no means without risk to the baby, may have to be repeated if the haemoglobin level continues to drop or that of the serum bilirubin to rise. General nursing care of the delicate, premature infant is also of the greatest importance and should take place in a Special Care Unit in charge of a consultant paediatrician.

Prevention

The measures to prevent the development of haemolytic disease consist of destroying the Rh. positive cells in the mother's blood by means of Anti-D Gamma Globulins, injected intramuscularly within three days of delivery. In the case of all Rh. negative patients, therefore, as soon as labour is over, a specimen of cord blood is sent to the laboratory. If this shows that the baby is Rh. positive the mother's blood is examined for the presence of foetal red cells. If these are found her chances of becoming sensitised and of developing antibodies are extremely high. By giving the mother Anti-D Globulin, however, these foetal cells will be destroyed before they can do any harm and the development of Rhesus incompatibility in a subsequent pregnancy will be prevented.

The Large-for-Dates Uterus

In the course of her work in the ante-natal clinic the midwife will often see a patient whose uterus is larger than would be expected from the menstrual history. This can sometimes cause confusion from the point of view of estimating the precise duration of pregnancy, especially if induction of labour is being considered as a means of treatment. Whenever such a discrepancy arises, therefore, it is important to consider its possible causes and to decide which of these is most likely to be present.

The Causes of a Large-For-Dates Uterus are:

1   Wrong dates

2   Multiple pregnancy

3   Hydramnios

4   Hydatidiform mole

5   Fibroids

6   An abnormally large foetus.

1 Wrong Dates

This is perhaps the most usual reason for the fundal height being greater than expected. It is usually due to the patient failing to note the exact date of her last period. Occasionally bleeding from implantation or an early threatened abortion may be misinterpreted as a period and pregnancy dated from that time.

It is usually impossible to clarify these points after the twenty-eighth week, since at this distance the patient's memory can seldom be relied upon. If, however, a vaginal examination has been carried out in early pregnancy, the relation of the size of the uterus to the period of amenorrhoea will have been established at that time and later confusion is less likely.

2 Multiple Pregnancy

The diagnosis of multiple pregnancy is discussed on page 286. Here it need only be said that whenever the uterus is larger than expected the possibility of twins must always be remembered.

3 Hydramnios

Hydramnios is defined as a demonstrable excess of liquor amnii. The condition may be present in either an acute or a sub-acute form. Acute Hydramnios is rare. It tends to occur in comparatively early pregnancy, e.g., before the twenty-fourth week and is usually although not invariably associated with uniovular twins. It is characterised by a rapid accumulation of liquor, the uterus becoming greatly enlarged and extremely tender and tense. Dyspnoea may be marked. In the sub-acute form the volume of liquor increases more slowly and although the final degree of uterine distension may be considerable, less discomfort is experienced. Although sub-acute hydramnios is sometimes associated with a major congenital defect of the foetus, other than Hydrocephalus, this is by no means invariable and the foetus or foetuses – twins are often present in these cases – are usually normal in all respects.

The complications of hydramnios, other than those mentioned above, are pre-eclampsia, premature rupture of the membranes, premature labour and malpresentations. These last are due to the fact that owing to the great amount of space available to the foetus, it is less likely to assume a correct lie, presentation and position than when only a normal volume of liquor is present.

Diagnosis

Hydramnios is diagnosed by noting that the uterus is larger than expected and that the lie and presentation of the foetus cannot easily be determined. A fluid thrill may sometimes be felt but this is less constant a sign than is usually taught. Difficulties may arise in distinguishing a case of hydramnios from one of multiple pregnancy, where often the same physical signs may be present. For this reason, an X-ray is often necessary to establish the diagnosis as well as to exclude any gross congenital malformations.

Management

Where hydramnios gives rise to symptoms severe enough to distress the patient, admission to hospital for rest and sedation may be necessary. The withdrawal of liquor by amniocentesis rarely brings more than temporary relief since the fluid rapidly reaccumulates. Furthermore, such a procedure carries the risk of inducing premature labour. When the patient is at or near term, or if pre-eclampsia is present, it is often best to induce labour by rupture of the membranes. In such cases it is important to check the lie and presentation of the foetus at frequent intervals, especially at the onset of labour, and to exclude a prolapse of the cord at this time. When the foetus is grossly malformed, labour should be induced as soon as is safely possible.

4 Hydatidiform Mole
This is discussed on page 86.

5 Fibroids
Although uterine fibroids tend to become flattened and less prominent as pregnancy advances, they may nevertheless be a cause of abnormal uterine enlargement near term. If the patient has

been seen and examined vaginally in early pregnancy, their presence will have been detected at that time and no confusion will arise later. When, however, this has not been done, a correct diagnosis may be more difficult. In such cases the fibroids may at times be felt as protuberances on the surface of the uterus, resembling in some respects small foetal parts save, of course, that their position never varies.

6   An Abnormally Large Foetus

The diagnosis of an abnormally large foetus is reached in part by excluding all other causes of undue uterine enlargement and in part by abdominal palpation. In addition, where the patient is a multipara there may be a past history of large babies. The importance of this condition lies both in its relation to maternal pre-diabetes and diabetes mellitus and in the possibility of disproportion complicating labour (page 290).

In all cases where the uterus is larger than the duration of amenorrhoea would suggest, the midwife should inform the doctor in charge of the case since the management of the various causative conditions is of medical rather than of nursing concern.

Prolongation of Pregnancy

A pregnancy which has lasted for more than forty-two weeks is usually regarded as being abnormally prolonged. The main importance of such pregnancies is that the associated perinatal mortality is above the average, although it must be stressed that in the great majority of instances a healthy living baby is delivered without any particular difficulties or dangers.

Relation to Postmaturity

Provided that the patient's menstrual history is reliable, prolongation of pregnancy is easy to diagnose. Postmaturity, often wrongly used as a synonym, is not. This latter condition may be defined as one in which the foetus has reached a stage of development in advance of that usually seen. Such a foetus is said to be of above average weight and to have an unduly well-ossified head, a dry, wrinkled skin and nails that extend beyond the finger-tips. While such a combination of physical signs may occasionally be encountered, it is by no means as common as simple prolongation of pregnancy, nor indeed is it necessarily associated with it. Moreover, since a diagnosis of postmaturity must necessarily await the delivery and subsequent examination of the baby, its detection and treatment during pregnancy are both impossible.

The Causes of Perinatal Death in Prolonged Pregnancy

It is commonly believed that after a prolonged pregnancy the baby will be overweight at birth and that, in consequence of this, difficulties may arise over its delivery. This is rarely if ever the case. The mean weight of such babies is only marginally increased while many are actually smaller than average. The main foetal danger is thus not dystocia but placental insufficiency, the functional capacity of the placenta being reduced to a level at which foetal life can no longer be maintained. Since such a reduction in efficiency is usually a gradual process, its effects on the development of the foetus will be noticeable for a considerable time. The foetus will therefore be smaller than would be expected and its rate of growth will be slowed down or arrested. It is thus the small-for-dates foetus which is at a particular risk in a prolonged pregnancy rather than one which is of average or above average size.

The Time of Foetal Death

Where placental function has become grossly defective the foetus may die in utero before the onset of labour. At other times the stress of uterine contractions may precipitate foetal distress under conditions where such a complication would not normally be expected. If this distress is not promptly detected and treated

F

it may lead to foetal death either during labour or immediately after delivery.

Associated Conditions of Particular Danger to the Foetus

Any condition predisposing to or associated with placental insufficiency will, if pregnancy is allowed to become prolonged, present a heightened risk to the foetus. This point must be remembered where pre-eclampsia, essential hypertension, antepartum haemorrhage or even bleeding in early pregnancy have been encountered, or where a history is obtained of a previous unexplained perinatal death, especially if this occurred after term. In cases of this sort care should be taken to ensure that pregnancy is not allowed to go beyond forty weeks.

The Management of Prolongation of Pregnancy

It should now be clear that it may be dangerous to allow pregnancy to become abnormally prolonged. In consequence, in many instances, delivery should be effected before forty-two weeks. For this reason, any patient in whom pregnancy has lasted over forty weeks must be referred to a doctor. The subsequent management of these cases may be summarised as follows:

1   Where pregnancy has otherwise been normal and the foetus is of good size, pregnancy may be allowed to continue until twelve days past term in the hope that labour will start spontaneously. Where this does not happen, admission will be arranged for induction of labour.

2   Where pregnancy has been complicated by any condition predisposing to placental insufficiency, immediate induction of labour is usually necessary.

3   Where the foetus is small, even in the absence of other evidence of placental insufficiency, it is dangerous to temporise or

to hope that further intra-uterine growth will take place. In these patients, therefore, labour should be induced at term.

4 Where doubt exists regarding the patient's dates and where the foetus is of good size and still growing, it may be best to await the spontaneous onset of labour since the duration of pregnancy cannot be accurately determined.

The conduct of labour in patients in whom pregnancy has been prolonged follows the pattern set out on page 193. It is, however, necessary to carry out frequent and regular checks of the foetal heart rate in view of the heightened possibility of foetal distress developing for no apparent reason. It need scarcely be added that at the first sign of such a complication medical aid must be sent for since the immediate delivery of the foetus may be its only hope of survival.

Summary

Effect on the Foetus of Drugs given during Pregnancy

Many patients are concerned about the possible effect upon the foetus of drugs administered during pregnancy. In the great majority of instances such fears are groundless.

In general, the action of any drug upon the foetus depends upon its toxicity and the period in pregnancy in which it is given. The earlier this is, the greater is the effect likely to be.

With regard to specific groups of drugs, those given in the treatment of malignant disease may kill the foetus, although this risk has probably been over-emphasised. Certain progesterone-like substances may produce masculinisation of a female foetus. This, however, is uncommon nowadays. Long-acting sulphonamides may damage the foetal liver with resultant jaundice and kernicterus, while the tetracyclines may affect the foetal teeth and the epiphyses of the long bones.

It must be remembered, in assessing this problem, that the number of foetuses actually affected by such drugs is extremely small in relation to the number of patients taking them.

In general, if any drug is really necessary for the safety of the patient it should be given. If reasonable and safer alternatives exist they should be preferred.

Rhesus Incompatibility

Apart from the A, B and O blood groups, many others exist, of which the Rhesus groups are the most important.

If a foetus is Rh. positive while its mother is Rh. negative, there is a chance that some of its red cells may pass into its mother's blood stream and cause antibodies to be formed. These antibodies can then pass back into the foetal circulation and cause Haemolytic Disease.

For various reasons, first-born children are unlikely to be affected in this way and even in subsequent pregnancies the chances are *against* rather than *for* any foetus developing Rhesus incompatibility.

Haemolytic disease can assume one of three forms:

a   *Hydrops Foetalis.* Invariably fatal

b   *Icterus Gravis.* Giving rise to anaemia, jaundice and kernicterus

c   *Anaemia of the Newborn.* The least serious form.

Diagnosis during pregnancy is made by finding an increasing titre of antibodies in the maternal blood.

Diagnosis after delivery depends upon clinical examination of the baby together with laboratory findings of anaemia and affected red cells.

Treatment during pregnancy rests on early diagnosis by blood examination and amniocentesis and consists either of premature delivery or of intra-uterine transfusion.

Rhesus incompatibility may be prevented by injecting a Rhesus negative woman whose blood contains foetal red cells with Anti-D Gamma Globulins. To be effective this injection must be made as soon after delivery as possible.

Large-for-Dates Uterus

A large-for-dates uterus can sometimes cause difficulties from the point of view of establishing the precise duration of pregnancy.

The causes of this condition are wrong dates, multiple pregnancy, hydramnios, hydatidiform mole, fibroids and an abnormally large foetus. Of these conditions, multiple pregnancy and hydatidiform mole are considered elsewhere.

Wrong dates are the most usual reason for the fundal height being greater than expected. If, however, the size of the uterus has been carefully assessed in early pregnancy, later confusion on this score need not arise.

Hydramnios may be either acute or sub-acute. The former is uncommon. It occurs relatively early in pregnancy and is usually associated with uniovular twins. The uterus is greatly distended, tense and tender. In the sub-acute variety the liquor accumulates more slowly and the symptoms are less urgent. Severe congenital malformations of the foetus are sometimes seen in these cases.

The complications of hydramnios are pre-eclampsia, premature rupture of the membranes, premature labour and malpresentations. Treatment consists of rest and sedation, followed by induction of labour if the patient is at or near term or if pre-eclampsia is present. After such a procedure it is important frequently to check the lie and presentation of the foetus and to exclude a prolapse of the cord.

Fibroids are an occasional cause of undue uterine enlargement. Although they usually become flattened as pregnancy progresses, at times they may project from the surface of the uterus and closely resemble foetal parts.

An abnormally large foetus is diagnosed partly by excluding the other conditions mentioned above and partly by abdominal examination. Its importance is due to its relation to maternal pre-diabetes and diabetes mellitus. It may also be associated with disproportion during labour.

Prolongation of Pregnancy

A pregnancy lasting for more than forty-two weeks is said to be abnormally prolonged. Despite the fact that such a pregnancy is associated with increased perinatal hazards, in the great majority of cases a healthy, living baby is delivered.

Postmaturity, often regarded as synonymous with prolonged pregnancy, is in fact far less common and need not necessarily be associated with a pregnancy of abnormal length.

The cause of perinatal death in prolonged pregnancy is usually placental insufficiency, dystocia from an overlarge foetus being uncommon.

Conditions which themselves contribute to placental insufficiency, such as pre-eclampsia, essential hypertension, bleeding in early pregnancy and ante-partum haemorrhage, present a greatly increased risk to the foetus when pregnancy is prolonged beyond term. In such cases, therefore, labour should always be induced at or before the expected date of delivery.

In all other cases, where the duration of pregnancy is known, delivery should be effected at or before the end of the forty-second week. In these patients it is particularly important to keep a careful check upon the foetal heart rate throughout labour in view of the increased possibility of the development of foetal distress.

PART THREE

Normal Labour

Introduction

Labour is defined as the process whereby the foetus is expelled from the uterus through the birth canal. It owes its importance in part to the fact that it is associated with certain dangers to the mother and to the foetus and in part to the fact that it represents to the former the culmination of the hopes and expectations built up during pregnancy. The proper conduct of labour should therefore take into account the mother's well-being as well as concerning itself with the bodily safety of the foetus. These requirements present a midwife with two problems:

1 In the first place she must understand the anatomy and physiology of labour so that she may detect any departures from normal whose management calls for medical assistance or advice.

2 Secondly, she must appreciate the physical and mental stresses to which a patient is subjected at this time and ensure that these are kept to a minimum.

While much can be learned from reading about labour, both normal and abnormal, knowledge gained in this way can never replace that derived from practical experience in the labour wards and from the careful observation of women during labour. Only in this way is it possible to understand the difficulties, dangers and stresses to which they are subjected and the manner in which these are dealt with.

Parts Three and Four of this book, in which first normal and then abnormal labour are considered, have been written with this realisation in mind. They cannot replace practical learning and are intended merely to serve as a guide to the nature of labour and to indicate some of the problems encountered during this process. Although every midwife must evolve for herself a code of conduct best suited to her own temperament and abilities, in all labours, whether normal or abnormal, certain fundamental requirements must be observed:

1   The safety of the patient and of the foetus must always be under close and constant review.

2   No patient should be allowed to suffer pain or discomfort if means exist for alleviating this without increasing the maternal or foetal dangers.

3   Any departure from the normal must be recognised as soon as possible and a doctor informed without loss of time.

These requirements cannot always be met, but if they are always remembered there will be few occasions when the well-being of the patient or of the foetus will be seriously at risk.

CHAPTER SEVEN

General Considerations

Normal Labour: General Aspects: The Anatomy of the Pelvis and of the Foetal Skull

Since a midwife is usually responsible only for the conduct of a normal labour, it is important that she should understand what this implies, otherwise she will be unable to tell when abnormalities have arisen. In seeking an acceptable definition of normal labour, the following factors must be taken into account:

1   The duration of labour

2   The state and maturity of the foetus

3   The manner in which the foetus presents

4   The way in which the foetus is delivered

5   The presence or absence of complications.

The following definition meets these requirements:

Normal labour is labour lasting between two and twenty-four hours in which a living mature foetus, presenting by the vertex, is delivered spontaneously without complications other than an episiotomy or a first- or second-degree perineal laceration.

The problems raised by this definition, the understanding of the terms it contains and the appreciation of the criteria it has to satisfy, must now be considered.

The essential problem of all labours is whether the foetus will safely negotiate the maternal pelvis when passing from the uterus to the outside world. Here, two facts are of relevance:

1   If the foetal head will pass through the pelvis the rest of the body will almost certainly follow.

2   If the foetal head can enter the pelvis from above it will be able to emerge from below.

The outcome of labour thus depends upon whether the foetal head can enter the pelvis.

In order to know not only whether this can happen but also the manner in which it may best do so, it is necessary to have some knowledge of the shape and size of the maternal pelvis and of the foetal head. For that reason the anatomy of the pelvis and of the foetal skull must now be considered.

The Maternal Pelvis

Basically, the maternal pelvis is a ring composed of three bones, the Ilium, the Ischium and the Pubis. These, although developing separately, soon fuse into the two Innominate Bones which meet anteriorly at the Pubic Symphysis. Posteriorly, the Innominate bones articulate at the Sacro-Iliac joints with the Sacrum, a flat, triangular bone consisting usually of five fused vertebrae. Above the Sacrum lies the fifth Lumbar Vertebra; below, it meets the Coccyx, which is formed of three or four small vertebrae, at the Sacro-Coccygeal joint.

Apart from providing attachments for various large muscles both of the trunk and of the lower limb, the Innominate bones and the Sacrum support the entire weight of the body and transmit it to the legs through the two Femoral heads.

The part of the pelvis which is of obstetric importance is called the True Pelvis. This is essentially a bony canal formed by both Innominate bones, the Sacrum and the Coccyx. This canal is curved, being shorter anteriorly than posteriorly, and the plane of its *entry* is thus at a different angle from that of its *exit* or *outlet*, an arrangement which raises certain problems in relation to the birth of the foetal head (Fig 20). For descriptive as well as for practical purposes the pelvic canal may be regarded as having a Brim, a Cavity and an Outlet, each of which requires separate consideration.

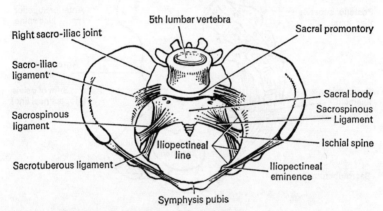

Fig. 19   Antero-posterior view of the pelvis

The Brim includes posteriorly the upper, anterior border of the Sacral Promontory, the two wings or Alae of the Sacrum, the Ilio-Pectineal line and the Ilio-Pectineal Eminence on the Ilium laterally and the Superior Pubic Rami and the upper part of the Pubic Symphysis anteriorly.

The Cavity is bounded posteriorly by the anterior aspects of the Sacral vertebrae, laterally by the Sacro-Sciatic notch and the inner walls of the Ilium and Ischium, and anteriorly by the posterior surface of the Superior and Inferior Pubic Rami, the Body of the Pubis and the Pubic Symphysis.

The Outlet is limited posteriorly by the Sacro-Coccygeal joint, laterally by the Ischial Spines and Ischial Tuberosities and anteriorly by the Inferior Pubic Rami and the lower part of the Symphysis Pubis.

The bony outline both of the Cavity and of the Outlet is incomplete owing to the large Sacro-Sciatic Notch posterolaterally and the Obturator Foramen between the Superior and Inferior Pubic Rami anteriorly. The Obturator Foramen is closed

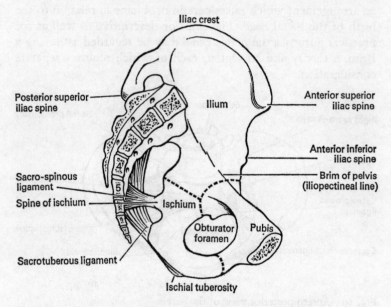

Fig. 20   Section of the pelvis showing brim cavity and outlet

by the Obturator Membrane and the Obturator muscles. The Sacro-Sciatic Notch is converted into the Sacro-Sciatic Foramen by two ligaments, the Sacro-Spinous Ligament and the Sacro-Tuberous Ligament. These run from the lower part of the Sacrum laterally and anteriorly to the Ischial Spines and Ischial Tuberosities respectively.

The Pelvic Measurements

In order to provide information about the three subdivisions of the pelvic canal, various measurements or *diameters* are described which connect certain well-defined landmarks. A knowledge of these diameters allows the midwife to visualise the actual shape and size of the pelvis much as a builder can visualise the size and shape of a house from certain standard measurements. Ideally, to gain an accurate picture of the Brim, the Cavity and the Outlet

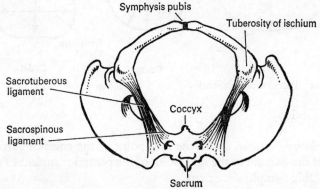

Fig. 21   The pelvic outlet

requires antero-posterior, transverse and oblique measurements. This is possible for the Brim and the Cavity but in the case of the Outlet no oblique diameters exist. This is because, owing to the presence of the Sacro-Sciatic Notch, the necessary bony points from which all diameters must be taken are lacking.

The diameters of the Pelvis are as follows:

The Brim

1   *Antero-Posterior or True Conjugate*. From the upper anterior border of the Sacral Promontory to the top of the back of the Symphysis Pubis. 11·5 cm.

2   *Transverse*. The widest transverse measurement cutting the True Conjugate at right angles. 13 cm.

3   *Oblique*. From the upper border of the Sacro-Iliac Joint of one side to the opposite Ilio-Pectineal Eminence. 12 cm.

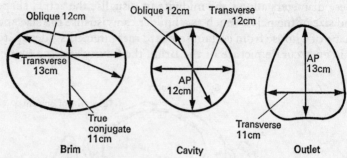

Fig. 22   Pelvic measurements

The Cavity

1   *Antero-Posterior.* From the mid-point of the anterior surface of the Sacrum to the mid-point of the posterior surface of the Pubic Symphysis. 12 cm.

2   *Transverse.* The widest transverse measurement of the cavity which cuts the antero-posterior diameter at right angles. 12 cm.

3   *Oblique.* From the middle of the Sacro-Iliac Joint of one side to a point one inch below the middle of the opposite Ilio-Pectineal Eminence. 12 cm.

The Outlet

1   *Antero-Posterior.* From the Sacro-Coccygeal Joint to the lower border of the Symphysis Pubis. 13 cm.

2   *Transverse.* Between the posterior ends of the inner surfaces of the Ischial Tuberosities. 11 cm.

These measurements show that:

1   The brim is roughly an oval, longer transversely than antero-posteriorly

2   The cavity is circular, all diameters being equal

3 The outlet is again an oval with an antero-posterior diameter longer than the transverse.

For ease of learning, the Pelvic Measurements can be set out as follows:

	Antero-Posterior	Oblique	Transverse
Brim	11.5 cm	12 cm	13 cm
Cavity	12 cm	12 cm	12 cm
Outlet	13 cm	NIL	11 cm

The Assessment of the Pelvis by Vaginal Examination

Precise clinical measurement of the pelvic diameters is not usually practicable. However, by recognising certain well-defined landmarks and by deciding whether these are normal in size, shape and position, it is possible to gain an accurate impression of the dimensions of the pelvic cavity and outlet.

The most important landmarks are the two Ischial Spines, which are situated low down on either side-wall of the pelvis. These spines vary in size and shape being at times blunt and difficult to feel and at others sharp and prominent, projecting into the cavity of the lower pelvis and reducing its width. The position and shape of the Ischial Spines are thus guides to the transverse diameter of the Pelvic Cavity.

Next, the Sacro-Spinous Ligaments must be felt for. These pass backwards and medially from the Ischial Spines to the lower part of the Sacrum, closing the lower end of the Sacro-Sciatic Notch. Their length, which should be slightly more than two fingers-breadth, allows a further impression of the width of the lower cavity to be gained. The lower part of the Sacrum must now be palpated. This is normally convex; if straight, it suggests a reduction in the antero-posterior diameter of the cavity which may give rise to difficulty in the later stages of labour. An attempt should then be made to feel the Sacral Promontory, but this will be possible only if the pelvis is abnormally small, the distance involved being otherwise too great.

The fingers must now be swept around the fore-pelvis to note the slope of the side-walls, which is normally vertical. They should then be passed backwards to the Sacro-Coccygeal joint and the mobility of the Coccyx tested. The distance between the lowest part of the Sacrum and the lower border of the Symphysis Pubis must now be estimated, as this is the important Antero-Posterior diameter of the Outlet. Lastly, two fingers should be placed under the Symphysis itself to estimate the Sub-Pubic Angle, which is normally wide. If it is narrow it will reduce the space available for the foetal head. To measure the Transverse Diameter of the Outlet the hand must be made into a fist which should be placed between the two Ischial Tuberosities to estimate whether they are close together or wide apart.

It must be emphasised that the ability to carry out this type of pelvic assessment with accuracy and to recognise confidently the various landmarks concerned can be gained only by practice and that experience alone will allow a midwife to gather a true idea of the size, shape and nature of the pelvis she is examining.

The Foetal Skull

A knowledge of the anatomy of the female pelvis is of little value unless the size and shape of the foetal skull which has to pass through it is also known. Although anatomists divide the skull

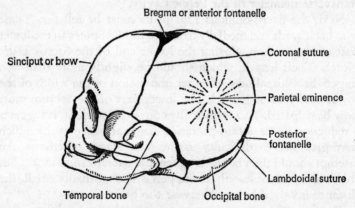

Fig. 23   Lateral view of the foetal skull

into a base, a face and a vault, from an obstetric point of view only the vault is of real importance. The reason for this is that it is the largest part of the skull and thus occupies the most space in the pelvic canal. In addition, it contains the delicate and vital brain which at all costs must not be injured during labour.

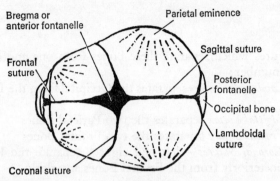

Fig. 24   The foetal skull seen from above

The vault is made up of several thin, plate-like bones, separated from one another by gaps or *sutures* which in the adult have joined to form a rigid structure. In the foetus, however, such rigidity would be a disadvantage since in order to meet the stresses imposed on it during delivery the skull must alter in shape. The degree of movement necessary for this alteration, which is known as *Moulding*, is made possible in part by the sutures and in part by the pliability of the bones themselves. The result is a change in the *shape* but not in the *size* of the foetal skull. This allows it to pass through a smaller pelvis than would otherwise be possible. Moulding naturally implies that the *contents* of the vault, i.e., the brain, also change in shape, but provided that such an alteration is not excessive it can be safely tolerated.

The Bones of the Vault

These are seven in number and consist of:
One Occipital Bone.
Two Parietal Bones.

Two Frontal Bones.
Two Temporal Bones.
Of these, the only ones normally felt on vaginal examination are the Occipital, the Parietals and the Frontals.

Sutures

The sutures which separate these bones from one another are four in number:

The Lambdoidal Suture separates the Occipital from the Parietal Bones

The Sagittal Suture separates the two Parietal Bones

The Frontal Suture separates the two Frontal Bones

The Coronal Sutures – left and right – separate the Parietal Bones posteriorly from the Frontal Bones anteriorly.

The Fontanelles

Where three or more bones meet, the gaps between the sutures widen to form what are called *Fontanelles*. Although several fontanelles exist, only two are of obstetric importance:

1 *The Posterior Fontanelle or Lambda* is situated just above the bony prominence of the Occiput, at the junction of the two Lambdoidal sutures with the posterior end of the Sagittal suture. Being small, it is best recognised by the fact that it is placed at the meeting-point of *three* sutures.

2 *The Anterior Fontanelle or Bregma* is a large, lozenge-shaped gap at the junction of the Sagittal suture posteriorly, the Frontal suture anteriorly and the two Coronal sutures laterally. It is thus a meeting-point for *four* sutures. Unlike the Posterior Fontanelle, it is always open at birth and closes only after some months of extra-uterine life.

The Vertex

The Vertex can now be defined. It is an area on the top of the head, bounded anteriorly by the Anterior Fontanelle, posteriorly by the Posterior Fontanelle and laterally by the two Parietal Eminences. These last are two raised areas on each side of the skull in the middle of each parietal bone. Their significance lies in the fact that the distance between them is the *widest* part of the foetal skull. This is the Biparietal Diameter, which measures 9·5 cm.

The importance of the Vertex is that in a normal labour it is the leading or *presenting* part and as such, is lowest in the birth canal.

The Diameters of the Foetal Skull

The antero-posterior diameters of the foetal skull are:

1 *The Sub-Occipito Bregmatic.* 9·5 cm.
   This is one of the smallest antero-posterior diameters. It extends from the nape of the neck to the middle of the anterior fontanelle.

2 *The Sub-Occipito Frontal.* 10 cm.
   This extends from the nape of the neck to the midpoint of the Frontal suture. It is thus slightly larger than the Sub-occipito-Bregmatic diameter.

3 *The Occipito Frontal.* 11 cm.
   This is an even larger diameter, extending from the Occiput to the mid-point of the Frontal suture.

4 *The Mento Vertical.* 13·5 cm.
   This is the largest antero-posterior diameter of the skull and extends from the point of the chin to the mid-point of the vertex.

5 *The Sub-Mento Vertical.* 11 cm.
   This diameter extends from the angle between the chin and the neck to the mid-point of the vertex.

6   *The Sub-Mento Bregmatic.* 9·5 cm.

This, the other of the two smallest diameters of the foetal head, extends from the angle between the chin and the neck to the mid-point of the Anterior Fontanelle.

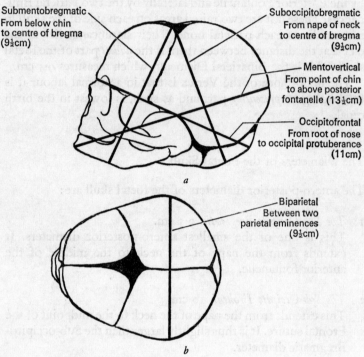

Submentobregmatic
From below chin
to centre of bregma
(9½cm)

Suboccipitobregmatic
From nape of neck
to centre of bregma
(9½cm)

Mentovertical
From point of chin
to above posterior
fontanelle (13½cm)

Occipitofrontal
From root of nose
to occipital protuberance
(11cm)

a

Biparietal
Between two
parietal eminences
(9½cm)

b

Fig. 25   Diameters of the foetal skull
(*a*) antero-posterior (*b*) transverse

Diameters of Engagement

The ease with which the foetal head enters the pelvis depends among other factors upon which of the various diameters described above presents at the pelvic brim. This in turn depends upon the degree of flexion of the foetal head upon the trunk. In full flexion the *presenting diameter* is the Sub-Occipito Bregmatic of only 9·5 cm. If deflexion of the head occurs progressively larger diameters such as the Sub-Occipito Frontal (10 cm), the

Occipito Frontal (11 cm) and finally the Mento Vertical (13·5 cm) are encountered. This last diameter is seen in the very unfavourable Brow presentation. Further extension, however, into an attitude which allows the *Face* to present, once more involves smaller diameters such as the Sub-Mento Vertical (11 cm) and the Sub-Mento Bregmatic (9·5 cm). These presenting or engaging diameters are therefore those antero-posterior measurements of the foetal head which lie parallel to the plane of the Brim when the head is entering the pelvis.

The practical value of this information is that it provides a means of determining both the *position* and the *degree of flexion* of the foetal head in the pelvis and hence of allowing an estimate to be made of the probable course and outcome of labour.

The Engagement of the Foetal Head

It has already been pointed out that once the foetal head has entered the pelvis it will usually emerge safely from below and that if the head can pass through the pelvis the remainder of the foetus will do so as well. It is therefore of the greatest importance to be able to tell whether the foetal head has entered or has *engaged* in the pelvis. By definition, engagement has occurred when the broadest part of the head, the Biparietal Diameter, has passed below the level of the Pelvic Brim. Clinically, there are three ways of determining whether this has happened:

1 By Abdominal Examination
If, when palpating the foetal head in the lower part of the uterus the fingers can be passed around its widest part to give the impression of meeting together below it, the head is *not engaged*, although it may be *fixed* in the pelvic brim in the same way as a large egg is fixed in a small egg-cup.

If, on the other hand, the head can be felt but the fingers cannot be passed around its greatest width, it is *engaged*. If the head cannot be felt at all in the lower part of the uterus and if it is certain that it is not elsewhere, then it is likely to be *deeply engaged*, a possibility that must be checked by vaginal examination.

2   By Vaginal Examination

If doubt arises as to whether the head is engaged or not, a vaginal examination *must* be carried out to decide this point. When the vertex is presenting, as is the case in all normal labours, the head is engaged when its lowest bony point is at or below the level of an imaginary line joining the two Ischial spines. There are few exceptions to this rule. Occasionally excessive moulding may distort the head so greatly that a vaginal examination may suggest that engagement has occurred when this is not really so. Here, careful abdominal examination will clarify the situation. Again, undue swelling of the soft tissues of the scalp, the Caput Succedaneum, may give a false impression of engagement by making the head appear to be lower than it really is. Once again an abdominal examination should reveal the true state of affairs. It should be pointed out that examples of this sort are rarely seen in modern obstetrics and then only in labours which are in some way abnormal and thus no longer the direct responsibility of a midwife.

3   By X-ray Examination

A lateral X-ray of the Pelvis will show whether the foetal head is engaged or not. Such an examination, however, is a medical and not a nursing matter and need not be discussed further.

The Position of the Foetal Head

The *position* of the foetal head is best made out by feeling the sutures and fontanelles, of which the most important is the Sagittal suture. At one end of this will be found the Posterior Fontanelle. As already stated, this may be recognised by the fact that it lies at the junction of three sutures. At the other end of the Sagittal suture the Anterior Fontanelle can be identified by its shape and size and by the fact that it is situated at the meeting-point of *four* sutures. If the Sagittal suture runs transversely across the pelvis with the posterior fontanelle to one side and the anterior to the other, the position of the head will be either Left or Right Occipito-Lateral – L.O.L. or R.O.L. – depending on the side towards which the occiput is directed. If the Sagittal suture lies in one of the oblique diameters of the pelvis with the occiput *anterior*, the position will be either Left or Right Occipito-Anterior – L.O.A. or R.O.A. If the Sagittal suture is in an oblique diameter with the occiput *posterior*, the position will be either Left or Right Occipito-Posterior – L.O.P. or R.O.P. Finally, if the Sagittal suture lies in the antero-posterior diameter of the pelvis, the occiput may be either directly *anterior* – O.A. – or directly *posterior* – O.P. Depending upon the position of the occiput there are therefore eight positions of the foetal head, namely:

L.O.L., R.O.L., L.O.A., R.O.A., L.O.P., R.O.P., O.A. and O.P.

The Degree of Flexion of the Foetal Head

It is important to estimate the degree of *flexion* of the foetal head since the more marked this is the smaller will be the diameter of engagement and the easier the descent of the foetal head into the pelvis. Flexion is determined by comparing the levels of the two fontanelles with each other; the lower the posterior fontanelle the greater the degree of flexion. In good flexion the anterior fontanelle is felt only with difficulty, if at all, while the posterior can easily be reached. If deflexion is present both fontanelles will be at the same level and both will be as readily palpable. In extended attitudes of the head, the anterior fontanelle can be felt without difficulty while the posterior will probably be out of reach of the examining fingers.

Labour is the most important moment in the obstetric life of a woman and it is therefore important for it to be properly understood and managed. Without a working knowledge of the anatomy of the pelvis and of the foetal skull, tedious though this may be to acquire, questions concerning the engagement, the position and the degree of flexion of the foetal head, all essential to the correct management of labour, can never be answered. Time taken in mastering the principles of anatomy so far as these are related to purely obstetric problems, and in gaining experience in the practical aspects of vaginal examination as outlined in this chapter, is always well-spent since it provides an understanding of some of the most basic features of midwifery.

Summary

Normal Labour: General Aspects

Normal Labour is labour lasting between two and twenty-four hours in which a living, mature foetus, presenting by the vertex, is delivered spontaneously without complications other than an episiotomy or a first or second degree perineal laceration.

The essential problem of any labour is to secure the safe passage of the foetus through the pelvis. In this context, if the head will enter the pelvis from above, it will emerge from below and if the head will pass, so will the foetal body.

The outcome of labour thus depends upon whether the head will enter the pelvis.

The pelvis is a ring composed of three bones, the Ilium, the Ischium and the Pubis, which are fused into the Innominate Bone. Posteriorly, the Innominate Bone articulates with the Sacrum at the Sacro-Iliac Joints. Above the Sacrum is the Fifth Lumbar Vertebra, below it is the Coccyx.

The True Pelvis is a curved canal, shorter anteriorly than posteriorly and sub-divided into a Brim, a Cavity and an Outlet.

The diameters of the Brim are the True Conjugate (11·5 cm), the Transverse (13 cm) and the Oblique (12 cm). Those of the Cavity are the Antero-Posterior, the Transverse and the Oblique, all of 12 cm and those of the Outlet are the Antero-Posterior (13 cm) and the Transverse (11 cm).

The shape of the Brim is an oval, longer in the transverse diameter, that of the Cavity a circle and that of the Outlet an oval, longer in the antero-posterior diameter.

The pelvic landmarks to be looked for on vaginal examination are the Ischial Spines, the Sacro-Spinous Ligaments, the shape of the lower Sacrum, the slope of the Pelvic Side-Walls and the Sub-Pubic Angle. The antero-posterior and transverse diameters of the Outlet should also be estimated.

Obstetrically speaking, the Vault is the most important part of the Foetal Skull. This is made up of seven thin, plate-like bones; one Occipital, two Parietal, two Frontal and two Temporal, separated by four sutures – the Lambdoidal, the Sagittal, the Frontal and the Coronal. The pliability of the bones and the presence of the sutures allow alteration in shape but not in size to occur. This is known as Moulding.

In addition to the sutures, two Fontanelles are present – the Posterior or Lambda and the Anterior or Bregma.

The Vertex is an area bounded anteriorly by the Anterior Fontanelle, posteriorly by the Posterior Fontanelle and laterally by the Parietal Eminences. In normal labour, it is that part of the head which is lowest in the birth canal.

The widest transverse diameter of the foetal head is the Biparietal Diameter (9·5 cm). The antero-posterior diameters are the Sub-occipito Bregmatic (9·5 cm), the Sub-occipito Frontal (10 cm), the Occipito Frontal (11 cm), the Mento Vertical (13·5 cm), the Sub-mento Vertical (11 cm) and the Sub-mento Bregmatic (9·5 cm).

The Diameter of Engagement is that antero-posterior measurement of the head which is parallel to the plane of the Brim when the head enters the pelvis.

The greater the degree of flexion of the foetal head, the smaller the Diameter of Engagement and the easier the engagement and descent of the head.

Engagement of the head has occurred when the Biparietal Diameter is below the plane of the Brim. This may be determined by Abdominal, Vaginal or X-ray examination.

The Position of the foetal head may be discovered by palpating the Sagittal suture and the two Fontanelles and comparing the relationship of these to one another and to the maternal pelvis.

The Degree of Flexion of the foetal head is assessed from the relation of the levels of the two Fontanelles to each other.

Since essential questions regarding the engagement, the position and the degree of flexion of the foetal head cannot be answered without a knowledge of the anatomy of the maternal pelvis and of the foetal skull, time spent in mastering this aspect of obstetrics is never wasted.

CHAPTER EIGHT

The Anatomy and Physiology of Labour

Normal Labour: First Stage

As already explained, the essential problem of labour consists in getting the foetus safely from the uterus into the outside world through the birth canal. This problem may be subdivided as follows:

1 The cervix must first dilate to allow the foetus to enter the lower birth canal.

2 The foetus must then pass through this birth canal.

3 Lastly, the placenta and membranes must be expelled from the uterus.

Each of these subdivisions represents one of the three *stages* of labour which are:

1 *The First Stage.* In which the cervix dilates.

2 *The Second Stage.* In which the foetus is born.

3. *The Third Stage.* In which the placenta is delivered.

The present chapter is concerned with the first of these three stages.

As described on page 64, the uterus at term is a muscular bag, closed at its lower end and containing the foetus, placenta, membranes and liquor. These contents, being incompressible, cannot be reduced in mass or volume, neither can they be subjected to any marked alteration in shape, since their main component, the foetus, is to all intents and purposes solid. For this reason, the uterus cannot expel its contents merely by relaxing a sphincter in the way that the urinary bladder evacuates its purely liquid contents. Some alternative mechanism is therefore needed which will enable the cervix to dilate to the large extent necessary for the passage of the foetus.

The mechanism which has been developed to meet this requirement is one which is peculiar to the uterus and closely resembles that resorted to in pulling a roll-necked sweater over one's head. This is usually done in two movements:

a By *pulling* the sweater over the head

b By *pushing* the head through the sweater.

To understand cervical dilatation, it is merely necessary to substitute for the wearer's head the foetal head and for the roll-necked sweater the cervix and cervical canal.

It will be remembered that the uterine muscle is not uniform throughout but is thickest in the region of the fundus and the upper part of the body and considerably thinner below this, while the cervix contains virtually no muscle at all. Since the thicker the muscle the greater its strength, it follows that the uterus is stronger in its upper half than in its lower. When it contracts, therefore, the stronger body and fundus do so at the expense of the lower segment and cervix. These structures stretch and thin out since the uterus cannot become any smaller, owing to the presence of its contents within it.

If the uterine muscle behaved in the same way as all other muscle, this stretching of the lower segment would be useless, since once a contraction was over and relaxation had occurred everything would return to its original position and no progress would have been made. Uterine muscle, however, is unusual in that not only can it contract and relax but it can also *retract*. This last property is an ability, even when relaxed, of remaining slightly shorter *after* a contraction than *before* it, and this allows the muscle fibres not only gradually to shorten but also to *remain* shortened. Since, initially at least, the volume of the uterus is unaltered, all its muscle cannot behave in this manner and retraction

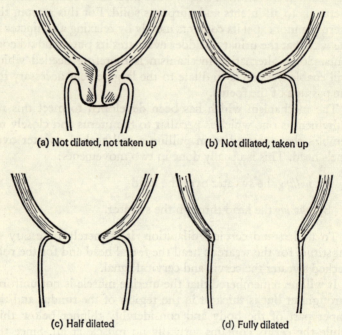

(a) Not dilated, not taken up   (b) Not dilated, taken up

(c) Half dilated   (d) Fully dilated

Fig. 26   The cervix in labour

therefore involves only the stronger muscle of the body and the fundus, which thus becomes progressively shorter and thicker while the lower segment is gradually stretched and thinned. In its turn, this lower segment muscle stretches and thins the cervix, converting it into a thin cap of tissue tightly drawn over the head of the foetus and obliterating the cervical canal. At this point, further contraction and retraction of the uterine muscle starts to pull this cap of cervix over the foetal head in precisely the same manner as the roll-necked sweater is pulled over the wearer's head. The effect of this is to cause the External Os of the cervix to enlarge or *dilate*.

At the same time, with each contraction the pressure within the uterus rises, much as when we squeeze a tennis ball we raise the tension within it. This increase in pressure tends to force the foetal head through the dilating cervix just as in the case of the roll-necked sweater the wearer's head is pushed through the hole at the top of the neck.

At this early stage, the foetal membranes are still intact and it is therefore not the head alone but the head covered by membranes containing some liquor amnii – the forewaters – which is pushed through the cervix and which helps to dilate it further.

Thus, by a combination of intermittent uterine contractions, retraction of the stronger muscle of the upper part of the uterus, thinning of the weaker lower segment, pulling of the cervix over the foetal head and forcing the head through the cervix, the external os slowly dilates until it has become sufficiently enlarged to allow the head to pass through it. At this stage dilatation is said to be *complete*, the first stage of labour is over and all is now ready for the foetus to be forced out of the uterus into the pelvic canal.

Practical Considerations

Certain practical considerations relating to the first stage of labour must now be discussed:

1   The Duration of the First Stage
Depending as it does upon a number of factors, the duration of the first stage of a normal labour varies considerably between limits of two and twenty-four hours, the average time being thirteen hours.

2   The Start of Labour
The start of the first stage of labour is signalled by progressive cervical dilatation. Unless therefore vaginal examination shows that the cervix is, in fact, dilating, it would be unwise to assume that labour has started.

3 The Assessment of Cervical Dilatation

Since rectal examination has by now been given up in obstetrics, the progress of cervical dilatation can be estimated only by vaginal examination. The degree of dilatation present is usually expressed either as 'fingers' or as 'fifths', both of which are largely subjective impressions and thus vary from person to person. For that reason it is better to express dilatation in centimetres. By this method, one centimetre corresponds to a cervix which has just started to dilate, five centimetres represents between two-fifths and three-fifths dilatation – about half dilated – eight centimetres corresponds to a four-fifths dilated cervic, nine centimetres to a 'rim' of cervix still just to be felt around the presenting part, while ten centimetres represents full cervical dilatation, no cervix at all being felt by the examining fingers.

4 Rupture of the Membranes

Although at the start of the first stage of labour the forewaters rather than the foetal head are pushed through the cervix, as dilatation proceeds, the force exerted upon these relatively thin membranes becomes so great that they eventually burst. This event is represented by a sudden gush of liquor from the vagina. It is often said that the dangers of a Prolapse of the Cord are very high at this moment. However, since such an accident may occur when the presenting part is high or fits the pelvis badly, it is much less likely when the head is well-fitting and engaged. This is because in such circumstances the necessary amount of room between the foetal head and the side-walls of the pelvis is lacking.

Following rupture of the membranes, further cervical dilatation is effected by direct pressure from the foetal head.

5 The Nature of the Uterine Contractions

Weak uterine contractions occur throughout pregnancy, becoming more frequent as term approaches. These Braxton Hicks contractions are never powerful enough either to dilate the cervix or to cause pain. The start of labour is characterised by much stronger contractions which raise the pressure within the uterus to the level of consciousness and thus result in a sensation of discomfort or pain. As a general rule, the stronger these contractions, the quicker will the cervix dilate. Strong uterine contractions, therefore, although more unpleasant to the patient, are preferable to weak since they mean that labour will be shorter. Although the rate of cervical dilatation is primarily related to the *strength* of the contractions, it is also dependent upon their *frequency* for the following reasons:

1   Since a fixed amount of cervical dilatation results from each contraction, the more frequent these contractions are the more rapidly will the cervix dilate

2   The intrinsic elasticity of the cervix encourages it to reform slowly between contractions, to some extent undoing the work of the uterus. The greater the interval between one contraction and the next, the more will the cervix revert to its previous state and the longer will dilatation take.

The Criteria of Good Uterine Contractions

The criteria of good uterine contractions may now be defined. These are:

1   The contractions should be *regular*

2   The contractions should be *strong*

3   The contractions should be *frequent*

4   To allow the uterine muscle time to recover, good *relaxation* should occur between contractions

5   *Fundal dominance* should be present. This means that the fundus should contract more strongly than the lower part of the uterus, since this favours more rapid cervical dilatation.

In the presence of such contractions the pattern of the first stage of labour is as follows:

1   Cervical dilatation will initially be slow since the contractions are at first relatively weak and infrequent.

2   Once labour is well-established and the contractions stronger and more frequent, dilatation will be rapid.

3   Towards the end of the first stage, owing to the increasing resistance of the maternal tissues, the time taken to reach full cervical dilatation is often unexpectedly long.

Normal Labour: Second Stage

The second stage of labour is concerned with the passage of the foetus through the maternal pelvis. It may conveniently be sub-divided as follows:

1   The engagement of the foetal head

2   The descent and delivery of the foetal head

3   The delivery of the shoulders and of the rest of the foetus.

Before describing these three separate but interrelated events, it is necessary to consider three important aspects of labour, namely the forces acting on the foetus, the attitude of the foetal head and the anatomy of the pelvic floor.

1   The Forces acting on the Foetal Head
The force required for the descent and the delivery of the foetus is provided partly by the uterine contractions and partly by expulsive efforts on the part of the mother. These two components work together and it is doubtful whether in a strictly normal labour either alone would be strong enough to complete the delivery of the foetus.

The uterine contractions, although similar to those seen in the first stage of labour, are stronger, more frequent and of longer duration. Their action is solely to force or squeeze the foetus through the birth canal. The expulsive efforts which accompany these contractions are to some extent involuntary but their effectiveness is always improved if the patient co-operates in their voluntary control. They consist first in raising the intra-abdominal pressure by holding the breath and then in straining or *bearing down* in an attempt to expel the foetus from the body. Together, these two components produce an extremely powerful expulsive effect which usually results in the rapid advance and delivery of the foetus.

2   The Attitude of the Foetal Head

Although it is usually taught that in a normal labour the foetal head is fully flexed, this is probably seldom the case. The powerful ligaments at the back of the neck resist the stretching imposed on them by extreme flexion and extend the head upon the trunk whenever this becomes possible. On the other hand, the narrow confines of the birth canal favour an attitude of flexion since this requires a smaller area for engagement (page 166). A compromise is therefore reached between these two opposing demands which results in the slightly greater sub-occipito frontal diameter of 10 cm being preferred to the sub-occipito bregmatic of 9·5 cm. This arrangement allows some deflexion of the head without too great an increase in the amount of room required.

3   The Anatomy of the Pelvic Floor and of the Perineal Body

Since in its descent through the birth canal the foetus will meet and pass through the pelvic floor, this structure must now be described.

The Pelvic Floor or Pelvic Diaphragm is a thin, curved layer whose function is to close off the outlet of the pelvis, converting it from a canal into a bucket. Consisting mainly of muscle, it also contains a certain amount of fat and connective tissue. Superficially it is covered by subcutaneous fascia and skin. As it supports the entire weight of the abdominal contents, it is particularly liable to herniation or *prolapse*. This tendency is encouraged by the fact that the pelvic floor contains three holes which form areas of special weakness. These, from before backwards, are the Urethra, the Vagina and the Anal Canal. Much of the design of the pelvic floor, as well as its behaviour during labour, is directed towards reducing as far as possible this intrinsic weakness and at preventing any tendency to give way under the stresses imposed on it.

Since connective tissue and fat lack elasticity and strength, the

G

main support for the pelvic floor comes from its muscles, principally the two Levatores Ani. These are paired, thin sheets, convex downwards and joined to each other in the midline to form a complete floor to the pelvis. Both Levatores Ani consist

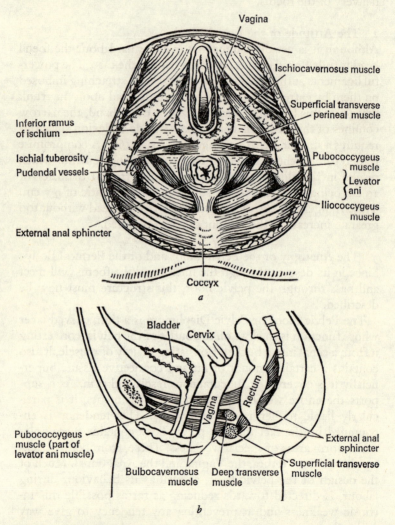

Fig. 27 The pelvic floor
(a) from below (b) lateral section

of three muscles, each of which runs from one of the components of the Innominate bone to be inserted into the Coccyx. These muscles are the Pubo-Coccygeus, the Ischio-Coccygeus and the Ilio-Coccygeus.

It has just been said that the pelvic floor is pierced by the Urethra, the Vagina and the Anal Canal. Since the greatest amount of stretching occurs in the region of the posterior vaginal wall, the Levator Ani muscles are strengthened at this point by a number of fibres which cross from one side of the midline to the other between the vagina and the anal canal. A further condensation of muscle fibres is present around the lower part of the anal canal and forms the Internal Anal Sphincter.

More superficially, between the Levatores Ani and the skin of the perineum, some added support is provided by two small muscles which run across the pelvic outlets from one side to the other. These are the Deep and the Superficial Transverse Perineal muscles. Immediately posterior to these is the External Anal Sphincter. The combined mass formed by that portion of the Levator Ani between the vagina and the anal canal, the Transverse Perineal Muscles and the two Anal Sphincters, is known as the *Perineal Body*. Its importance lies in the fact that although it is vital to the structure of the entire pelvic floor, it is extremely liable to be damaged during labour. If not adequately repaired after such damage it may be permanently weakened and predispose to prolapse in later life.

The Engagement of the Foetal Head

Normally the foetal head is engaged before the onset of labour. However, for the sake of simplicity and in order to view the descent and delivery of the foetus as a whole, it is assumed that engagement has been delayed until the start of the second stage of labour.

It has already been explained that the foetal head normally presents by the sub-occipito frontal diameter rather than by the slightly smaller sub-occipito bregmatic. In these conditions the presenting shape of the head is an oval, longer antero-posteriorly than transversely. Since the outline of the pelvic brim is also an oval, the foetal head will fit the pelvis best when its own oval coincides with that of the brim. In this condition the sagittal suture will lie in the transverse diameter of the brim with the foetal occiput directed laterally to the left or to the right. Since the foetal back is turned towards the maternal left rather more

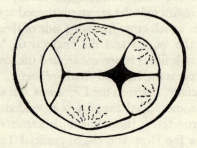

Fig. 28   Presenting shape of the flexed head and pelvic brim

frequently than towards the right, the foetal head engages more commonly in the Left Occipito-Lateral position – L.O.L. – than in the Right Occipito-Lateral position – R.O.L. In this position, and under the force of the uterine contractions, the head descends into the pelvis until its biparietal diameter is below the level of the brim, at which point it is engaged.

The Descent and the Delivery of the Foetal Head

Further downward pressure upon the foetus causes the head to continue its descent until it reaches the lower part of the pelvic cavity and the muscular pelvic floor. At this point two difficulties must be overcome:

1   In the first place, owing to the forward curve of the sacrum and the presence of the levator ani muscle, no further downward progress is possible. A change in the *direction* taken by the head must therefore be made.

2 Secondly, since the oval shape of the pelvic outlet is different from the circular shape of the cavity, the head must adapt itself to this difference. This it does by altering its *position*.

This double change both in *direction* and in *position* is brought about by the occiput turning *forwards*, the sagittal suture moving from the transverse into the antero-posterior diameter of the outlet. This *Anterior Rotation* is assisted by the muscular action of the pelvic floor which tends to guide the occiput anteriorly.

Once anterior rotation has occurred, the forward curve of the birth canal allows the head freedom to extend. The effect of this is to bring the sub-occiput under the symphysis pubis, the rest of the head gradually stretching the posterior part of the introitus, the perineal body and the anal canal in a movement which eventually allows the vertex, the brow and the face to emerge in turn from the now fully distended vulva.

Once free, the head resumes a more normal attitude and the extreme extension which characterises its actual delivery now disappears.

The Delivery of the Shoulders and of the Rest of the Foetus

The shoulders enter the pelvic brim while the head is being delivered. Although they would obviously fit best in the transverse diameter, since the foetal back is usually directed laterally this would involve too great a twisting movement in a uterus which at this point is often firmly contracted around the foetus. A compromise is therefore reached and the shoulders engage in the oblique diameter of the brim. This still provides adequate room and requires less alteration in the position of the foetus. The foetal head, now outside the vulva, follows this rotation of the shoulders by turning slightly laterally, a movement known as *Restitution*.

The shoulders now pass through the pelvis and in doing so turn into the antero-posterior diameter of the outlet, since this larger measurement provides them with more space. In following this, the head rotates still further laterally so that the occiput is directed towards one of the mother's thighs. This is known as *External Rotation*.

The importance of Restitution and External Rotation is that they are outward evidence of the engagement and descent of the shoulders.

The anterior shoulder now escapes from under the symphysis pubis, after which the posterior is born over the perineum. This arrangement allows a somewhat smaller diameter to distend the vulva than would be the case if both shoulders were to be born simultaneously.

Once the delivery of the shoulders is complete, the trunk, abdomen and legs follow without any special pattern.

Perineal Lacerations

Owing to the distension of the vulva and perineum by the foetus, perineal lacerations are common. These are of three types or *degrees*:

1 *First Degree Lacerations* involve only the skin of the vulva, the lower vagina and the perineum.

2 *Second Degree Lacerations* are more extensive and involve not only the vaginal and perineal skin but also the superficial muscles of the perineum. Both First and Second Degree Lacerations are usually repaired under local infiltration analgesia.

3 *Third Degree Lacerations* extend backwards and upwards into the Levator Ani muscle and the External Anal Sphincter as well as involving the mucosa of the Anal Canal. Unless adequately repaired, a process usually requiring a general anaesthetic, anal continence may be impaired.

It need scarcely be said that a perineal laceration should always be anticipated and forestalled by deliberately cutting the perineum, an operation known as an Episiotomy. This cut, which may be made in either a posterior or a postero-lateral direction, is easily carried out under local infiltration analgesia, such as obtained with Lignocaine, 0·5 per cent. Its advantages are that it can be more firmly repaired than a ragged and extensive perineal tear which often involves much bruising and damage to under-lying tissues.

Normal Labour: Third Stage

The third stage of labour is in many respects the most critical since its various complications, some of which present serious risks to the patient, often appear with dramatic speed. As these complications usually represent some deviation from the normal and as their treatment involves the correction of these devia-tions, an understanding of the principles of the Third Stage of Labour is essential if its abnormalities are to be effectively dealt with.

The physiology of the third stage of labour is best considered under two separate but closely related headings:

1   The separation and the delivery of the placenta.

2   The control of haemorrhage from the placental site.

1   The Separation and the Delivery of the Placenta
The placenta is separated and delivered as follows:
After the birth of the baby the size of the uterus is much reduced, its walls becoming very much thicker while its inner surface area is greatly decreased. This decrease includes the placental site which thus becomes considerably smaller. The placenta, however, being relatively inelastic, is unable to adapt itself to this reduced area and is therefore partly sheared off its attachments. The actual plane of placental separation is not in the intervillous space but lies in the decidua, which is thus split into two layers. One of these remains on the lining of the uterus, the other forms the maternal surface of the separated placenta. This splitting of the decidua tears open those maternal vessels running to and from the intervillous space. Bleeding from these vessels forms a haematoma behind the placenta which forces it still further off its attachments and normally completes its separation.

Once the area of separation has extended to the margin of the placenta the blood behind it is free to escape and runs out of the uterus into the vagina. As in the case of accidental and inevitable

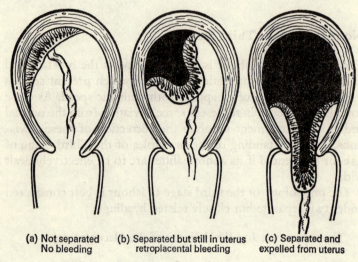

(a) Not separated   (b) Separated but still in uterus   (c) Separated and
   No bleeding   retroplacental bleeding   expelled from uterus

Fig. 29   Stages in the separation of the placenta

ante-partum haemorrhage, vaginal bleeding is therefore a sign that the placenta has separated either partly or completely from its uterine attachments.

The uterus now treats the separated placenta like a foreign body and by a series of contractions forces it out into the vagina, its smooth foetal surface being the first to present at the vulva.

This method of placental separation, often referred to as the Schultze method, is the one normally seen. At times, however, separation starts at the edge rather than in the middle of the placenta and proceeds inwards towards the centre. This process, known as the Matthews Duncan method, is less efficient, as the effect of the retroplacental haematoma is largely lost, the blood extravasated behind the placenta escaping too easily into the cavity of the uterus. When this happens both post-partum haemorrhage and retention of the placenta, two of the most common abnormalities of the third stage of labour, are liable to occur. Where, however, separation and expulsion of the placenta by the Matthews Duncan method are successful, it usually presents at the vulva either by an edge or by its rough maternal surface.

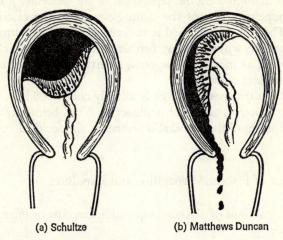

(a) Schultze   (b) Matthews Duncan

Fig. 30   Types of placental separation

2   The Control of Haemorrhage

This is brought about in three separate ways:

1   It has already been said that once the placenta has separated it is expressed into the vagina. Following this the uterus remains contracted for some minutes and during this time the criss-cross bundles of myometrial fibres squeeze the blood vessels passing through them on their way to the placental site. The effect of this is to reduce very considerably the blood flow through these vessels.

2   The increased thickness of the uterine wall causes the blood vessels which run between the placental site and the surface of the uterus to be stretched to several times their original length.

This stretching causes the vessel walls to come into apposition, still further reducing the blood flow through them.

3   The blood still remaining in these constricted and stretched vessels now clots. This is due to the fact that the decidua, which has been disrupted by the separation of the placenta, gives off Thromboplastin, one of the main elements in the clotting of blood. The clot thus formed is sufficiently strong in normal circumstances to withstand any further flow of blood which may occur when, as inevitably happens, a certain amount of uterine relaxation later takes place.

It follows that haemorrhage is initially controlled by a firmly contracted uterus, any later tendency to bleed being prevented by the clotting of the blood still present in the decidual vessels.

The Signs of Placental Separation and Expulsion

The classical signs of placental separation can now be interpreted as follows:

1   *Vaginal Bleeding.* If bleeding is from the placental site it will present as a series of intermittent gushes, corresponding to the uterine contractions which are forcing the blood into the vagina.

2   *Lengthening of the Cord.* If the cord appears to lengthen at the vulva this can only mean that the placenta has not only *separated* but that it has also *left the uterus* and is now in the lower genital tract.

3   *The Level of the Fundus Rises.* This is a sign that the placenta is now in the vagina, displacing the empty uterus upwards into the abdomen.

4   *The Uterus becomes Smaller and more Mobile.* This means that the uterus, being empty, is smaller and can therefore be moved more easily.

5   *The Uterus is Hard*. This merely means that the uterus is well contracted.

It should now be clear that the only sign of placental separation, either partial or complete, is *bleeding from the placental site*, since a placenta that is still completely attached to its uterine site obviously cannot give rise to bleeding. The other so-called 'signs of separation' are either indications that the placenta has left the uterus to enter the vagina or are merely evidence that the uterus is contracted.

It is important to remember this distinction since upon it depends to a large degree the safe management of the many abnormalities which complicate the third stage of labour.

Summary

Normal Labour: First Stage

Labour is divided into three stages:

a   The First Stage of cervical dilatation.

b   The Second Stage of the birth of the foetus.

c   The Third Stage of the delivery of the placenta.

Since the contents of the uterus cannot appreciably alter in shape, they cannot be expelled by means of some simple sphincter mechanism. Dilatation of the cervix is therefore achieved by a double movement of drawing it up around the foetal head on the one hand and forcing the foetal head through it on the other.

Retraction of the muscle fibres of the fundus and upper part of the body of the uterus prevent complete return of the cervix to its original state between contractions.

The cervix is fully dilated when the External Os is sufficiently wide to allow the presenting part to pass through it.

The duration of the first stage of a normal labour lasts between two and twenty-four hours, the average being about thirteen hours.

The start of labour is characterised by the onset of cervical dilatation. This can be recognised only by vaginal examination.

Dilatation of the cervix is estimated in centimetres, from one to ten. The latter measurement represents full dilatation.

Rupture of the membranes usually occurs during the first stage of labour. Although the danger of Prolapse of the Cord at this moment is said to be great, this is not so when the presenting part is well-fitting and is engaged.

The rate of cervical dilatation is related both to the strength of the uterine contractions and to their frequency.

The criteria of good uterine contractions are that they should be regular, strong and frequent. It is also important that there should be good relaxation between contractions and that Fundal Dominance should be present.

In normal labour cervical dilatation is initially slow but later becomes more rapid as the strength of the contractions increases. Owing to the resistance of the maternal tissues, the final stages of dilatation often take longer than expected.

Normal Labour: Second Stage

Three important aspects of the second stage of labour are the forces acting on the foetus, the attitude of the foetal head and the anatomy of the pelvic floor.

The forces acting on the foetus consist of strong and frequent uterine contractions supplemented by voluntary expulsive efforts on the part of the mother. *The attitude of the foetal head* is one of moderate flexion, the diameter of engagement being the sub-occipito frontal. This allows for some deflexion without too great an increase in the amount of space needed by the head. *The pelvic floor* consists of the Levator Ani muscles and Transverse Perineal muscles, together with a covering of skin and connective tissue. A criss-cross arrangement of muscle fibres provides additional support between the vagina and the anal canal. The *Perineal Body*, which is situated in this area, is made up of fibres of the levator ani muscle, the transverse perineal muscles and the external anal sphincter.

Engagement of the foetal head usually takes place with the

occiput directed laterally, more often to the left than to the right. The reason for this is that in this position the shape of the head and of the pelvic brim coincide.

Downward pressure on the foetus causes the head to descend to the level of the pelvic floor, at which stage the occiput rotates anteriorly under the pubic arch. Extension of the head upon the trunk now takes place, which allows the vertex, the brow and the face to emerge through the distended vulva.

The shoulders enter the brim in the oblique diameter but rotate at the outlet into the antero-posterior diameter. The anterior shoulder is then delivered under the symphysis pubis and the posterior over the perineum. Restitution and External Rotation of the foetal head are evidence of the engagement and descent of the shoulders.

Perineal lacerations are of three degrees. The first involves only the skin of the perineum and lower vagina, the second includes the superficial perineal muscles while the third produces damage to the levator ani, the external anal sphincter and the anterior wall of the anal canal. This last variety of tear usually requires a general anaesthetic for its repair.

Where a perineal laceration appears inevitable, an Episiotomy should be performed under local infiltration analgesia.

Normal Labour: Third Stage

The physiology of the third stage of labour is best considered under two headings:

a The separation and the delivery of the placenta

b The control of bleeding from the placental site.

Separation of the placenta is started by a reduction in the area of the placental site. This causes the centre of the placenta to be sheared off its attachments. Separation is completed by the action of the retroplacental haematoma.

Once separated, the placenta is expelled into the vagina by uterine contractions.

Occasionally one edge of the placenta separates first. In such cases the effect of the retroplacental haematoma is largely lost and in consequence the placenta may remain partly attached to the uterine wall. Post-partum haemorrhage and retention of the placenta are often seen in such cases.

Haemorrhage is arrested primarily by the constricting effect of the bundles of uterine muscle fibres upon the blood vessels running through them on their way to the placental site. Stretching of these vessels from thickening of the uterine wall contributes to this result. Any later tendency to bleed is controlled by clotting of the blood which remains in the vessels.

The only sign that the placenta has either partly or completely separated is bleeding from the placental site. Most of the so-called signs of separation indicate that not only is the placenta no longer attached to the uterine wall but that it has also been expelled into the lower genital tract.

CHAPTER NINE

Practical Aspects of Normal Labour

Management of Normal Labour

Since the management of labour is a subject which can only be properly learnt by observation and practical instruction, it is pointless to include in any text-book a step-by-step description of the conduct of a normal delivery. There are, however, certain principles which should be observed in all labours if the well-being and safety of the patient and of the foetus are to be assured and it is with these principles that the present chapter is concerned.

The First Stage

The obstetric care of a woman in the first stage of labour involves consideration of the following points:

1   The Comfort and Well-Being of the Patient

All women in labour must be reassured that if they consider it necessary they can quickly summon a midwife. This point must always be borne in mind and arrangements made accordingly. Once made, these arrangements must on no account be broken, since to do so would destroy the patient's confidence both in herself and her attendants.

Careful attention must be paid to the patient's personal comfort, especially in respect of the state of her clothing and of her bed, the temperature of her surroundings and the availability of fresh air and clear but subdued lighting.

2 Bowels and Bladder
Since an enema is usually given at the start of labour, the lower bowel is usually empty and requires no further attention. The bladder, however, is liable to refill in the course of even a short labour. Since distension not only causes discomfort but also interferes with the normal progress of labour, it must always be watched for and, if necessary, be relieved by means of a catheter.

3 Diet
It is often taught that a light diet may be given during the first stage of labour. This is dangerous since digestion is greatly delayed at this time and the stomach therefore retains its contents far longer than might be expected. As it is never possible to be certain that an anaesthetic, often at short notice, may not be required during labour, the presence of undigested food in the stomach presents a very real risk to the patient's life. In view of the relatively short duration of most labours, it is probably unnecessary to provide nourishment of any sort in the great majority of cases. When, however, it is felt that some form of oral feeding is desirable, small quantities of puréed foods are probably most easily absorbed and hence least dangerous from the point of view of possible anaesthetic hazards.

These restrictions do not apply in the same way to fluids, as these are somewhat more readily absorbed, especially if taken in small quantities. It is important, however, to make sure, from study of the patient's fluid balance chart, that these fluids are not merely accumulating in the stomach. This can be done by comparing the oral fluid intake with the urinary output. If fluids are being normally absorbed, the two readings should be approximately equal. If the urinary output is considerably less than the oral intake it is probable that fluids are remaining in the stomach.

4 Sedation and Analgesia

In early labour, when the uterine contractions are weak and infrequent, the patient is not in pain and needs no analgesics. On the other hand, she is often tense and apprehensive and may thus require a sedative such as Chloral, 2 grammes, Trichloryl, Tabs 2 or Welldorm, Tabs 2. Barbiturates, being both stronger and longer acting, are best avoided in a normal labour and in any event can be prescribed only by a doctor.

As the contractions increase in strength and frequency, pain begins to be felt and analgesics are needed. Here the drug of choice is Pethidine, the initial dose being either 100 or 150 mg by intramuscular injection. If it seems necessary, a further 100 mg may be given by the midwife in three or four hours' time, but should it appear desirable either to exceed this amount or to give additional doses, medical aid must always be sought.

Pethidine has a strong depressant effect upon the foetal respiratory centre if given within three or four hours of delivery. For this reason it is always wise to check by vaginal examination the stage to which labour has progressed before this drug is administered.

Towards the end of the first stage inhalational analgesia is preferable to that given either orally or intramuscularly. Either nitrous oxide and oxygen, given by the Entonox apparatus, or Trilene, from an approved inhaler, being in common use. Since both nitrous oxide and Trilene are usually self-administered, there is much to be said for every patient receiving instruction in the use of the special apparatus involved during the last weeks of pregnancy.

5 The Assessment of the Progress of Labour

It is not enough merely to attend to a patient's comfort and to ensure adequate sedation and analgesia. It is also necessary to keep a constant watch upon her progress during labour. While careful observation of the strength, duration and frequency of the uterine contractions is undeniably of use in estimating the course of labour, this cannot replace direct assessment of progress by vaginal examination. Although it can be argued, in theory, that this may cause a genital tract infection, in practice this risk is very small and is far outweighed by the advantages of the procedure.

In a normal labour a vaginal examination should be carried out at the following times:

a At the start of labour or on the patient's admission to the Labour Ward Suite in order to obtain a base-line from which further progress may be estimated

b When the membranes rupture, to establish the progress already made and to exclude a prolapse of the cord

c To confirm that the second stage has been reached

d Whenever it is necessary to give further sedation or analgesia in order to avoid the risk of depressing the foetal respiratory centre.

In addition, a vaginal examination should be carried out in the following *abnormal* circumstances:

a Where foetal or maternal distress develop, in order to discover, if possible, the cause of this distress and to assess the degree of cervical dilatation, since this may influence the subsequent management of labour

b Where labour is abnormally prolonged. In such a case a vaginal examination should be carried out every four to six hours to determine what progress, if any, is taking place.

If it is thought that these indications are unrealistic, two points should be remembered:

a A vaginal examination provides the only certain means of measuring progress in labour

b In a normal labour it should not be necessary to carry out more than three or four such examinations, a small expenditure of effort and time for a great return in terms of reliable information.

6   The Safety of the Patient and of the Foetus
In order to assure the safety of the patient and of the foetus the following observations should be made in the first stage of labour:

a The maternal pulse and foetal heart rate should be recorded hourly

b The maternal blood pressure and temperature should be taken four-hourly

c All specimens of urine passed must be tested for ketone bodies

d A fluid balance chart must be kept.

Provided that these records remain within normal limits, neither the patient nor the foetus will be at risk. On the other hand, an alteration in the foetal heart rate, a rise in the maternal pulse rate or temperature, the development of ketonuria or a reduction in the volume of urine passed despite a satisfactory fluid intake, suggest the development of some maternal or foetal danger and require immediate medical attention.

The Second Stage

As an understanding of the management of the second stage of labour comes almost entirely from practical experience, only certain points related to it need be emphasised.

1 Preparations for the actual delivery of the foetus must be made in good time and all unnecessary hurry avoided. For this reason the patient should be moved to the delivery suite as soon as it is certain that the cervix is fully dilated.

2 At no time during the second stage may the patient be left unattended, even if only for a few minutes.

3 Since it is important to enlist the active co-operation of the patient in the birth of her child, inhalational analgesia should be used in a manner which allows the patient to remain conscious of the events taking place around her and of the part she has to play in them.

4 During the second stage, foetal and maternal distress are liable to arise with little or no warning. The foetal heart rate and

the maternal pulse must therefore be checked at five-minute intervals.

5   As progress is normally rapid during the second stage, any delay, such as failure of the presenting part to advance over a period of twenty minutes, must at once be reported to a doctor. Progress is usually estimated by watching the foetal head advance with each contraction. If the presenting part is not visible, a vaginal examination is necessary to assess progress in terms of the level and position it occupies.

6   It is important to maintain a correct amount of flexion during the crowning of the head in order to avoid undue distension of the vulva and the possibility of severe vaginal and perineal lacerations. At the same time, extension must not be prevented for too long, for fear of forcing the head too far back. Finally, in protecting the perineum, care must be taken to avoid pushing the head too far forwards since damage to the anterior part of the vagina and vulva often results, causing severe bleeding and later painful scarring. The course which must be steered between these three extremes can be learnt only from practical experience.

7   If the perineum appears to be in danger of tearing, an episiotomy should be performed under local analgesia (page 184).

The Third Stage

Points of importance in the management of the third stage are as follows:

1   In order to reduce the incidence of abnormal bleeding from the placental site, an oxytocic is usually given at the end of the second stage. At present, those in common use are Ergometrine (0·5 mg), Syntocinon (5 units) or preferably, Syntometrine (1 ml), this last being a combination of Ergometrine (0·5 mg) and Syntocinon (5 units). These drugs, which have the effect of increasing the power and duration of uterine contraction, are given either intravenously or intramuscularly with the crowning of the foetal

head or the birth of the anterior shoulder. If, owing to lack of opportunity, this becomes impracticable, little will be lost by delaying the injection until after the birth of the foetus. It should always, however, be given *before* the delivery of the placenta.

2   *The Delivery of the Placenta.* Once the signs of its separation and descent are present, the placenta may be delivered by any means with which the midwife is familiar, that of choice being Controlled Cord Traction. For this to be effective the uterus must be well-contracted and firmly anchored by one hand placed below it on the abdomen. If this method fails at its first attempt it should be repeated after a short interval, when it may well succeed, provided that it is carried out on a firmly-contracted uterus and that traction is applied in the correct direction. If delivery of the placenta still cannot be achieved, medical aid must be called without delay. Failure of the placenta to separate within twenty minutes of the start of the third stage is also a reason for summoning a doctor. The other abnormalities of the third stage are considered on page 303.

3   If doubt exists as to whether the placenta has, in fact, separated, a vaginal examination should be carried out to check this point and to see if the placenta is in the vagina or is protruding through the cervix.

4   Bleeding after the delivery of the placenta should *not* be treated by pushing the uterus downwards into the pelvis, as is usually taught, since this increases venous engorgement and encourages oozing. It is better to raise the uterus up out of the pelvis, thus reducing its blood supply by stretching the uterine arteries. This is best done either by pushing the uterus up with the help of two fingers in the anterior fornix or by placing a hand on the abdomen below the uterus and then raising it upwards, holding it in this position for a few minutes.

5   At the end of the third stage the vulva, vagina and perineum must be inspected for lacerations. Any tears, however small, must be repaired, partly because they may prove to be larger than was first suspected and partly because they may otherwise

heal badly and leave a tender scar which will predispose to dyspareunia. Perineal suturing must always be carried out as soon after the end of the third stage as possible. The practice of deferring this operation until a suitable moment later in the day is, in normal circumstances, indefensible.

6 Observations after Delivery

The following observations should be made before the patient is sent to the post-natal ward.

a Her temperature, pulse and blood pressure must be recorded

b The fundus must be felt to make certain that the uterus is firmly contracted

c The vulva must be inspected to exclude any undue blood loss

d An estimate of the amount of blood lost during delivery must be entered in the patient's case notes.

7 The Examination of the Placenta, Membranes and Cord

Retention of a placental cotyledon or succenturiate lobe is a common cause of post-partum haemorrhage. The placenta must therefore be carefully examined at the end of labour to make certain that it is complete. This examination is best carried out by holding the placenta, with its maternal surface uppermost, in the cupped hands and noting if any cotyledon appears to be missing. Next, the edges of the placenta must be examined for the presence of torn blood vessels, indicating a possible connection with a succenturiate lobe still retained in the uterus.

The membranes should then be inspected to ensure that they are complete, as a portion of the amnion or chorion may have torn free and remain in the uterine cavity.

Lastly, the umbilical vessels in the cord must be counted since an abnormal number – one artery or two veins – suggests the presence of congenital foetal malformations.

Where the possibility exists that any part of the placenta or of the membranes is retained in the uterus, or if a vascular abnormality of the cord is discovered, a doctor must be informed without delay.

Analgesia and Anaesthesia

Labour is in most cases accompanied by some degree of pain. It is the duty of those in attendance on the mother to alleviate so far as possible the discomforts of normal delivery and to minimise the dangers of the anaesthetic procedures which may be necessary for an operative delivery.

Before considering these two topics in detail, it is important that we should define clearly some of the terms which we will use:

Anaesthesia. A state of temporary poisoning of the nervous system in which all the senses are absent. The patient is unaware of her surroundings and can neither hear, feel nor remember anything that has happened. Drugs which produce anaesthesia are known as anaesthetics.

Analgesia implies an absence of one specific sensation, that of pain. Local or Regional analgesia can be produced in specific parts of the body by local analgesics. General analgesia implies absence of pain sensation over the whole body, following administration of a drug which interferes with the appreciation of pain impulses in the brain.

Amnesia is the absence of memory for a specific period or event. No drug can be characterised as being specifically amnesic, but some analgesics produce more amnesia than others.

Hypnotics are drugs which induce sleep. It is worth noting at this point that many anaesthetic and hypnotic drugs are poor analgesics.

Analgesia for Normal Delivery

Theocritus described the summons for one 'Lucina, the friend of women in travail, who possessed the gift of alleviating pain. She, with kind favour, stood by the daughter of Antigone and in sooth poured down her whole limbs an insensibility to pain, and so a lively boy, like to his father, was born'.

Alas, the modern midwife cannot in most cases wholly emulate Lucina. She can however by intelligent use of the drugs and techniques at her disposal do much to alleviate the pain of child-birth.

The emphasis in this chapter will be on analgesic methods which can be used by midwives without reference to a doctor. Most normal deliveries in the United Kingdom are conducted by midwives. A high percentage happen in hospital but a midwife's drug or technique must be as safe by the light of a paraffin lamp in a snowbound cottage as it is in the delivery room of a modern district hospital. Brief mention only will be made of the excellent regional analgesic techniques which produce superb analgesia and which will undoubtedly become increasingly popular as resources become available.

The techniques available for analgesia in normal delivery can be divided into three groups:

1 Antenatal preparation, education and mental conditioning

2 The use of general analgesic drugs

3 Local and regional analgesic techniques.

1 Antenatal Preparation and Education

Other methods of analgesia will work best against a background of preparation for labour. There have been many exponents of various techniques of preparation. The extreme attitudes taken by some of these people must not blind the midwife to the fact that much can be done to help the parturient patient by conditioning her mental attitude to labour, whether the technique be called relaxation, natural childbirth, psychoprophylaxis or simple humanity.

Grantly Dick Read in his early work on 'natural childbirth' stressed that the three pain-producing factors in labour are ignorance, fear and tension.

It is easy for doctors and midwives to forget how ignorant many patients are of the anatomy and physiology of pregnancy and childbirth. In their first pregnancy, many women have a very confused idea of how things will develop and of what will happen during labour. Education and information are potent analgesics.

Much can be done to help if the patient is told in simple terms what will happen. It is in the antenatal period that the techniques of analgesia can be discussed with the patient and that she can be shown the equipment which she will meet in the labour ward. Now is the time to show the patient how properly to apply an anaesthetic mask to her face and to discuss and describe what will happen in the various stages of labour.

Ignorance breeds fear for which the analgesic is reassurance based on information. The midwife must impress her personality on the patient and gain her confidence.

Fear breeds tension which in turn causes pain and more fear, setting up a very unpleasant train of events. The cure for tension is relaxation, and properly conducted relaxation classes where patients are taught to relax are an invaluable preparation for labour. The patient can be taught at the same time breathing and other exercises which will help her when the time comes to push in the second stage of labour.

Other more sophisticated psychiatric methods are in vogue. Psychoprophylaxis depends on modifying the patient's response to labour by inducing conditioned reflexes. Hypnosis is also used by some practitioners who are able to produce this state in their patients.

Antenatal preparation is a stage which should merge naturally into the first stage of labour. Nothing is more likely to produce a frightened non-co-operative patient than a cold 'production line' welcome from the midwife in the first-stage room or a similar inhuman approach in domiciliary practice.

Some patients who have been well prepared can go through labour without need of analgesic drugs; they are uncommon, and most mothers need some form of drug analgesia. There is an unfortunate attitude in some circles which suggests that a mother has in some way failed who has had to receive the slightest help during her labour from analgesic drugs. Drug analgesia is enormously helped by antenatal preparation, but it is unkind to ruin the mother's joy in the birth of her baby by suggesting at any stage that a resort to drug analgesia is in some way disreputable.

2 General Analgesic Drugs

An ideal drug technique which is used for obstetric analgesia should have the following properties:

a Analgesia must be adequate.

b The effect on the mother must be fairly quickly achieved. Events follow each other quite rapidly in some phases of labour, and promise of pain relief at some time in the future can do little to enhance the patient's confidence in her attendants.

c The method must not endanger the life or well-being of the mother, and there must be a minimum of unpleasant side-effects.

d Equally, it must not affect the unborn infant's well-being. Ideally, the perfect analgesic drug would produce pain relief in the mother without crossing the placenta into the infant's circulation. Such a drug has yet to be discovered.

e There must be no interference with uterine action. Labour must not be prolonged nor must the technique cause an increase in the incidence of operative deliveries.

f There must be no interference with the patient's powers of intelligent co-operation with her attendants.

g The method must be simple to use and must not distract the midwife from her obstetric duties.

h In domiciliary practice, the equipment associated with the analgesic technique must be as light and portable as possible.

It needs very little knowledge of pharmacology to realise that no drug exists which will fit in with all these criteria. However, much can safely be done by drugs if they are used intelligently. Every drug which can depress the activity of the central nervous system has been tried at some time as an obstetric analgesic. Of these, some have proved themselves less dangerous and more useful than others. A few have become established as 'midwives' drugs', that is, drugs which can safely be given by a trained midwife without reference to a doctor. These drugs can conveniently be classified according to their route of administration whether orally, by injection or by inhalation.

a Drugs Given by Mouth

This is not an ideal route because the rate of absorption of the drug is unpredictable, particularly from the intestinal canal of a parturient woman. It is however of some use in the early part of the first stage of labour.

Chloral given as a syrup in a dose of 5 to 10 ml (1 to 2 grammes of Chloral Hydrate) has been used for many years as a sedative in early labour. Chloral has very little analgesic effect in this dosage, but it helps to soothe and calm the anxious patient. It should not be given more often than two-hourly and the patient should not have more than five doses in any period of twelve hours. Chloral is a very safe drug and can do little harm to mother or infant. Its main disadvantage is that in many patients, it tends to cause nausea and vomiting, whatever attempts are made to disguise its taste.

Recently, this problem has been overcome by the introduction of *Tricloryl* tablets containing 500 mg of Triclofos. This compound acts in exactly the same way as Chloral and one or two tablets can be given to patients who cannot tolerate syrup of chloral.

Welldorm tablets have also been used. These combine Chloral with another hypnotic called phenazone. Unfortunately, in a very small percentage of cases, phenazone can produce an unpleasant rash. As the combination in this application has no advantage over Chloral, it is best avoided.

b Drugs Given by Injection

Two drugs will be discussed: Sparine and Pethidine.

Sparine. Drugs given by mouth in the early stages of labour are absorbed to varying degrees and it is a disadvantage of Chloral and its analogues that the blood level following a given dose is unpredictable. The injection route is much more certain in its effect and of the injectable drugs which have been used at this stage of labour, Sparine (Promazine) has gained considerable popularity. Like Chloral, it produces sedation and allays anxiety. It is also a useful anti-emetic and can be used to prevent or treat nausea or vomiting. It has little or no demonstrable effect on the baby's breathing in the dosage used: 50–100 mg by intramuscular injection.

Sparine is not a powerful analgesic. It does however tend to add to the effect of other analgesics such as Pethidine given later in labour; it is therefore wise to reduce the dose of such drugs in patients who have been given Sparine early on in their labour. In some centres, Sparine is given in combination with Pethidine during the latter part of the first stage of labour.

At present, Sparine is not officially recognised as a drug which can be used in all circumstances without a doctor's prescription. It is possible however that the Central Midwives Board may in the future consider adding it to the midwife's armamentarium.

Pethidine (Meperidine, Demerol)

As labour progresses and pain becomes more of a feature, the calming effect of Chloral or Sparine is not sufficient and the patient needs the more potent analgesic effect of Pethidine which is the injectable drug most commonly used by midwives. It is a powerful analgesic with a mild sedative effect. A qualified midwife is not required to call for a doctor's prescription before giving Pethidine.

If it is given too early, Pethidine tends to interfere with the progress of labour. It is therefore important to make sure that labour is well established before giving the patient her first dose of Pethidine. The contractions should be regular and strong enough to cause discomfort. On vaginal examination, a patient having her first baby should have her cervix dilated to three fingers (5 cm) and a multiparous patient's cervix should be two fingers (3 cm) dilated. These are approximate rules which may be modified in the light of experience but they are useful guidelines which will prevent unnecessary delay in the progress of labour with its train of complications.

The first dose of Pethidine varies from 100 mg to 150 mg given intramuscularly. The dose depends on the weight of the patient, the severity of her pain and on the presence in her body of other drugs which may have been given. It is important for the patient's confidence that the first dose produces good analgesia and it is therefore best to err at this stage towards the larger dose. Pethidine can be repeated in doses of up to 100 mg when the effect of the first dose wears off. The total maximum dose that a midwife may administer varies from centre to centre, but it is suggested that after a total of 250 mg has been given, and the patient has not been delivered, the time is approaching to call for a medical opinion on obstetric grounds.

The main disadvantage of Pethidine is that it is a powerful depressant of respiration. This is of no consequence to the mother in the doses used, but it crosses the placenta and an infant with a high level of Pethidine in its blood may be slow to start breathing at birth. There is a wide variation in the rate at which Pethidine crosses the placenta but the infant's blood level is usually at its maximum about one hour after administration to the mother. Attempts should therefore be made to time the last dose of Pethidine so that there is at least one hour before the baby is born.

In the last few years, a group of drugs has appeared which act as antagonists to the respiratory depressant effects of Pethidine. Of these, the most useful is *Lorfan* (Levallorphan tartrate). The preparation Pethilorfan consists of a mixture of Pethidine 100 mg and Lorfan 1·25 mg. Some authorities advocate the routine use of Pethilorfan instead of Pethidine alone. There is a suggestion that Lorfan not only antagonises the effect of Pethidine on respiration but that it also reduces the analgesic effect. For this reason, the total dose of Pethilorfan may be greater than that of Pethidine alone. Despite this, the infant is at less risk of being born with a reluctance to breathe. If Pethidine alone is being used and labour progresses more quickly than expected, a dose of 1 mg of Lorfan to the mother before delivery will help considerably. Failing this, the newborn infant can be given a neonatal dose of 0·25 mg of Lorfan by injection.

Pethidine is a drug of addiction and comes under the regulations of the Dangerous Drugs Act. Stocks must be kept under lock and key and an accurate register must be maintained.

In most cases, the use of Pethidine is completely free of complication. Some patients however react adversely. The commonest complaint is of nausea and vomiting. In a very small percentage of patients, this may go on to a more severe sensitivity reaction with a fall in the patient's blood pressure and a cold and clammy skin. Pethidine is not compatible with the antidepressant drugs known as mono-amine-oxidase inhibitors. There are several of these drugs such as Marplan, Actomol,

Cavodil, Drazine, Eutonyl, Marsilid, Nardil, Niamid, Parnate, Parstelin and Tersavid. Administration of Pethidine to patients under treatment with these drugs can produce a catastrophic reaction potentially fatal to the mother or the baby or both. If a patient is under drug treatment for a mental illness, it is therefore prudent to find out if the drug is a mono-amine-oxidase inhibitor. Drugs in this group should be withdrawn for at least a fortnight before it is safe to give Pethidine.

c Drugs Given by Inhalation
The inhalational route is ideal in many ways for obstetric use because the analgesic drug can be rapidly introduced into the patient's circulation and almost equally rapidly removed when the need for it is past. In the latter part of the first stage and during the second stage, the midwife has in her hands an analgesic which can be introduced when pain is at its height and withdrawn when the added analgesia is not needed. The inhalational route for drug administration is not normally taught to nurses during their training and although it is no more difficult than giving an injection, it sometimes takes time for a pupil midwife to accustom herself to the technique.

Three drugs are recognised by the Central Midwives Board as being suitable for administration by trained midwives without reference to a doctor: Entonox, Trilene and Penthrane.

Entonox is a mixture of equal parts of nitrous oxide gas and oxygen. Nitrous oxide is an excellent analgesic, although a weak anaesthetic. It is non-inflammable, odourless and non-irritant to the throat and trachea. It is not very soluble in body fluids and therefore acts quickly. It does not interfere with uterine contractions and is non-toxic to all body systems provided it is given with a high enough percentage of oxygen.

Nitrous oxide was first accepted for use by unsupervised midwives in 1936 when Dr Minnitt invented his apparatus which delivered a mixture of equal parts of nitrous oxide and air. This equipment was used for many years and gave excellent analgesia but at the cost of halving the oxygen percentage available to the mother and her unborn infant. In addition, it was demonstrated that the accuracy of many gas and air machines could not be relied on so that the gas mixture delivered to the patient might produce either inadequate analgesia or a dangerous lowering of the available oxygen. For these reasons gas and air became unpopular and research was carried out to discover techniques which would allow midwives safely to administer nitrous oxide with oxygen instead of air.

The first attempt was the Lucy Baldwin apparatus. This machine is equipped with cylinders of nitrous oxide and of oxygen and can be set to give mixtures of the two gases down to 30 per cent oxygen. It is fitted with a mechanism which cuts off the nitrous oxide supply if the oxygen supply fails. Its main disadvantage is that it is very non-portable and the 'cut-off' mechanism failed in one of the prototype machines. It therefore remains a piece of hospital equipment and has not gained complete acceptance for use by unsupervised midwives.

Entonox on the other hand can be used in all circumstances by unsupervised midwives, provided certain conditions are fulfilled. This is a mixture of 50 per cent nitrous oxide and 50 per cent oxygen packed in a blue cylinder with white quarterings on its shoulders. The cylinder is attached to the special miniaturised demand valve. The gas mixture in the cylinder is at a high pressure of approximately 2000 lb per square inch. This is reduced by the valve to a much lower pressure just sufficient to ensure that the gas flows to the patient. When the patient takes a breath, she distorts the sensing diaphragm which opens another valve allowing the gas to flow to the patient. Entonox will therefore flow to the patient only when she breathes from the equipment and the exhaled gas is vented through the exhalation valve. The equipment can be used in domiciliary practice with a small 500-litre cylinder giving a total weight of $13\frac{1}{2}$ lb. In hospital practice, the larger trolley mounted 2000-litre cylinder is more convenient.

The physical characteristics of the Entonox gas mixture are such that the gases will be delivered in a 50/50 concentration provided the cylinder has not been cooled below 0°C. If such cooling happens, the gases separate out and the patient will not receive the correct gas mixture. Remixing of the gases can be ensured by keeping the cylinder on its side in a warm room for 24 hours and inverting or rolling the cylinder a few times, depending on its size. It is a good policy to treat all Entonox cylinders in this way – a cylinder being used in midsummer may well have been in store since the winter.

The Entonox inhalation unit has on it a pressure gauge which gives an exact indication of the cylinder contents.

Entonox gives excellent analgesia in a high percentage of cases. It can be given to cover the pain of each contraction and as it is rapidly removed from the body, its use can be started quite early in the first stage of labour if the patient needs it.

The following practical points in the use of Entonox are worth noting:

i   Make sure that the cylinder contains gas. Check frequently by looking at the contents gauge and have a spare full cylinder ready.

ii   Learn to change cylinders quickly and efficiently. There should be no hissing leak when the cylinder is turned on. If there is a leak and the apparatus has been correctly fitted, check and change the Bodok seal washer.

iii   Remember that the apparatus is a demand valve; it will not work unless the patient breathes from it. The patient must therefore apply the mask accurately to her face without any leakage around it. There must also be no kink in the tube connecting the patient to the equipment. This can happen if the patient keeps twisting the mask in between inhalations.

iv   Develop the habit of listening for the proper functioning of the equipment. If all is in order, there will be a soft rushing noise each time the patient breathes and draws gas from the machine. A loud hiss means a high-pressure leak. Silence may mean an empty cylinder, a badly fitted mask or a kinked tube.

v   In the average patient, it takes about 40 seconds to obtain the maximum analgesic effect. The administration should therefore be so timed that maximum analgesia is attained when the pain is at its height. During the first stage, this can usually be done by starting the administration when the palpating hand feels the uterus beginning to contract. During the second stage, the patient must breathe in the analgesic mixture between contractions because she has to hold her breath to push when the contraction comes. Contractions at this stage are fairly regular and the administration can be timed so that the patient has at least 40 seconds of inhalation before she has to bear down. For the actual delivery, the patient can inhale the mixture continuously, and if she is encouraged to breathe in and out with her mouth open, it will reduce the danger of her pushing at the wrong moment and damaging the perineum.

vi Encourage the patient to take reasonably deep breaths. Very shallow panting respirations slow down the rate at which the gas enters the circulation.

vii Some patients may tend to become restless and uncooperative. This usually happens in patients who are less resistant than normal to the effects of nitrous oxide. In fact, they reach the excitement stage of anaesthesia. In these cases, the start of inhalation should be delayed until the contraction is under way, so that the duration of inhalation is reduced.

The Central Midwives Board has laid down rules which must be adhered to by midwives administering Entonox or any other recognised inhalational analgesic:

A practising midwife must not, except on the instructions and in the presence of a Registered Medical Practitioner, administer an inhalational analgesic unless:

i She has, either before or after enrolment, received at an institution approved by the Board for the purpose, special instruction in the essentials of obstetric analgesia and has satisfied the institution or the Board that she is thoroughly proficient in the use of the apparatus.

ii The patient has at some time during the pregnancy been examined by a Registered Medical Practitioner who has signed a certificate that he finds no contra-indication to the administration of the analgesic by the midwife and, if any illness which required medical attention subsequently developed during pregnancy, the midwife obtained confirmation from a Medical Practitioner that the certificate remained valid; and

iii One other person, being any person acceptable to the patient, who in the opinion of the midwife is suitable for the purpose, is present at the time of the administration in addition to the midwife.

H

Trilene is the trade name for the drug Trichloroethylene. It exists as a liquid which has added to it a blue dye. It must be converted to a vapour before being administered to the patient.

Two forms of apparatus are recognised by the Central Midwives Board for use by midwives when giving Trilene. They are the Tecota Mk 6 and the Emotril. These are complicated vaporisers which compensate automatically for changes in airflow through the equipment and for any temperature change between 12°C and 37°C. Within these limits, a patient breathing from one of these machines will receive a mixture containing 0·35 per cent to 0·5 per cent of Trilene vapour in air depending on whether it is set low or high. At this percentage, there is no appreciable reduction in the available oxygen.

Trilene is an excellent analgesic and most patients accept its rather sweet smell quite happily. It does not interfere with the course of labour and in these concentrations it has no toxic effect on any other of the body systems.

The main way in which Trilene differs from Entonox is that it tends to have a cumulative effect. The vapour absorbed during one contraction may not be completely eliminated before the onset of the next. It crosses the placenta and if therefore it is administered for too long there is a danger that the baby may be born with a fairly high blood concentration of Trilene and in a rather sleepy state. Its administration should not therefore be started as early in the first stage as with Entonox and the midwife should aim at a maximum of four hours of Trilene analgesia.

Apart from this, there are few practical differences between the use of Trilene and that of Entonox. The Trilene inhalers are draw-over machines and it is therefore as important as with Entonox to ensure that there is no leak between the mask and the patient's face. Unlike Entonox, there is no sound of gas flowing through a Trilene vaporiser; if, however, the expiratory valve is heard to hiss when the patient breathes out, all is probably well during inspiration.

Trilene is slightly more potent as an analgesic than is Entonox. If, therefore, a patient is not responding to Entonox in the later stages of labour, it may be worth switching to Trilene if it is available. For domiciliary work, Trilene also has the immense advantage of portability.

The vaporisers used for Trilene must be sent annually to a British Standards Institute Test Centre. There, the instruments are checked to ensure that they are delivering the correct vapour concentrations. A date stamp is applied to the equipment at the time of testing and a document is issued to certify that the tests have been carried out.

In anaesthetic practice, Trilene must not be administered through a closed-circuit apparatus. If, therefore, a patient comes to anaesthesia who has been inhaling Trilene vapour, the anaesthetist should be informed of the fact.

Penthrane (Methoxyflurane) is an anaesthetic agent with some similarities to Trilene. Recent work has shown that Penthrane can safely be used as an analgesic for normal delivery in a concentration of 0·35 per cent in air. It can be administered in this concentration through the Cardiff inhaler and its use in this apparatus by unsupervised midwives is sanctioned by the Central Midwives Board.

The mechanism and outward appearance of the Cardiff Penthrane inhaler is very similar to that of the Tecota. It differs in that it is painted a pale green colour and can be filled only by attaching it directly to a Penthrane supply bottle.

Experience is being gained in the use of this drug. Some patients and midwives dislike its sweetish pervasive odour, but patient-acceptance is on the whole good. It produces excellent analgesia and is probably marginally more potent than Entonox and Trilene. Whereas the other inhalational analgesics tend to produce restlessness and non-co-operation in overdose, Penthrane tends to produce a sleepy state. Even without overdosage, patients who are being given Penthrane tend to lie quietly with their eyes closed, although conscious and co-operative. Its main indication seems to be in the later stages of labour, particularly in apprehensive and noisy patients.

Penthrane shares with Trilene the immense advantage of portability. Against this, it is said to be at present 45 times more expensive than an equal dose of Trilene.

The recent introduction of Penthrane illustrates the fact that the search continues for improved analgesics which midwives can safely use in all circumstances. Much has been done in this direction but there are many women who do not receive from the methods at present available the relief to which they are entitled. The ideal midwife's drug and technique is still to be found.

Other Analgesics and Hypnotics

The drugs so far discussed are the ones which can generally be considered as suitable for use by midwives without reference to a doctor. There are however centres where other drugs are used, the following of which are some examples:

Barbiturates. The barbiturates with a medium duration of action (e.g., Seconal, Nembutal) can be given by mouth in doses of 100 mg to 200 mg. They are generally used to sedate patients early in labour and as they are very poor analgesics, they are not suitable for use in the presence of severe pain. These drugs produce quite good amnesia but if given late in labour they produce restlessness, impaired co-operation and prolongation of the second stage with its attendant obstetric complications. They are fairly powerful respiratory depressants and therefore tend to produce asphyxia in the new-born baby.

Morphine (10 mg to 15 mg by intramuscular injection) is in many ways similar to Pethidine. In addition to its powerful analgesic properties, Morphine and the similar drug Omnopon produce a very pleasant state of euphoria. Unfortunately, morphine cannot be relied on not to depress uterine activity whatever the stage of labour and it is the author's opinion that the midwife should always share responsibility for its administration with a doctor. It is a powerful respiratory depressant and crosses the placenta to the infant. Its respiratory depressant effect can be reversed by Lorfan, but even so, it is prudent not to use Morphine as a routine analgesic unless there is available a full infant resuscitation service.

Pentazocine Fortral is under investigation as an analgesic in labour in doses of 30 mg to 60 mg. It is a slightly less powerful analgesic than Pethidine and its effect on the infant's respiration is not reversible by Lorfan. Much research needs to be carried out on Fortral in this application. If it should prove useful for routine use in obstetrics, it would be an advance as it is non-addictive and its use does not call for the administrative complications surrounding a substance controlled by the Dangerous Drugs Act.

Scopolamine. This drug, given in doses of 0·4 mg by injection, produces some sedation and excellent amnesia. However, as this is accompanied by a high incidence of maternal excitement and non-co-operation, it is not now widely used as the drug of choice.

Avertin or Bromethol is quoted as an example of the many drugs which have been administered by rectum in obstetric practice. A dose of 0·075 grammes per kilo injected slowly in about 30 ml of warm saline will produce sleep for 1½ to 2 hours. It is alleged to cause prolonged labour and respiratory depression in the infant. It is however used in some departments as the drug of choice in patients suffering from pre-eclamptic toxaemia or eclampsia.

3 Local and Regional Analgesic Techniques

The midwife acting alone may use local analgesia to reduce the pain which she causes in performing an episiotomy. She can infiltrate the site of incision with either 10 ml of 0·5 per cent Lignocaine solution or 5 ml of a 1 per cent solution of the same substance. It is suggested that the larger volume of the weaker solution is the more useful.

In using this local analgesic, the following points should be borne in mind:

i All possible precautions must be taken to maintain sterility. The equipment used must be sterile and the area through which the injection is to be made must be carefully prepared with an antiseptic solution.

ii Injection into a blood vessel even of this small dose can prove fatal in a patient who is sensitive to the drug. To avoid any appreciable amount of the drug entering a vein or artery, the needle should be kept constantly in motion while the injection is being made.

iii Local analgesics do not take effect instantaneously. It is upwards of five minutes after a local injection of Lignocaine before the maximum effect is obtained. It therefore helps if the decision to perform an episiotomy can be made in good time so that the local injection has time to take effect before the operation is performed.

Other more complicated methods of using local analgesic drugs can be applied to obstetrics. The most effective is that of continuous epidural analgesia, the technique which provides the nearest approach to completely painless labour. Its efficiency depends on the anatomical fact that pain impulses from the uterus and birth canal enter the spinal cord at the eleventh dorsal segment and below. The nerves which produce uterine contraction leave the cord above this level. It follows that a block by local analgesia up to and including the eleventh dorsal segment of the spinal cord will block all the pain pathways while not interfering with uterine contraction. The local analgesic is placed in the epidural space where it affects nerves entering and leaving the spinal cord. The solution is injected either at the sacral end of the spinal column or into the epidural space in the lumbar region. Using an indwelling tube, analgesia can be maintained by adding increments of analgesic solution as labour proceeds. This technique demands a relatively high degree of medical supervision and the other minor penalty of the excellent analgesia is that there is an increased incidence of low forceps deliveries. The midwife who is involved with this technique will be asked to monitor very carefully the mother's physical state, and aseptic preparation of the environment, the equipment, and the site of injection must be of the highest standard.

Two other local analgesic techniques are in use – paracervical and pudendal blocks. Paracervical block, which is usually carried out at four to six cm dilatation of the cervix, involves injection of local analgesic solution into each lateral fornix of the vagina. This blocks most of the pain arising from uterine contraction and cervical dilatation. It can be followed by a local block of the pudendal nerve, which carries pain sensation from the lower birth canal and the perineum.

Care of the Mother Undergoing Operative Delivery

In cases where local and regional analgesic techniques are used for operative deliveries, the midwife's task is largely an extension of her usual monitoring role.

A large number of operative deliveries in this country are however carried out under general anaesthesia, a procedure which carries particular dangers for the parturient woman. It is presumed that the midwife, as a practical nurse, does not need reminding of the routine procedures that should always be followed in a patient about to undergo operation such as obtaining consent, removing dentures and emptying the bladder.

Three particular points in pre-operative care will be stressed:

i   *Gastric Contents.* The commonest anaesthetic cause of mortality and morbidity in parturient women is the inhalation of vomited or regurgitated stomach contents. The stomach of such patients empties very slowly and it is very dangerous to act on the usual criterion that the stomach is likely to be empty four hours after the last meal. Therefore, if there is any likelihood of an operative delivery, patients in early labour should be fed either intravenously or with a light gruel-like diet (not sugar or glucose). In an emergency, or if there is any doubt about the stomach contents, the stomach must be emptied either by the passage of a large stomach tube or by the injection of apomorphine, a drug which induces vomiting.

It has been shown that complications following aspiration of stomach contents are minimised if the acidity of the stomach contents is reduced. This can be accomplished by giving Mist. Mag. Trisil., in doses of 10 ml to 15 ml four-hourly. As all parturient patients are potential candidates for operative delivery, every woman in labour should be given this mixture every four hours from admission to delivery.

ii   *Premedication.* It is important to avoid respiratory depression in the infant, particularly if the mother is to undergo Caesarean Section. For this reason, no potent depressants of respiration such as Morphine, Pethidine or Omnopon should be included in the premedication. Many anaesthetists confine their premedication to Atropine 0·6 mg with or without 50 mg or so of Sparine. Others use Scopolamine (0·4 mg) which has been shown to reduce the dangers of awareness during the very light level of anaesthesia used before the birth of the infant. The patient will therefore need even more comfort and reassurance than the usual pre-operative patient who has had a euphoric or sedative pre-medication.

iii   *The Mother's Blood Pressure.* It sometimes happens that a pre-operative parturient patient will show a fall of blood pressure with or without a change in pulse rate and for no apparent reason. It has been shown that in many of these cases the apparent shock is due to a reduction in the volume of blood returning to the heart because of pressure by the uterus on the inferior vena cava. If this situation develops, it can be resolved by turning the patient on to her left side.

Post-operative Care

During anaesthesia, the presence of a cuffed endotracheal tube usually protects the patient from any danger of obstructed breathing or inhalation of stomach contents. As soon as the operation is completed and the tube is withdrawn, the patient is again at risk, however light a level of anaesthesia she may appear to have reached.

She should therefore be nursed in a position where any vomited or regurgitated gastric contents will flow out of the mouth, that is, on her side with the foot of the bed or trolley raised. The patient must never be left unattended and meticulous attention must be paid to the maintenance of her airway. Suction and Oxygen must be immediately available, and the pulse and blood pressure should be monitored at ten to fifteen minute intervals for the next few hours.

If the patient complains of pain, she should be given an analgesic of adequate strength in adequate dosage having been assured if it be the truth that all is well with her infant.

Too many lives have already been lost through accidents occurring before, during and after operation. It is only by meticulous attention to detail at all stages that obstetric operative mortality and morbidity can be reduced. The midwife has a very important part to play in this.

Summary

Management of Normal Labour

The management of labour can be learnt only by practical experience. Certain principles, however, must be observed in all labours.

Obstetric care during the first stage includes consideration of the comfort and general well-being of the patient as well as attention to the state of the bladder, a catheter being used if necessary. No solid food should be given during labour for fear of inhalation of vomit should an anaesthetic be necessary. Small amounts of puréed foods may be allowed. Fluids should be given sparingly provided that the urinary output is maintained.

In early labour sedatives such as Chloral, Trichloryl or Welldorm are useful. When the strength of the contractions causes pain or discomfort an analgesic such as Pethidine must be given. At the end of the first stage inhalational analgesia is preferable to that given orally or intramuscularly.

Progress can be accurately assessed only by vaginal examination. Such an examination is needed at the start of labour, when the membranes rupture, before giving analgesics and when it is thought that the cervix is fully dilated. A vaginal examination must also be carried out when maternal or foetal distress develop or when labour becomes abnormally prolonged.

The safety of the mother and of the foetus must be checked by regular observation of the rates of the foetal heart and maternal pulse, recording the maternal temperature and assessing the maternal fluid balance. Any deviation from the normal requires immediate medical attention.

Preparations for the delivery of the foetus must never be unnecessarily hurried. The patient must never be left alone at any time during the second stage, and her active co-operation must always be enlisted.

Owing to an increased liability to maternal or foetal distress during the second stage, the foetal heart and the maternal pulse must be checked at five-minute intervals.

Medical aid must be summoned if the head fails to advance over a period of twenty minutes.

In delivering the head, care must be taken to maintain flexion and to prevent damage to the anterior part of the vagina and vulva. If the perineum is at risk of tearing an episiotomy should be performed.

To reduce the incidence of bleeding from the placental site, an oxytocic – usually Syntometrine – should be given at the end of the second stage. If this is impracticable, it should be administered *after* the birth of the foetus but *before* the delivery of the placenta.

Once the placenta has separated its delivery usually presents no problems. If retained in the uterine cavity, its removal may prove more tedious. If there is any undue difficulty in this respect or if there is delay in separation, medical aid must be called at once.

Any tendency to further bleeding after the delivery of the placenta is best managed by raising the uterus upwards out of the pelvis.

At the end of the third stage, the vulva, vagina and perineum must be inspected for lacerations. These must be sutured without any unnecessary delay.

Before warding the patient her temperature, pulse and blood pressure must be checked, the uterus must be firmly contracted and there should be no undue vaginal bleeding. An estimate of the total blood loss must be entered in her case notes.

The placenta and membranes must be examined to make certain that they are complete. The cord must be inspected to exclude an abnormal number of umbilical vessels.

Analgesia for Normal Delivery

Antenatal Preparation – the need to combat ignorance, fear and tension and to gain the patient's confidence.
General Analgesic drugs.

The ideal technique: produces adequate analgesia
    acts quickly
    is safe for the mother
    is safe for the infant
    does not interfere with labour
    does not interfere with the patient's co-operation
    is simple to use
    is portable.

a   Orally Administered Drugs
Chloral Hydrate (1–2 grammes) or Tricloryl ($\frac{1}{2}$–1 gramme) in the early first stage – sedation and little analgesia.

b   Injected Drugs
i   Sparine (50–100 mg) in the early first stage – sedation and control of vomiting.

ii   Pethidine (100–150 mg) when labour is well established and the cervix dilated 3–5 cm.
Maximum total dose for a midwife – 250 mg.
As Pethidine depresses the infant's breathing, there should be more than 1 hour between the last dose of Pethidine and delivery.
Lorfan in a dose of 1–1·25 mg per 100 mg of Pethidine antagonises the respiratory depressant effect.
Pethidine must not be given to depressive patients on treatment with mono-amine-oxidase inhibitors.

c   Inhaled Drugs
i   Entonox – 50 per cent nitrous oxide/50 per cent oxygen.
Ensure that the gases are mixed by keeping in a warm place for twenty-four hours and rolling or inverting the cylinder.
Make sure that the cylinder is loaded, that the mask fits the patient's face and listen to make sure that gas flows when the patient breathes from the machine.
   It takes 40 seconds for the full analgesic effect to occur – the rhythm of administration in various stages must tie in with this.
   Entonox is non-cumulative, therefore its administration can be started as early as necessary.

The C.M.B. rules on using inhalational agents:

1   Adequate instruction of the midwife

2   A doctor's certificate

3   A third person present, acceptable to midwife and patient.

ii   Trilene – 0·35 per cent to 0·5 per cent in air from the Emotril or Tecota inhaler.
Tends to accumulate in the body, therefore do not use for longer than four hours.

iii   Penthrane – 0·35 per cent in air from the Cardiff Inhaler. Very like Trilene, but slightly more potent.
   Other drugs are used, but the midwife should share with a doctor responsibility for their use.

Local and Regional Techniques

Midwives can use Lignocaine infiltration before episiotomy. It is important to maintain sterility, to keep the needle moving and to give the analgesic time to work.
   Other more sophisticated regional and local methods are in use. The midwife's part in these is to ensure sterility and to monitor the patient's condition.

Care of the Anaesthetised Patient

Preoperative. In addition to other routines:

i   Ensure an empty stomach. Give *all* patients Mist. Mag. Trisil. 10–15 ml four-hourly.

ii   Premedication must avoid respiratory depressant drugs.

iii   If the blood pressure falls, turn the patient on her left side.

Postoperative

i   Maintain the airway.

ii   Guard against vomiting or regurgitation.

iii   Monitor the patient's condition.

iv   Ensure adequate postoperative analgesia.

PART FOUR

Abnormal Labour

Introduction

It will be remembered from p. 155 that a normal labour is one lasting between two and twenty-four hours in which a living, mature foetus, presenting by the vertex, is delivered spontaneously without any complications other than an episiotomy or a second or third degree perineal tear.

It follows, therefore, that any labour in which there occurs some departure from these criteria must be regarded as abnormal. Such a labour is of importance in that it almost invariably presents an increased risk both to the mother and to the foetus and that, in addition, it may demand specialised obstetric management, either to overcome these dangers or to effect delivery. Furthermore, the complications developing in abnormal labours may occasionally be of so urgent a nature as to require the midwife's immediate intervention pending the arrival of a doctor.

The midwife's responsibilities are therefore as follows:

1   She should be able to anticipate the development of an abnormality

2   Once an abnormality has developed, she must be in a position to discover its presence without undue loss of time

3   With certain exceptions, once the abnormality has been discovered she must inform a doctor immediately

4   She must then carry out whatever emergency measures may be necessary for the safety of the patient or of the foetus.

The Classification of the Abnormalities of Labour

1 Abnormalities Involving Primarily the Foetus
   Malpositions and malpresentations
   Prolapse of the umbilical cord
   Multiple pregnancy
   Foetal distress in labour.

2 Abnormalities Involving Primarily the Patient
   Prolonged labour
   Precipitate labour
   Maternal distress in labour
   Post-partum haemorrhage and other complications of the
   third stage.

3 Abnormalities Involving Both the Mother and the Foetus
   Premature labour
   Disproportion
   Obstructed labour.

It should be emphasised that these subdivisions are rarely as
clear-cut as this and that seldom indeed is one partner alone involved. In addition, in many cases more than one abnormality is
present. In such an event both the mother and the foetus may be
at risk for different reasons. Here a good working rule is to
decide upon the major complication present and to plan the
management of the case accordingly rather than to attempt the
often impossible task of evolving a complex schedule of treatment designed to deal simultaneously with all aspects of the
situation.

In every case, however, whatever the particular complications
or abnormalities present, the following three questions must be
answered:

1 What is the *main* complication present?

2 What risks does this present to the patient and to the foetus?

3 How may these risks best be overcome?

CHAPTER TEN

Malpositions and Malpresentations

General Remarks

A malposition is a vertex presentation in which the position of the foetal head is abnormal. A malpresentation, on the other hand, is any presentation other than a vertex. Both malpositions and malpresentations may arise either during pregnancy or during labour. Those arising during pregnancy may either persist into labour or be converted spontaneously or artificially into a normal vertex presentation before or after the onset of labour. Malpresentations encountered during labour may either have been present from pregnancy or, less commonly, have arisen after the onset of labour, the presentation until then having been normal.

Malpositions and Malpresentations Encountered During Pregnancy

These may be classified in a manner which represents increasingly greater departures from a normal vertex presentation.

1 Abnormal Positions of the Vertex
The only malposition of any obstetric importance is the *Occipito-Posterior Position*. Here the occiput, instead of pointing laterally is

directed posteriorly, either completely or somewhat to the left or to the right.

2 Abnormal Presentations of the Head

Here the head still presents but owing to extension having occurred the vertex is replaced either by the face or by the brow.

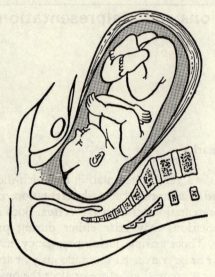

Fig. 31 Occipito-posterior position

3 Abnormal Presentations of the Breech

Here, although the *lie* of the foetus is still longitudinal the head no longer presents, its place having been taken by the *Breech*. Two subdivisions of this malpresentation are recognised, depending upon whether the foetal legs are extended or flexed.

4 Abnormal Lies

In such cases the lie of the foetus is no longer longitudinal but instead is either *Transverse* or *Oblique*, the long axis of the foetus being at an angle to that of the mother. Although under such conditions the presenting part may not always be clearly defined, it is often accepted as being the *Shoulder*.

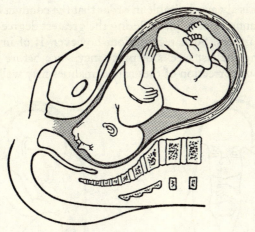

Fig. 32   Face presentation

The Diagnosis of Malpositions and Malpresentations in Pregnancy

Since abnormal positions or presentations which complicate labour are invariably associated with some increase in the risks presented to the patient or to the foetus, their recognition during

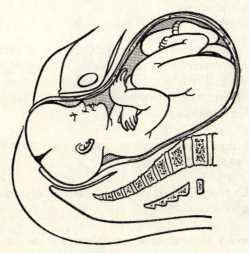

Fig. 33   Brow presentation

pregnancy is always desirable in order that the conduct of labour may be planned along lines offering the greatest degree of safety to both partners. Such recognition, however, is of importance only during the last weeks of pregnancy since before this time spontaneous correction of these abnormalities may well occur.

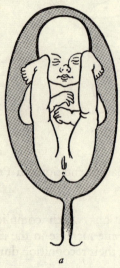 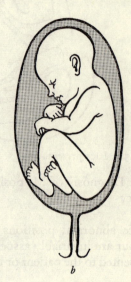

a   *b*

Fig. 34 Breech presentation
(*a*) extended (*b*) flexed

Owing to the fact that the very great majority of presentations are normal, a correct mental approach is essential if the occasional abnormality is not to be missed. This means, in effect, that the midwife, when examining a patient, should ask herself the following questions:

1 Is there more than one foetus present or is there only one? This excludes a *Multiple Pregnancy*.

2 Is the lie transverse or oblique or is it longitudinal? This excludes an *Abnormal Lie*.

3 Is the breech lowermost in the uterus or is the head presenting? This excludes a *Breech Presentation*.

4   Is the head extended or is it flexed? This will exclude a *Face* or *Brow Presentation*.

5   Is the occiput posterior or is it lateral? This excludes an *Occipito-Posterior Position*.

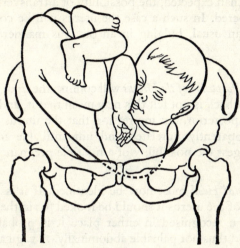

Fig. 35   Transverse lie

In principle it is best, wherever possible to:

1   Exclude a multiple pregnancy by the twenty-eighth week.

2   Exclude a transverse or oblique lie by the thirtieth or thirty-second week.

3   Exclude a breech presentation by the thirty-second week.

4   Confirm that the foetal head is normally flexed and in the correct position by the thirty-sixth week.

The above questions can be answered correctly only if the examination of the patient is carried out carefully and methodically, especially with regard to abdominal palpation.

1   *The Height of the Fundus* must first be checked. If greater than normal this suggests wrong dates, multiple pregnancy, hydramnios or a large foetus (page 145). If smaller, this may once again be due to wrong dates or, alternatively, to a small-for-dates foetus (page 116).

If the foetus seems to be of normal size but the fundal height is still lower than expected, the possibility of a transverse lie must be remembered. In such a case the uterus will be considerably broader than usual, bulging in an obvious manner into both flanks.

2   *Lateral Palpation of the Uterus* will confirm the *lie* of the foetus. If the foetal back is not felt this may mean that it, and hence the occiput, is posterior. An impression that the uterus contains a mass of apparently unrelated and unidentifiable foetal parts should suggest the possibility of a multiple pregnancy.

3   *The Foetal Head* must now be identified. If it is not in the lower part of the uterus it should be looked for in the fundus. If it cannot be recognised in either place it is probably deeply engaged and thus not palpable abdominally. A vaginal examination will clarify this point.

4   Lastly, if the head is in the lower part of the uterus but is not engaged, its size should be estimated since this will provide a good indication of whether it is well-flexed – in which case it will feel relatively small – or extended – when it will appear large owing to the fact that greater antero-posterior diameters are being felt. If the foetal head feels abnormally large the possibility of hydrocephalus must be remembered.

Whenever a midwife suspects, from her findings on examination, that any abnormality involving the foetus or the patient is present, she should at once inform the doctor in charge of the case in order that her suspicions may be confirmed and that the correct management of the patient may be decided in good time.

Malpositions and Malpresentations Discovered During Labour

It has already been said that in some instances a malposition or a malpresentation may first be discovered during labour, the presentation having apparently been normal throughout pregnancy. Although this by no means applies to all varieties of malpresentations, breech presentations, for example, being almost invariably established before the onset of labour, certain others are particularly liable to arise in this manner, examples of this being occipito-posterior positions and face and brow presentations. It is now necessary to consider how this may happen.

On page 181 it was explained that when engagement takes place the presenting plane of the foetal head, which is longer antero-posteriorly than transversely, normally coincides with that of the brim, which is longer transversely than antero-posteriorly. The head thus engages with the occiput directed laterally, either to the left or to the right. It will also be remembered that once the foetal head reaches the pelvic floor the altered shape of the outlet favours anterior rotation of the occiput at this level.

These two points should make it clear that the factor influencing most decisively the way in which the foetal head engages, descends and is delivered is the shape of the maternal pelvis and that any pronounced variation in this shape will tend to alter the normal mechanism of labour.

Variations in the Shape of the Maternal Pelvis

It is generally agreed that there are three main or 'parent' types of pelvis, each of which, to a greater or lesser extent, is subject to individual variations in shape and size. These three types are known as Gynaecoid, Anthropoid and Android.

1   The Gynaecoid Pelvis

This variety of pelvis which has been described on page 156 is that most usually seen in this country. The brim is oval, widest in its transverse diameter, the cavity is circular and the outlet is once again oval, the antero-posterior diameter now being longer than the transverse. In such a pelvis the descent and delivery of the foetal head takes place as set out in page 182, the occiput being directed laterally on engagement and rotating anteriorly on reaching the pelvic floor. In other words, both the pelvis and the mechanism of labour are normal.

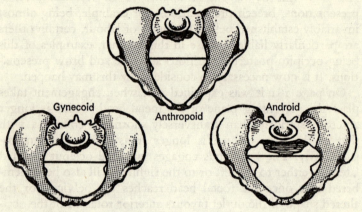

Fig. 36   Pelvic types

2   The Anthropoid Pelvis

This is a large pelvis, having an oval brim which, unlike the gynaecoid pelvis, is longer in its antero-posterior diameter than in its transverse. This shape, moreover, is retained in both the cavity and the outlet. Engagement therefore tends to take place with the occiput pointing either directly anteriorly or, far more commonly, directly posteriorly. This latter position is favoured by the wide angle made by the pelvis with the maternal trunk. Once engaged, there is no tendency for the head to alter its position since the shape of the pelvis is the same at all levels. The head therefore descends to the pelvic floor with the occiput directly posterior and is delivered in this position.

3   The Android Pelvis

While the Anthropoid Pelvis is one which as a rule is *larger* than normal, the reverse is true of the Android Pelvis, which is unsatisfactory from the point of view of its shape as well as from that of its size, most if not all of its diameters being considerably reduced. The *Brim* is triangular, the anterior part being narrow and the widest transverse diameter being situated very far back. The *Cavity* is narrow in all its measurements and the pelvic side-walls slope inwards, progressively reducing the amount of space available to the descending head. In consequence, the *Outlet* is narrow, the ischial tuberosities being close together while the lower part of the sacrum is curved forwards and the sub-pubic angle is reduced. In such a pelvis the head tends to engage late, the occiput being directed laterally and posteriorly, thus making most use of the greater amount of space available in one or other of the sacral bays. Owing to the small size of the cavity of this pelvis, the foetal head is often arrested at this level, either with the occiput still pointing postero-laterally or after a certain amount of rotation has occurred, the sagittal suture being then in the transverse diameter, resulting in what is called Deep Transverse Arrest of the head.

On other occasions the head fails to engage, the occiput remaining above the brim in a postero-lateral position. In such a situation the force of the uterine contractions acting upon the foetus may very occasionally cause the head to extend into a *Brow* or a *Face* presentation.

The Aetiology of the Three Pelvic Types

Although it used to be believed that the three parent pelvic types were inherited, it is now thought that they are related to the nutritional status of the woman during her childhood and early adolescence. Evidence favouring this view is that women with anthropoid pelves are usually taller and come from a better social background than those whose pelves are of the gynaecoid type, while the android pelvis is most likely to be found in women of short stature whose economic status has always been bad. It could thus be argued that the anthropoid pelvis is the true parent type, while the others represent departures from this attributable to a greater or lesser degree of impaired nutrition and growth during the formative years. A further observation in favour of this theory is that the proportions of the three types of pelvis has much altered since the 1939–45 war made necessary fairer food distribution and better nutrition of the population as a whole and of children in particular. Possibly owing to this, the android pelvis, which even twenty years ago was by no means uncommon, is now a rarity while the anthropoid is at present far more frequently seen than might be supposed from the study of some text-books. In addition, the *average* measurements of the pelvis have somewhat increased over the past two decades while a contracted pelvis – one whose diameters are much smaller than normal – is nowadays a rarity. Rapid changes of this sort would be impossible if pelvic status were determined solely on a genetic basis.

Disproportion

Although Disproportion, a condition in which the pelvis is too small for the passage of the foetus, is considered on page 290, it should perhaps also be mentioned here, since it is occasionally associated with an abnormal lie. In such a case, owing to the discrepancy between the size of the pelvis and that of the foetal head, engagement fails to occur and the head remains above the brim. If, when this happens, the abdominal muscles are abnormally lax, or if there is an excess of liquor amnii, the head may slide away from the brim into one or other iliac fossa, producing an oblique or a transverse lie. It should be stressed, however, that such cases are nowadays rare.

Occipito-Posterior Positions

An occipito-posterior position of the head is one of the most common of all malpositions and malpresentations and may be encountered either during the later weeks of pregnancy or during labour. Its importance lies in the fact that the associated maternal and foetal hazards, although by no means as high as in other malpresentations, are still greater than those of a normal delivery. Since these dangers are directly related to the course taken by labour in such a case and since this course is largely dependent upon the type of pelvis through which the foetus has to pass, it follows that the size and shape of the maternal pelvis must always be kept in mind when considering the management of an occipito-posterior position.

Aetiology

In the last chapter the suggestion was made that occipito-posterior positions in labour were associated with either an Anthropoid or an Android pelvis, the occiput turning directly posterior in the former and postero-laterally in the latter. During pregnancy, however, the malposition is probably due in most instances to an *extended attitude* of the foetus, when it is best accommodated in the uterine cavity if its relatively straight back is nearest to the maternal spine. This arrangement is responsible for two important clinical features:

1   Since the foetal back is posterior, the limbs come to occupy the anterior part of the uterine cavity

2   As extension of the back is rarely present without deflexion of the head, the presenting diameters are larger than normal. Engagement therefore rarely occurs before the onset of labour.

Diagnosis in Pregnancy

1   *Inspection.* Although inspection of the abdomen can frequently be misleading, an occipito-posterior position may at times be suspected during pregnancy if it is noted that the usual smooth curve of the uterus is absent. Instead the contour of the abdomen rises abruptly at the Xiphisternum and then gradually slopes away towards the pubis.

2   *Palpation:* When the occiput is posterior, abdominal palpation during the last weeks of pregnancy will reveal the following points:

a   The height of the fundus is greater than normal. This is due in part to the fact that the foetus when extended is longer than when it is flexed and in part to the fact that the head is not usually engaged

b The back being posterior is felt far round in one or other flank, if indeed it can be felt at all, while foetal limbs may be made out anteriorly

c The head is deflexed and not engaged and is therefore easily palpable. As the sinciput is anterior it is more readily felt than the occiput and owing to its rather indefinite and less well recognised shape may easily be mistaken for an extended breech.

3 *Auscultation.* In occipito-posterior positions the foetal heart sounds are most easily heard at a higher level and further out in the flank than when the occiput is anterior or lateral. However, in view of the wide variation that normally exists regarding the site of maximum intensity of these sounds, this sign is of limited clinical value.

Management in Pregnancy

In the past an attempt was sometimes made to correct an occipito-posterior position discovered during pregnancy by means of pads and binders. This was usually unsuccessful and is rarely practised today.

The Occipito-Posterior Position in Labour

The course of labour in a woman in whom the foetus has presented with the occiput posterior during the last weeks of pregnancy presents certain dangers. These depend upon the deflexed attitude of the head and upon the type of pelvis through which the head must pass. There are thus two main factors which must be considered in these cases:

1 The strength of the uterine contractions

2 The shape of the maternal pelvis.

1 The Strength of the Uterine Contractions
It has already been explained that when the occiput is posterior
the back of the foetus is extended and the head deflexed, offering
presenting diameters which are considerably larger than normal.
For the head to engage it is therefore necessary both for it and
for the foetal back to become flexed. This process usually requires strong uterine contractions. If these are present, little
difficulty or delay will be incurred in securing the amount of
flexion needed to produce smaller presenting diameters. Unfortunately, however, the deflexed head is a badly fitting presenting part and tends to stimulate only weak and infrequent contractions. A vicious circle is thus established, the deflexed head
leading to poor uterine activity which in its turn fails to correct
the deflexion. As a result, engagement of the head may be delayed and labour become abnormally prolonged. In consequence,
the incidence of operative delivery, either abdominal or vaginal,
is very high in this type of case.

2 The Shape of the Maternal Pelvis
The influence of the shape of the maternal pelvis upon the position of the foetal head has already been considered on page 231.
From what was said there it should be clear that if the occiput is
posterior at the start of labour, provided that the uterine contractions are strong, the head may pursue one of the following
courses:

a Where the pelvis is *Gynaecoid* the head will flex and the occiput rotate somewhat laterally before engaging, more room being
available in this position. Once the head reaches the pelvic floor,
further anterior rotation will bring the occiput under the symphysis pubis. The occiput will thus have turned forwards
through a total of three-eighths of a circle from its original position.

b Where the pelvis is *Anthropoid* the occiput will turn backwards to a directly posterior position, engagement, descent and
delivery then occurring without further rotation.

c Where the pelvis is *Android* engagement, if it takes place at
all, will occur with the occiput posterior and lateral. Descent
will be slow and arrest at any level is liable to complicate labour.

Diagnosis in Labour

This is based in part upon abdominal findings, as described earlier, and in part upon vaginal examination. In early labour, when the head is high, the precise situation may be hard to interpret since the level of the head and the limited amount of cervical dilatation together make recognition of the sagittal suture a matter of some difficulty. In such circumstances an occipito-posterior position may be suspected if the head is not engaged and the cervix badly applied, thick and poorly taken up.

Later in labour, when the head is lower in the pelvis and the degree of dilatation greater, a definite diagnosis may be reached by feeling the direction in which the sagittal suture is running in relation to the anterior fontanelle. This, owing to the deflexion of the head so commonly present, will be particularly easy to recognise. It usually lies either near to or directly beneath the symphysis pubis. The posterior fontanelle, on the other hand, being far back and relatively high up, will in many cases be out of reach of the examining fingers.

Management in Labour

1   If the occiput is postero-lateral but the pelvis feels normal in size, the fore-pelvis being wide and the outlet adequate, a spontaneous delivery may be expected following long anterior rotation of the occiput. Such a case should be managed, at least initially, as a normal labour, although the uterine contractions are often weak and time may be required for flexion and engagement of the head. Labour may therefore be somewhat prolonged. There is thus a slightly increased risk of foetal or maternal distress. In addition, as the membranes may rupture before engagement of the head has occurred, prolapse of the cord is rather more common than in a normal labour (page 260). If anterior rotation eventually occurs, however, delivery usually proceeds uneventfully.

2   If the occiput is directly posterior and the pelvis feels very large, delivery as a Persistent Occipito-Posterior – P.O.P. – may

be expected. In such a case labour will often be straightforward although difficulties may arise over the delivery of the foetal head. The reason for this is that the mechanism of labour is different from that observed when the occiput is anterior in that the head, in negotiating the forward curve of the birth canal,

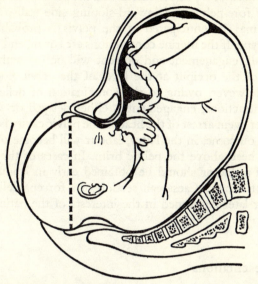

Fig. 37   Occipito-posterior position in labour

presents the longer occipito-frontal diameter (11 cm) to the antero-posterior diameter of the outlet. Considerable distension of the vagina thus occurs, resulting at times in tearing and bleeding before the head appears at the vulva, a diagnostic point of some value. Further progress of the head brings the anterior part of the vertex to present at the introitus, following which the occiput slips over the perineum, the brow, face and chin then emerging from under the symphysis pubis.

Although the long antero-posterior measurements of the anthropoid pelvis provide ample room for the larger diameters involved in such a delivery, difficulties may arise from the undue distension of the lower birth canal. Arrest of the foetal head on the pelvic floor is often seen, requiring for its management either a wide episiotomy or a forceps or ventouse extraction. If the uterine contractions are sufficiently strong to overcome this resistance on their own, severe vaginal and perineal lacerations may result. For these reasons a doctor should be informed if either of these complications seems liable to arise.

3   If the occiput is postero-lateral and the pelvis feels small with a narrow fore-pelvis and inward-sloping side-walls, a difficult delivery may be anticipated as the pelvis is probably of the android type. If the uterine contractions are strong and the foetal head small, engagement and descent will occur, with anterior rotation of the occiput at the level of the pelvic floor. More usually, however, owing to the combination of deflexion and weak contractions, engagement is either delayed or absent. In the former event arrest of the head in the pelvic cavity is the most probable outcome, in the latter, labour will become obstructed with the head above the pelvic brim. In cases of this sort the advice of a doctor should be obtained early in labour as it is likely that either a Caesarean section or a forceps delivery will sooner or later be needed in the interests of the patient or the foetus.

Face Presentations

Face presentations differ from occipito-posterior positions in that the deflexion attitude of the foetal head is replaced by one of extreme extension, the presenting diameter being either the sub-mento vertical (11 cm) or even the sub-mento bregmatic (9·5 cm). As in the case of occipito-posterior positions, face presentations may either arise during the last weeks of pregnancy or develop spontaneously after the onset of labour, the presentation until then having apparently been normal.

Aetiology

1   In Pregnancy
Extension of the foetal back leads, as a rule, merely to deflexion of the head. For full head extension to be present, something

more than a simple extended foetal attitude is therefore required. At times the head of the foetus is forced backwards by some tumour of the neck – a goitre or a bronchocele. At others, gross congenital malformations such as Anencephaly or Iniencephaly are present. Twisting of the cord around the neck of the foetus is also said to predispose to a face presentation, the tense cord forcing the head backwards. While it is impossible to prove or to disprove this contention, it must be remembered that it is very common for the cord to be around the neck but very rare for the face to present. Lastly, there may be no obvious reason for the malpresentation, in which case it could be argued that the extension of the head was congenital in origin.

2   In Labour

When the pelvis is of the android type, the head tends to engage with the occiput postero-lateral. In such circumstances it sometimes happens that the occiput catches on the brim of the pelvis and is thus prevented from descending. Continued pressure on the foetus by the contracting uterus is transmitted to the head which is forced to extend into a face presentation. If the dimensions of the pelvis are adequate descent will ensue, otherwise arrest occurs at the brim. The clinical importance of this is that such a train of events strongly suggests that the pelvis is abnormal.

Diagnosis in Pregnancy

A face presentation is rarely discovered in pregnancy. This is because the diagnosis is difficult and also because the possibility of the malpresentation is not usually considered. The following features, however, should suggest that the face may be the presenting part:

a   The foetal head will not be engaged. As extension at this stage is rarely extreme, it will also appear large, the presenting diameter being the sub-mento-vertical of 11 cm.

b   The extended foetus thrusts its chest and abdomen forwards or laterally. On palpation these structures may be mistaken for the back, an error which may be avoided by noting the foetal limbs to be on the same side, an impossibility if it is the back which is really being felt.

Diagnosis in Labour

Vaginal examination in the early stages of labour is usually inconclusive as the face is too high to be felt clearly. Later in labour, if descent occurs, the situation will be less confusing. A common mistake in these circumstances is for the face to be confused with the breech (page 253). The points of difference which should be looked for are:

a   No feet or legs will be felt, thus excluding a flexed breech

b   The face is softer than the extended breech. Despite this the chin may be mistaken for the sacrum and the mouth for the anus. This error should not arise if it is remembered that the latter has no alveolar margins

c   The infra-orbital ridges and eyes may be recognised. These are both important landmarks but care must be taken to avoid injury to the latter.

Management in Pregnancy

Since the diameters involved in delivering a foetus presenting by the face are greater than when it presents by the vertex, difficulties are liable to arise if the pelvis is smaller than normal. For that reason an X-ray Pelvimetry is often carried out during pregnancy to allow the best method of management to be decided in advance. This apart, the malpresentation demands no special care during pregnancy save of course to ensure that arrangements have been made for a hospital confinement.

The Mechanism of Labour

The mechanism of labour in face presentations, although basically similar to that observed where the vertex presents, involves certain dangers which must be understood if the safety of the patient and of the foetus are to be assured. Engagement usually takes place in the Right or Left Mento-Lateral position – R.M.L. or L.M.L. – the chin instead of the occiput being the denominator. Descent to the pelvic floor then occurs, whereupon the chin rotates anteriorly and emerges under the symphysis pubis. The delivery of the head is completed by the face, the brow and the vertex passing over the perineum. The birth of the rest of the foetus is as in a normal labour.

The dangers that may be encountered are as follows:

1 Engagement of the head may never take place, owing to incomplete extension or to inadequate pelvic measurements.

2 Owing to the large diameters involved, arrest of the head in the pelvic cavity frequently occurs.

3 Owing to the long distance between the chin and the parietal eminences the head is not engaged until the face is on the perineum. Failure to appreciate this point may lead to premature attempts at instrumental delivery.

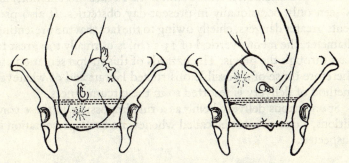

Fig. 38   Distance between lowest part of head and parietal eminences

4 If the chin turns into the hollow of the sacrum, vaginal delivery is impossible. This is because the pelvis, being deeper posteriorly than anteriorly, must contain not only the foetal head but also the shoulders when the chin is posterior. Sufficient room for this is not available. In such a situation, long anterior rotation

I

of the chin will not occur and on no account must be awaited. To do so can only lead to an obstructed labour with a Persistent Mento-Posterior Position, one of the most dangerous and difficult emergencies in obstetrics.

Obstetric Management

In view of the above dangers and difficulties, medical aid should be sought as soon as a face presentation is suspected. While anterior rotation of the chin followed by spontaneous delivery admittedly often occurs, owing to the possibility that the head may become arrested at any level and in any position, an operative delivery is required in a high proportion of cases. For this reason a face presentation must remain essentially a medical rather than a nursing problem and must always be managed as such.

Brow Presentations

A brow presentation is less common than a face presentation and is seen only occasionally in present-day obstetrics. It also presents greater dangers, chiefly owing to the fact that the presenting diameter, the mento-vertical of 13·5 cm, is normally too great to pass through the pelvis. The hazards of this malpresentation are therefore those of a possible obstructed labour and of whatever method of delivery is resorted to in the circumstances.

Spontaneous delivery being as a rule impossible in these conditions, a doctor must be called whenever a brow presentation is suspected.

Aetiology

The causes of a brow presentation are the same as those of a face presentation (page 240). It may arise either in the last weeks of pregnancy or after the onset of labour, the latter being the more usual occurrence.

Diagnosis

During pregnancy the incompletely extended foetal head, presenting its greatest antero-posterior diameter, seems abnormally large, so much so that at times Hydrocephalus may be suspected. An X-ray will, however, reveal the true state of affairs. In labour the same abnormal abdominal findings will be noted while on vaginal examination the presenting part will be high and reached only with difficulty. However, provided that the cervix is sufficiently dilated, it may be possible to identify the anterior fontanelle on one side and the supra-orbital ridges on the other, these two landmarks being joined by the frontal suture.

The Mechanism of Labour

No mechanism of labour exists where the brow presents, arrest of the foetal head occurring at the pelvic brim. On rare occasions spontaneous conversion to a face or, even less frequently, to a vertex, presentation may take place. This event must never be awaited.

Management in Labour

The management of a brow presentation in labour is entirely a medical concern. In general, an X-ray is taken to exclude any gross pelvic or foetal abnormality which may be the cause of the malpresentation. If the pelvis is normal and there are no other reasons for immediate interference, labour may be allowed to proceed, close watch being kept for the development of maternal or foetal distress or for any of the signs of impending uterine rupture (page 294). Once it is clear that conversion of the brow to a more favourable presentation is not likely to take place, Caesarean section is usually performed. On those rare occasions where the cervix becomes fully dilated and the pelvis is capacious it may be possible to convert the brow into a face or vertex presentation and to deliver the foetus with the forceps.

Breech Presentations

Breech presentations are, after occipito-posterior positions, the most common of all malpositions and malpresentations and make up about three per cent of all labours. Their importance is due in part to this relatively high incidence and in part to the hazards imposed by the malpresentation both on the patient and, in particular, on the foetus.

The dangers of any labour, regardless of the foetal presentation, are *least* in association with the delivery of the trunk and legs, *greater* with the delivery of the arms and *most marked* with the delivery of the head. In consequence, while in cephalic presentations the hazards *diminish* as the birth proceeds, the reverse occurs in breech presentations where the maximum risks and difficulties are encountered over the delivery of the after-coming head. A further disadvantage of this malpresentation is that due to lack of time moulding of the foetal head cannot take place and that in consequence it will not pass as safely through the pelvis as is the case when it constitutes the presenting part.

For all these reasons, the management of a breech delivery is a medical rather than a nursing responsibility.

The Foetal Hazards

The two chief foetal hazards of a breech delivery are Anoxia and Trauma, the latter being related in particular to the delivery of the after-coming head. The extent of these risks is reflected in the perinatal mortality which, for all such deliveries is in the region of eight to nine per cent, this figure dropping to between three and four per cent when mature foetuses only are considered.

Relation to Prematurity

The longer that pregnancy lasts, the more likely is a foetus to turn spontaneously from a breech to a cephalic presentation. A premature foetus is thus more liable to present by the breech than one which is mature. The incidence of premature breech deliveries is thus comparatively high. Although in such cases the foetus withstands delivery by the breech better than is usually taught, it is liable to perish during the first week of its life from complications related to its premature state. It is this rather than the hazards of labour which accounts for the high perinatal mortality associated with premature breech delivery. The practical implication of this is that the services of a Special Care Unit must be available if the high death rate among these babies is to be reduced.

Types of Breech Presentation

1 *The Extended Breech.* Here the spine of the foetus is extended, the head deflexed and the legs flexed at the hips but extended at the knees, the feet being placed alongside or in front of the face

2 *The Flexed Breech.* The foetal attitude here is one of flexion, similar to that seen in normal vertex presentations.

Of these two varieties, the extended breech is the more common, especially in primiparae.

Aetiology

The cause of a breech presentation depends upon the position of the foetal legs. When these are *extended* the shape of the foetus is such as to fit the uterus best when the smaller foetal pole, the breech, is accommodated in the lower uterine segment, the bulkier head and feet can then occupy the roomier fundus.

If the legs are *flexed*, either the capacity of the fundus is reduced by the presence in it of the placenta, thus forcing the smaller foetal pole, in this case the flexed head, to fit into it, or the lower uterine segment is unduly spacious, such as may occur in a multipara with lax abdominal walls. In such circumstances it most readily accommodates the larger breech and feet of the foetus. Lastly, where there is hydramnios the amount of space available to the foetus allows it to present in a variety of ways, a breech presentation in this case being merely fortuitous.

It should perhaps be stressed that neither a placenta praevia nor a contracted pelvis themselves *cause* the breech to present, although naturally the malpresentation may be seen in association with either of these abnormalities purely as a matter of chance.

Diagnosis in Pregnancy

This is based upon the following points:

1 *Abdominal Palpation* shows the uterus to be of normal size and shape. The head of the foetus may be felt in the fundus, but this is not always easy if the legs are extended as the feet may be in front of the face and the 'round, hard and ballottable' head of the text-books will not then be felt. An added difficulty is that the breech itself closely resembles an occipito-posterior position of the vertex.

2 Although the *foetal heart* may be heard at a slightly higher level than normal, this sign is of little absolute value since the site of maximum intensity of the heart sounds is subject to such wide variation.

3 A vaginal examination must always be carried out if any doubt exists regarding the presentation of the foetus. Its main purpose is to exclude a deeply engaged head. If the extended breech is engaged it may easily be mistaken for the head, although it may be possible to confirm the absence of sutures. When the breech is above the brim, as is usually the case when it is flexed, the pelvis will be empty and no foetal parts will be felt.

Management in Pregnancy

Once a breech presentation has been diagnosed in pregnancy it must be decided whether:

1   To leave matters as they stand, or

2   To convert the breech into a cephalic presentation.

Of these alternatives, the second is usually preferable since it will result in a normal presentation and thus reduce the maternal and foetal risks.

External Cephalic Version

The process of converting a breech into a head presentation is known as external cephalic version. Version itself means *turning*, Cephalic implies that the *head* is made to present and External signifies that the operation is carried out by purely *external* means. External Version is thus the opposite of internal version which requires a hand to be passed into the uterus and is thus possible only late in labour when the cervix is sufficiently dilated to allow this to be done.

Although the dangers of external cephalic version are often emphasised, in reality they are negligible provided that the operation is carried out carefully and gently and the following contra-indications borne in mind:

1   Where separation of the placenta is liable to occur, such as where bleeding has occurred either in early or in late pregnancy

2   Where rupture of the uterus is possible, such as where a previous Caesarean section or hysterotomy has been carried out.

If Caesarean section has already been decided upon as the method of delivery, version is unnecessary; if there is a multiple pregnancy it will be impossible.

It follows that the main dangers of version are separation of the placenta and rupture of the uterus, others being compound presentations – where more than one part of the foetus presents – and entanglement of the foetus in its cord.

The Time for Version

This is usually at or shortly after the thirty-second week. The malpresentation should therefore be diagnosed at or before this time. If version is carried out earlier, the breech presentation may recur, if delayed until later in pregnancy, the space available in the uterus may be insufficient.

If version is successful the patient should be seen in a week's time to ensure that reversion has not occurred; if unsuccessful, a further attempt may be made later in pregnancy.

Precautions which should always be taken after version, whether successful or unsuccessful, are:

1 Auscultation of the foetal heart to exclude abnormalities of rate or rhythm

2 Checking that no vaginal bleeding has started.

If version is either contra-indicated or has failed, the foetus must be delivered as a breech. Here the alternatives are:

1 *Vaginal Breech Delivery*. This should be contemplated only when the maternal and foetal dangers are known to be small

2 *Elective Caesarean Section*. This should be considered where the risks of vaginal delivery are high.

As already pointed out, the main foetal hazards of a breech delivery are anoxia and trauma. Of these the former can be anticipated if there is reason to believe that placental insufficiency may develop during labour while the latter is chiefly related to the capacity of the maternal pelvis and the size of the foetal head. In this connection it must be remembered that since moulding cannot occur, minor degrees of disproportion, easily overcome when the head is lowermost, are serious dangers when the foetus is presenting by the breech.

A vaginal breech delivery would therefore be relatively safe in the following circumstances:

1   Where the pelvis is of satisfactory shape and size

2   Where the foetus is small

3   Where there is a past history of easy, spontaneous deliveries

4   Where the course of pregnancy has not suggested the possibility of placental insufficiency.

By contrast, a vaginal breech delivery would be hazardous:

1   Where the pelvis is of unsatisfactory shape and size

2   Where the foetus is large

3   Where there is a past history of difficult labours or of still-births

4   Where pregnancy has been complicated by a condition associated with placental insufficiency

5   Where the patient is an elderly primigravida – over thirty-five years of age.

In such cases Caesarean section would offer the foetus a better chance of survival.

The Assessment of the Patient

In deciding upon the most suitable method of delivering a foetus presenting by the breech, attention should be paid to the following points:

1   The past obstetric history

2   The history of the present pregnancy

3   The estimated weight of the foetus

4 The size and shape of the maternal pelvis as determined by vaginal examination and X-ray pelvimetry.

Labour

The Mechanism of Breech Delivery

The extended breech is not circular but oval on cross-section, its widest diameter, the Bitrochanteric, measuring 11 cm and its circumference about 33 cm, almost exactly that of the well-flexed head. It follows, therefore, that if engagement, descent and delivery of the breech can be safely accomplished, little difficulty should be encountered over the birth of the after-coming head. On the other hand, if delay occurs with the delivery of the breech, the risks associated with the birth of the head may be considerable. Engagement of the extended breech usually occurs with the bitrochanteric diameter occupying the transverse of the brim. The breech descends to the pelvic floor and rotates to bring one hip under the symphysis and the other into the hollow of the sacrum. The breech is then born by lateral flexion around the symphysis pubis. Following the birth of the breech, the trunk appears, after which the shoulders descend to the pelvic floor, the anterior being delivered under the symphysis pubis and the posterior over the perineum. The after-coming head engages in the transverse diameter of the brim but later rotates into the antero-posterior diameter of the outlet. The sub-occiput then stems under the symphysis while the face, brow and vertex are born over the perineum.

It is important to bear this mechanism in mind when conducting a breech delivery since provided it is followed, serious complications are unlikely to arise.

The Management of Labour: First Stage

A hospital confinement is essential for all women in whom it is proposed to deliver the foetus by the breech. Moreover, owing to the various difficulties and dangers that may suddenly appear in the course of the second stage, a consultant or registrar obstetrician, an anaesthetist and a paediatrician should all be present at the actual birth of the baby.

Since anoxia and trauma must be avoided wherever possible, labour is usually induced at or shortly before term, thus reducing on the one hand the chance of an over-large foetus and on the other that of placental insufficiency from a prolonged pregnancy. In addition, since anoxia is liable to develop if the first stage is prolonged, careful and frequent auscultation of the foetal heart is necessary whenever labour lasts for over twelve hours.

It is often taught that the patient should be kept in bed during the whole of the first stage of a breech labour to avoid premature rupture of the membranes and prolapse of the cord. This advice is useless. On the other hand, the risk of cord prolapse is undoubtedly increased if the breech is flexed and consequently poorly-fitting. Cases of this sort need careful supervision if such an accident is not to pass unnoticed.

It is important to be sure of the nature and level of the presenting part as early in labour as possible. For this reason, a vaginal examination must be carried out in all breech labours on admission to the Labour Ward. Where the breech is extended this will reveal the smooth buttocks of the foetus, the natal cleft and the sharp projection of the lower sacrum and coccyx. If the legs are flexed, these landmarks are less definite but one or both feet may be felt. The breech is engaged when its lowest part is at or below the level of the ischial spines. If the breech remains high, or if the sacral hollow gives the impression of being peculiarly empty, it is best to assume that disproportion is present and to inform a doctor without delay.

The Second Stage

A foetus may be delivered by the breech in one of three ways:

1 By a *Spontaneous Breech Delivery*: Here delivery is effected entirely by the mother's own efforts, external assistance playing no part. Such cases are uncommon and are usually the result of abnormally rapid labours. In addition, the foetus is almost always premature.

2 By an *Assisted Breech Delivery*: Here the delivery of the legs, breech and trunk is left largely to the maternal powers, assistance being provided mainly for the birth of the shoulders and of the head. This is by far the best and safest method of breech delivery.

3 By *Breech Extraction*: Here delivery is entirely operative, the natural forces playing no part and the patient being under a general anaesthetic.

It follows that the only type of breech delivery which a midwife may have to conduct is an assisted breech delivery. In addition, this is likely to prove both rapid and easy, the foetus being small and the contractions strong, since otherwise there would be ample time for a doctor to arrive on the scene.

If a midwife finds herself having to take charge of such a case, she should bear the following points in mind:

1 That the main danger to be avoided is that of trauma to the foetus.

2 That although such trauma usually consists of cerebral haemorrhage from the rapid and uncontrolled delivery of the after-coming head, fatal damage may also be caused to the liver and supra-renals by squeezing the soft foetal abdomen. Fractures of long bones such as the femur or the humerus, which may occur in delivering the legs or arms, although unfortunate, are rarely fatal.

3 That in view of this the delivery must be conducted deliberately, slowly and gently. Speed is particularly dangerous, especially if foetal anoxia is present, since the congested cerebral vessels are liable to rupture at the slightest trauma.

4 That as in the case of a vertex delivery, the best result will be achieved if the natural mechanism of labour is followed as closely as possible.

The Conduct of the Second Stage

1 Full cervical dilatation may be suspected when the breech is seen to be distending the vulva. It should be confirmed by vaginal examination.

2 Medical aid must now be called.

3 If the breech is advancing so rapidly that the doctor is unlikely to arrive in time, the midwife should take steps to conduct the delivery herself.

4 The patient must be placed in the lithotomy position. When the vulva is widely distended by the breech an episiotomy must be carried out under local infiltration analgesia.

5 The Delivery of the Breech and Legs
The breech will usually be born spontaneously with the next contraction but even if this does not happen on no account should it be pulled down. This may cause extension of the arms and head and lead to later difficulties. It is best to await the spontaneous delivery not only of the breech but also of the legs.

6 The Delivery of the Trunk
Once the breech and legs are delivered the foetal back will turn anteriorly. At this stage a loop of cord should be drawn down to avoid subsequent traction upon it. It is unnecessary to feel for cord pulsation since if this is present all is well and if not, hurry will only make the situation worse. With the next contraction the trunk is usually born to the level of the scapulae.

7 The Delivery of the Arms
One hand supports the foetus by its feet, the other is passed up its ventral aspect and feels for the arms. If flexed, these will be folded across the abdomen and may easily be hooked down. If, however, they are extended, the foetus must be firmly grasped by its buttocks, the thumbs being directed upwards along the iliac crests. Held in this way the liver and supra-renals are in no danger. The foetus is then gently turned so as to bring one

shoulder anteriorly, when the arm may easily be delivered by hooking it down from behind the symphysis. The foetus is then turned to the opposite side, keeping the back anterior, and the second arm delivered by a similar manoeuvre.

8   The Delivery of the After-Coming Head

A doctor usually applies forceps to the after-coming head. A midwife cannot do this and must therefore adopt one of the several available alternatives. Of these, the most suitable is the method of jaw flexion and shoulder traction – the Mauriceau Smellie Veit manoeuvre. This is carried out as follows:

Once the shoulders and arms have been delivered, the foetus should be straddled over the left forearm, the fingers of the left hand being directed upwards over the face, and the middle finger passed into the foetal mouth and along one alveolar margin. By depressing this finger the jaw may be flexed. The index and fourth fingers of the right hand are then placed over the foetal shoulders, the middle finger pushing the occiput forwards and thus increasing flexion. Traction is then made upon the shoulders by the fingers of the right hand in a downward and outward direction until the sub-occiput appears under the symphysis pubis. The foetus should now be lifted slowly upwards, allowing the face, the brow and the vertex to slip gently over the perineum.

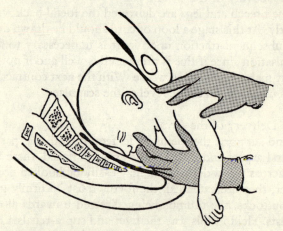

Fig. 39   Jaw flexion and shoulder traction

The Third Stage

Following the delivery of the head, Syntometrine (1 ml) is usually given either intravenously or intramuscularly, after which the third stage is conducted as in a normal labour.

The above description of an assisted breech delivery has been purposely written in an abbreviated form and cannot replace experience gained on the doll and pelvis, which are particularly suitable for learning this technique.

In conclusion, it must be emphasised once again that if a midwife is obliged to conduct a breech delivery, the case will almost certainly be one in which the pelvis is capacious, the foetus small and the contractions strong. In such circumstances delivery will be straightforward, easy and safe, provided that hurry and roughness are avoided and the normal mechanism of labour followed as closely as possible.

Transverse and Oblique Lie

In the various malpresentations already considered, the *lie* of the foetus has always been longitudinal, either the head or the breech presenting. In the type now to be discussed, the lie itself is abnormal – transverse or oblique – with the long axis of the foetus at or near a right angle to that of the mother. Although such a state of affairs is not uncommon before the thirtieth week of pregnancy, owing to the small size of the foetus and the relatively large amount of liquor amnii present until this time, after this date the lie usually becomes established as longitudinal.

The practical significance of a transverse or oblique lie is that unless the foetus is both dead and so small as to be capable of expulsion in a doubled-up attitude, spontaneous vaginal delivery is impossible.

Aetiology

The causes of such abnormal lies are:

1 *Congenital Uterine Abnormalities* such as a septate or subseptate uterus, where, owing to the structural defect, the foetus cannot assume a normal lie.

2 *Intra-uterine or Extra-uterine masses* such as a placenta praevia, fibroids or ovarian cysts. These produce their effect by pushing the head or the breech to one or the other side.

3 *Lax Abdominal Walls* which allow the uterus to fall forwards, altering the disposition within it of the foetus.

4 *Hydramnios* where, owing to the excessive amount of space available to the foetus an unstable presentation rather than a strictly transverse lie is apt to occur.

Although in the presence of any of the above conditions a contracted pelvis may, by preventing the engagement of the presenting part, encourage a transverse lie, it is not in itself a cause.

Diagnosis

A transverse lie is one of the reasons for the fundal height being lower than expected. In such a case, the uterus is also abnormally wide and the girth is greater than normal. On palpation the foetal head is found in one loin or iliac fossa with the breech on the opposite side. The lower part of the uterus feels empty. The foetal heart is often best heard above the umbilicus. A vaginal examination, although of value in confirming the diagnosis, should not be carried out unless a placenta praevia has been excluded. This restriction does not apply after the onset of labour if there is no vaginal bleeding. Such an examination shows the pelvis to contain neither head nor breech while at times an arm or shoulder may be identified.

Dangers

Since vaginal delivery is impossible as long as the abnormal lie persists, the *maternal dangers* are those of an obstructed labour (page 298), with the added risk that the over-distended lower segment may rupture. This accident may occur either spontaneously or as a result of unwise interference. The *foetal risks* are related to the maternal dangers and to difficulties associated with the delivery itself. A further hazard is prolapse of the cord due to the high and badly-fitting presenting part.

Management

Whether diagnosed in pregnancy or after the start of labour, a transverse lie is a complication which requires immediate medical attention. The management of this abnormality need thus only be summarised:

1 If discovered during pregnancy, the cause is sought. Depending on its nature, a decision is taken either to carry out version at once or to defer this procedure until later. Alternatively, it may be thought best to deliver the patient by elective Caesarean section at or near term.

2 If correction of the lie is impossible or inadvisable, the patient is usually admitted to hospital at about the thirty-fourth week. Once there, if spontaneous version occurs and the longitudinal lie is maintained, she may be sent home, further management being that of a normal pregnancy. If, as is usually the case, the lie remains uncorrected, a doctor must be informed both when the membranes rupture and when labour starts.

3 As a rule, choice of treatment now rests between correcting the lie with or without subsequent artificial rupture of the membranes, or immediate Caesarean section. Rarely, however, labour may be allowed to continue until the cervix is sufficiently dilated to allow an internal version to be performed, the foetus then being delivered by the breech. This procedure, however, carries

the risk of provoking a prolapse of the cord and of favouring uterine rupture and, in modern practice, is seldom indicated.

Presentation and Prolapse of the Cord

Prolapse of the cord is a most serious obstetric accident. It is also one in which the midwife can play an important part, not only in diagnosis but also in the first-aid treatment necessary to save the life of the foetus.

The dangers of prolapse of the cord are almost entirely foetal, what maternal hazards there are being related to the treatment of the condition. The chief effect on the foetus is that of oxygen

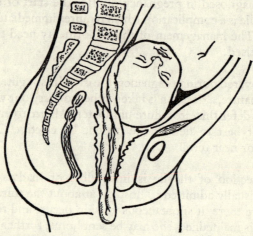

Fig. 40   Prolapse of the cord

deprivation through compression of the cord between the presenting part and the side-wall of the pelvis. A less serious risk is spasm of the umbilical vessels. This has the result of reducing the blood flow through them if it has not already been subjected to the effects of direct pressure.

The distinction between *Presentation of the Cord* on the one hand and *Prolapse of the Cord* on the other depends upon whether the forewaters are intact or ruptured. If intact, and the cord is in advance of the presenting part of the foetus, it is said to be *Presenting*; if ruptured, then the cord has *Prolapsed*. Since usually a smaller amount of cord is involved in presentation than in prolapse, the risks of the former condition are less than those of the latter.

Predisposing Conditions

For the cord to prolapse, sufficient space must be available between the presenting part and the pelvic side-walls. The predisposing conditions are therefore mainly related to a *badly fitting presenting part*, and include:

1 Cephalic presentations where the head is either too large to enter the pelvis, too small to fit snugly in it, deflexed, as in occipito-posterior positions, or extended, as in a face or brow presentation

2 Flexed breech presentations

3 Transverse or oblique lies

4 Hydramnios, since here the presenting part often remains high until after the onset of labour.

Although the cord may prolapse at any time throughout pregnancy or labour, it is most liable to do so when the membranes rupture *during labour*. Contrary to what is usually taught, rupture of the membranes before the onset of labour does not predispose to cord prolapse.

Diagnosis

The diagnosis of prolapse of the cord may be reached:

1 By *seeing* a loop of cord protruding from the vulva

2 By *feeling* a loop of cord on vaginal examination. This is less easy than might be imagined, the cord being sometimes mistaken for foetal fingers or toes or for an oedematous lip of the cervix

3   Cord prolapse should always be suspected if foetal distress develops suddenly during an otherwise normal labour. In any such case a vaginal examination must at once be carried out to exclude this accident.

Management

When prolapse of the cord has occurred the midwife should act as follows:

1   Medical aid must be called at once, the Emergency Obstetric Unit being alerted if the patient is in her own home.

2   Next, it must be decided whether the foetus is alive or dead. If it is dead only the patient's interests need be considered.

3   The state of the foetus may be assessed by feeling for pulsations in the cord or by listening to the foetal heart. In cases of doubt it is best to assume that the foetus is still alive.

4   In such a situation the guiding principle is that either delivery should be completed within ten to fifteen minutes or, if this is not possible, that pressure should be taken off the cord while awaiting active medical interference.

5   If the cervix is fully dilated, the presentation favourable, the presenting part low in the pelvis and the contractions strong and frequent, an episiotomy should be performed and delivery completed as rapidly as possible.

6   If the presenting part is high or if the cervix is not fully dilated, pressure must be taken off the cord.

This may be achieved as follows:

1   The foot of the bed must be raised on blocks or chairs.

2   The pelvis is raised still further by placing the patient either in the Knee-Elbow position or, preferably, in the exaggerated Sims' position.

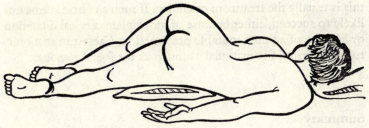

Fig. 41 Exaggerated Sim's position

3 Two fingers are passed into the vagina and pressure applied to the presenting part, especially during contractions. This pressure is maintained until the doctor's arrival.

Medical Management

This generally consists of immediate delivery, either vaginally or by Caesarean section, since further delay may prove fatal to the foetus. Attempts at reposition of the cord are rarely successful.

For these reasons, the patient is usually transferred as soon as possible to an operating theatre, all being in readiness for Caesarean section. A vaginal examination is then carried out under general anaesthesia and the position reviewed. If a straightforward vaginal delivery, either forceps or breech extraction with or without preliminary internal version, appears possible

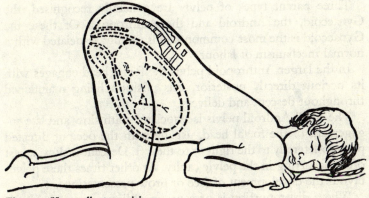

Fig. 42 Knee–elbow position

this is usually the treatment of choice. If such a course seems unlikely to succeed, either because of incomplete cervical dilatation or because of an unfavourable presentation, Caesarean section is to be preferred for maternal as much as for foetal reasons.

Summary

General Remarks

A malposition is a vertex presentation in which the position of the head is abnormal. A malpresentation is any presentation other than a vertex.

Both malpositions and malpresentations can arise either during pregnancy or after the onset of labour.

Diagnosis during the last weeks of pregnancy is desirable in order that the conduct of labour and the safest way of delivery may be planned in advance. Such a diagnosis may best be made by developing a correct mental approach and by the careful and methodical examination of every patient seen in the ante-natal clinic.

Malpresentations arising in labour do so primarily as a result of some abnormality of pelvic shape or size which adversely affects the normal process of engagement, descent and delivery of the foetal head.

Three parent types of pelvis are generally recognised, the Gynaecoid, the Android and the Anthropoid. Of these the Gynaecoid is the most common and is usually associated with a normal mechanism of labour.

In the larger Anthropoid pelvis the foetal head engages with its occiput directly posterior, this position being maintained throughout descent and delivery.

The small Android pelvis is associated with slow and late engagement of the foetal head, usually with the occiput directed postero-laterally to the right or to the left. Descent is slow, arrest often occurring in the pelvic cavity. At other times these pelves favour the development of face or brow presentations.

Where disproportion is present, an oblique or transverse lie may occasionally develop during labour if the abdominal walls are unduly lax or if hydramnios is present.

Occipito-Posterior Positions

An occipito-posterior position is the most common of all the malpositions and malpresentations. Its importance lies in the hazards it presents to the patient and to the foetus. These in turn depend upon the attitude of the foetus and the size and shape of the pelvis through which it must pass.

Diagnosis during pregnancy usually depends mainly on abdominal palpation, the fundus being somewhat higher than normal, the foetal limbs being felt anteriorly and the head being both deflexed and high.

Although in the past the correction of the malposition was often attempted during pregnancy, this is seldom advocated today.

When the occiput is posterior the course of labour depends upon the strength of the uterine contractions and the size and shape of the pelvis.

When the contractions are strong, flexion and engagement of the head usually take place. When they are weak, as is often the case, the necessary degree of flexion is obtained slowly, if at all. In such cases labour is often abnormally prolonged.

If the pelvis is Gynaecoid, long anterior rotation of the occiput through three-eighths of a circle, followed by the delivery of the head in the occipito-anterior position may be anticipated.

If the pelvis is Anthropoid, delivery as a Persistent Occipito-Posterior – P.O.P. – is the rule.

If the pelvis is Android, the occiput tends to engage in a postero-lateral position. In such a pelvis arrest of the head may occur at any level.

Diagnosis in labour is based upon abdominal findings and on vaginal examination, important landmarks being the sagittal suture and the anterior fontanelle.

If the occiput is directed postero-laterally at the start of labour but the pelvis feels adequate, labour usually proceeds uneventfully. If the occiput is directly posterior and the pelvis is large, delivery as a P.O.P. can be expected, although owing to the larger diameters involved arrest on the pelvic floor may occur. If the occiput is postero-lateral and the pelvis seems small and narrow a prolonged labour and an operative delivery are likely. Medical aid should be asked for early in such cases.

Face Presentations

In face presentations the head is in an attitude of extreme extension, the presenting diameter being either the sub-mento vertical or the sub-mento-bregmatic (11 cm or 9·5 cm).

Aetiological factors during pregnancy are tumours of the neck, gross congenital malformations and twisting of the cord around the neck. In many instances no obvious cause can be found.

Face presentations may arise in labour when the pelvis is Android in type and engagement is delayed. In such a situation pressure on the foetus by the contracting uterus may cause the head to extend into a face.

Diagnosis in pregnancy is difficult. Points of importance are the large non-engaged head and the palpable chest and abdomen. In labour, vaginal examination will reveal the chin, mouth, alveolar margins and eyes. Confusion with the more common breech often arises.

The hazards encountered during labour are those of arrest of the head either above the brim or in the pelvic cavity, premature attempts at instrumental delivery before engagement has occurred and posterior rotation of the chin into the hollow of the sacrum. In this last situation, delivery as a mento-posterior is impossible and long anterior rotation of the chin will not occur spontaneously.

In view of these dangers, a face presentation should always be regarded as a medical rather than a nursing problem.

Brow Presentations

Brow presentations are only rarely seen in modern obstetric practice. They present considerable dangers both to the patient and to the foetus. This is chiefly owing to the fact that the presenting diameter of the foetal head is too large to pass through the pelvis.

The causes of a brow presentation are similar to those of a face presentation.

Diagnosis during pregnancy is usually based upon the discovery of an abnormally large head above the pelvic brim. In labour the anterior fontanelle and the supra-orbital ridges, joined by the frontal suture, may be felt on vaginal examination if the cervix is sufficiently dilated.

Management in labour is entirely a medical matter. Although Caesarean section is usually performed once the diagnosis has been established, it may at times be justifiable to allow labour to proceed in the hope that spontaneous conversion to a face or to a vertex presentation may take place.

Breech Presentations

A breech presentation complicates about three per cent of all deliveries. The importance of this malpresentation is in part this high incidence and in part the dangers it presents to the foetus.

The foetal hazards are essentially anoxia and trauma. The latter is related in particular to the delivery of the after-coming head.

A high proportion of premature foetuses present by the breech. The increased perinatal mortality in this group of cases is, however, related more to the prematurity of the babies than to the delivery itself.

A breech presentation may be either extended or flexed. Of these two types the former is the more common, especially in primigravidae.

Diagnosis in pregnancy, which can at times be difficult, depends upon discovering the head at the fundus and noting its absence from the lower part of the uterus or from the pelvic cavity.

Unless contra-indicated, external cephalic version should be attempted at or shortly after the thirty-second week. The dangers of this operation, when it is carried out gently and carefully, are negligible.

Should version fail, the best method of delivery must be decided upon. Here account should be taken of the size and shape of the maternal pelvis, the estimated size of the foetus, the past obstetric history and the possibility of placental insufficiency.

A breech delivery must always be conducted in a hospital. A consultant or registrar obstetrician, an anaesthetist and a paediatrician should be present for the birth of the baby.

To avoid anoxia or an over-large foetus, labour is often induced at or shortly before term.

While it is unnecessary to keep such patients in bed during the whole of the first stage of labour, the possibility of a prolapse of the cord must be remembered, especially if the breech is flexed.

An assisted breech delivery is the safest method of vaginal breech delivery and should always be aimed at.

This procedure involves the spontaneous expulsion of the breech, legs and trunk, following a wide episiotomy, the assisted delivery of the arms and the delivery of the head by one of several methods, of which the most suitable is that of jaw flexion and shoulder traction.

Following the birth of the head an oxytocic should be given. The third stage should then be conducted as in a normal labour.

Transverse and Oblique Lie

In a transverse or oblique lie the long axis of the foetus, instead of being parallel to that of the mother, is at or near a right angle to it.

The practical significance of this abnormality is that unless it can be corrected, spontaneous vaginal delivery is to all intents and purposes impossible.

The causes of a transverse lie are congenital uterine abnormalities, placenta praevia, fibroids, ovarian cysts, lax abdominal walls and hydramnios.

Diagnosis is reached by finding the fundus to be lower and broader than normal. On palpation, the head is felt to one side and the breech to the other. The foetal heart may be heard above the umbilicus.

A vaginal examination should not be carried out in such cases until a placenta praevia has been excluded.

The maternal dangers associated with a transverse lie are obstructed labour and rupture of the uterus. The foetal hazards are related to the maternal dangers and also to the difficulties presented by the delivery itself. In addition, prolapse of the cord is apt to occur.

Management depends upon the cause. Where the abnormal lie persists after the thirty-fourth week, admission to hospital should be arranged. If the lie remains uncorrected at the onset of labour, either version or Caesarean section will usually be necessary. Rarely, labour may be allowed to continue until cervical dilatation is sufficiently advanced to allow an internal version followed by a breech delivery.

Presentation and Prolapse of the Cord

The dangers of prolapse of the cord are almost entirely foetal. They consist mainly of oxygen deprivation due to compression of the cord. Spasm of the umbilical vessels plays a less important part.

The distinction between presentation and prolapse of the cord depends upon whether the membranes are intact or ruptured.

Prolapse of the cord is most likely to occur when the membranes rupture *during* labour.

Predisposing conditions to this accident are a badly fitting presenting part and hydramnios.

Diagnosis is made by seeing or feeling the prolapsed loop. The condition should be suspected if foetal distress develops suddenly in the course of an otherwise normal labour.

Nursing management depends upon whether the foetus is alive or dead. If alive, either delivery should be completed within ten to fifteen minutes or steps should be taken to relieve the pressure upon the cord while awaiting medical assistance.

Medical management usually consists of immediate delivery, either vaginal or by Caesarean section, following examination under anaesthesia in an operating theatre. Attempts at reposition of the cord are rarely successful.

CHAPTER ELEVEN

Abnormal Uterine Action

General Considerations

It will be remembered from page 173 that an essential feature of normal uterine action is of contractions which start in the region of the fundus and extend downwards into the lower segment. Although each contraction is followed by a period of relaxation, the special property of *retraction* prevents a complete return of the muscle of the upper part of the uterus to its original length. As a result, the cervix is first *taken up* and then gradually *dilated*, the lower segment thinning and stretching while the fundus becomes progressively shorter and thicker. Such uterine action is often spoken of as 'well-co-ordinated', as showing 'normal polarity' or of revealing 'fundal dominance'. In addition, for labour to proceed smoothly and rapidly, the contractions must be regular, frequent and strong.

From this it follows that abnormal uterine action could be of three different types:

1   Where the contractions, although normal in respect of co-ordination and polarity, are both weak and infrequent. This is usually called *Hypotonic Uterine Inertia*.

2   Where the contractions themselves are poorly co-ordinated, with disturbed polarity and absent fundal dominance. This state

of affairs is variously referred to as *Hypertonic Uterine Inertia*, disordered uterine action, colicky uterus or uncoordinated uterine action.

3 Where the contractions show normal polarity but are so frequent and so strong that they endanger the safety of the patient and of the foetus. This is known as *Precipitate Uterine Action*.

1 *Hypotonic Uterine Inertia* is seen both in primigravidae and in multiparae and is characterised chiefly by slow cervical dilatation. Labour is therefore prolonged. The weak and infrequent contractions, however, being almost painless, produce little maternal distress or exhaustion and the pulse and temperature therefore remain within normal limits. Dehydration and ketosis, however, may eventually appear due to insufficient intake or absorbtion of fluids or carbohydrates. The long intervals between contractions allow the placental circulation to be adequately maintained and foetal distress is thus not often seen. It is sometimes said that infection is liable to complicate these labours, due either to the long interval elapsing between rupture of the membranes and the delivery of the foetus, or to repeated vaginal examinations. In practice this complication is rarely encountered.

As a rule, in these patients, the cervix eventually becomes fully dilated and labour ends with a spontaneous vaginal delivery. Occasionally, however, operative interference, either vaginal or abdominal, may be indicated for maternal or foetal distress.

2 *Hypertonic Uterine Inertia* is almost entirely confined to primigravidae and is characterised by uterine contractions which are abnormal both in their site of origin and in the manner in which they spread. In such a case, various parts of the uterus seem to contract at different times. This results in much expenditure of effort but little progress. Relaxation is poor, polarity is lost and fundal dominance is absent. The uterine contractions are usually abnormally painful and the uterus is extremely tender. These various features lead to slow and

irregular cervical dilatation. Dehydration and ketosis are common and foetal and maternal distress tend to appear at an early stage.

In a typical case of hypertonic uterine inertia, owing to the strain imposed on the patient and the foetus, it is seldom possible to allow labour to continue for more than a few hours. In less severe cases cervical dilatation may eventually be complete and here a vaginal delivery, usually with the help of the forceps or the ventouse, will be possible.

3 *Precipitate Uterine Action* is a rare abnormality in which the contractions are so strong that labour is completed in a dangerously short time. The maternal risks of this type of abnormal uterine action are either rupture of the uterus or extensive cervical, vaginal or perineal lacerations, which may cause severe haemorrhage and shock. The chief foetal hazard is intracranial haemorrhage from the forceful and rapid passage of the unmoulded head through the maternal pelvis.

The Causes of Abnormal Uterine Action

So long as the reasons for normal uterine action remain unknown, it will be impossible to discover the precise causes of the three types of abnormality described above. However, conditions such as disproportion, malpresentations – especially occipito-posterior positions – and over-distension of the uterus by twins or hydramnios are often associated with some form of uterine inertia, either hypotonic or hypertonic. In these cases the presenting part, being badly-fitting, stimulates poor uterine contractions. So far as precipitate uterine action is concerned, no cause or associated factors have ever been described.

Prolonged Labour

Prolonged labour may be defined as labour lasting over twenty-four hours. Such a labour is always associated with some degree of uterine inertia since where the contractions are normal labour is either completed within this time or maternal or foetal distress develop and make interference necessary. Either hypertonic or hypotonic inertia may be seen in a prolonged labour. The former, however, is usually of a mild type since otherwise, as already pointed out, it is rarely possible to allow labour to continue for more than a few hours.

The Dangers of Prolonged Labour

1 *Maternal.* Dehydration and ketosis, being associated with uterine inertia, are liable to arise when labour is prolonged. These abnormalities result in maternal distress, revealed by a rising temperature and pulse rate. In such a case trauma and blood loss are poorly tolerated. Long labours are also associated with an increased incidence of post-partum haemorrhage.

2 *Foetal.* The chief foetal hazards of a prolonged labour are anoxia from placental insufficiency and trauma from a difficult delivery. These two conditions frequently coexist.

Management

1 Investigations
These may be subdivided into three groups:

a Those concerned with the nature of the uterine contractions

b Those concerned with the progress of labour

c Those concerned with the development of complications.

a Investigations Concerned with the Nature of the Uterine Contractions
The following features related to the uterine contractions should be noted at either half-hourly or hourly intervals:

i Their strength

ii Their frequency

iii   Their duration

iv   Their regularity

v   The amount of associated pain.

b   Investigations Concerned with the Progress of Labour
Although the nature of the contractions often provides a clue to
the progress of labour, this can be accurately assessed only by
vaginal examination. This should be carried out every four to six
hours, or even more frequently should an indication for this
arise. At each of these examinations the following points should
be noted:

i   The state of the cervix

ii   The degree of cervical dilatation

iii   The level of the presenting part

iv   The position of the presenting part

v   The degree of flexion of the head if it is presenting.

c   Investigations Concerned with the Development of Complications

i   *Foetal Distress.* In order to detect foetal distress at an early
stage, an hourly record of the foetal heart should be kept. In
hypotonic inertia, however, if the patient is asleep and if the
foetal heart rate has so far caused no concern, it need only be
checked two-hourly.

ii   *Maternal Distress.* The maternal pulse should be taken hourly
unless the patient is asleep. Her temperature and blood
pressure should be recorded four-hourly.

iii   *Dehydration.* This may result from a reduced fluid intake,
from loss of fluid by vomiting or excessive sweating, or from
a failure to absorb ingested water. The last of these three
causes is the one most usually present in a prolonged labour.
Since an early sign of dehydration is a diminished urinary
output, a fluid balance chart is the best way of revealing its
presence.

iv   *Ketosis.* This is usually due to a reduced carbohydrate intake
or to impaired absorbtion of food from the gut. For it to be

detected as early as possible, all specimens of urine passed or obtained by catheter must be tested for ketone bodies.

2   Treatment

a   General Nursing

In a prolonged labour, especially one associated with hypertonic inertia, it is important to maintain the patient's morale. Such cases need constant reassurance and security and should never be left alone for more than a few minutes at a time. The patient's well-being and comfort must always be borne in mind, care being taken over her general hygiene and attention paid to the state of the mouth, the face and the skin. Bright lighting and an over-heated room are particularly distressing and must be avoided. The state of the bladder must also be noted, a catheter being passed if there is any suspicion of urinary retention. The presence at the bed-side of a sympathetic but sensible husband, relative or friend can be of value in relieving the nursing staff of some of the more simple of these duties.

b   Special Measures

i   *Dehydration.* If the volume of urine passed in twelve hours falls below 500 ml, dehydration is probably present. As this is almost always due to impaired absorbtion, oral fluids are useless and indeed, by remaining in the stomach, may prove dangerous should an anaesthetic be needed later in labour. In such cases, therefore, fluids such as Normal Saline, 1/5 Normal Saline in 4·5 per cent Dextrose, or 5 per cent or 10 per cent Glucose in water may be given intravenously. Although the choice of solution and of the actual volume required are a doctor's responsibility, as a rough guide the first litre should be administered in between two and three hours, after which the rate may be reduced to one litre every eight to twelve hours.

ii   *Ketosis.* If ketosis is present in the absence of dehydration, intravenous administration of 5 per cent or 10 per cent Glucose solution will probably be the best form of treatment and is certainly preferable to giving sugar by mouth. This latter course carries with it the danger of inhalation of

K

the extremely irritating gastric contents should a general anaesthetic be needed later in labour.

iii *Sedation and Analgesia.* In considering whether a sedative or an analgesic is needed, it must first be decided whether the patient stands in need of rest or of relief from pain. This distinction must be recognised for treatment to be of value. *Sedation* is usually required in cases of hypotonic inertia, Chloral (2 grammes), Welldorm (tabs 2–3) or, rarely, a Barbiturate being of value here. Analgesics are particularly necessary in hypertonic inertia, very large doses being at times required to bring adequate relief, e.g., Pethidine, 150 mg initially followed by 100–150 mg two- to four-hourly. Morphia (15 mg) or Omnopon (20 mg) may be used as alternatives since they may also help to provide sleep.

iv *The Stimulation of Uterine Contractions.* In hypotonic inertia Syntocinon, given either intravenously or as Buccal Pitocin,* may be useful in improving the strength and frequency of the contractions. In hypertonic inertia, on the other hand, this drug is, generally speaking, useless and may even prove dangerous. Other methods applicable to either type of inertia consist of an enema, of particular value if the rectum is full, and of digital stretching of the cervix. These measures have the advantage of simplicity and safety.

Where Syntocinon or Pitocin are being given, particular attention must be paid to the uterine contractions and to the foetal heart, the drip being slowed or the mouth washed out and medical aid called should any abnormality be noticed.

Premature Labour: Precipitate Labour

Premature Labour

A premature labour was originally considered to be one resulting in the delivery of a baby weighing 2·5 kg or less. Nowadays this definition is not entirely accurate since many such babies are

* Since writing this the use of Buccal Pitocin has been abandoned.

small-for-dates rather than premature, pregnancy having reached or even progressed beyond term. It is therefore better to regard a premature labour as one which takes place before the start of the thirty-seventh week. This concept is more in accordance with present obstetric teaching and is therefore preferable to the original definition, despite its disadvantage that it presupposes an accurate knowledge of the patient's menstrual history.

Incidence

Premature labour occurs in about five per cent of all deliveries. Of greater importance is the fact that it is especially liable to occur in certain types of case, such as elderly primigravidae, grand multiparae, patients of low social class, unmarried mothers and twin pregnancies. A patient in any of these categories should therefore be warned that her labour may start some weeks before term.

Dangers

a   *Maternal.* Strictly speaking, there are no maternal hazards associated with premature labour. However, as the lie and presentation of the foetus are more likely to be abnormal in earlier pregnancy, this itself may lead to increased maternal dangers.

b   *Foetal.* The foetal dangers are those of an abnormal lie or presentation as mentioned above, those associated with the neonatal progress of a premature baby, and those of the passage of a poorly ossified head through the birth canal. Here the risk of intracranial haemorrhage is particularly high, the soft skull being often grossly distorted by pressure either from the bony pelvis or from the muscles of the pelvic floor.

Management

1   Since the baby will almost certainly need treatment in a Special Care Unit, a home confinement must, wherever possible,

be avoided. Should labour start at home, the patient's transfer to a properly equipped Maternity Unit must be arranged as soon as possible.

2   A doctor must be informed of the patient's arrival in hospital as it may be possible to stop the uterine contractions either with heavy sedation or with some specific product such as Isoxuprine. Measures of this sort, however, are of value only in very early labour; once the first stage is well established they are unlikely to prove effective and indeed the action of such drugs on the foetus may well prove an added hazard.

3   The conduct of labour differs from normal in two respects. In the first place, as already suggested, sedatives should be given with caution owing to their effect upon the foetus. Secondly, special care should be taken over the delivery of the head in order to minimise the risk of cerebral damage. Here a prophylactic episiotomy is of great value.

4   The care of the premature infant is discussed on page 387. Here it need only be mentioned that an injection of Vitamin K analogue – Synkavit or Konakion – should always be given immediately after delivery to reduce the risk of cerebral bleeding.

Precipitate Labour

It is sometimes said that any labour lasting for less than two hours is precipitate. This view is unacceptable since the vast majority of such labours are otherwise perfectly normal. A precipitate labour, therefore, is one which occupies an even shorter space of time and which is characterised by extremely powerful contractions of which a very small number are sufficient to complete all three stages.

Incidence

While precise figures are not available, the incidence of precipitate labour is probably extremely low.

Dangers

1 *Maternal*. These are principally due to the abnormally strong contractions. To a lesser extent they are related to the hazards associated with the unusual and unsatisfactory places of confinement so often forced upon these patients. They may be summarised as follows:

a *Uterine Rupture*. Usually in the lower segment or in some previously weakened area of uterine muscle.

b *Cervical Lacerations*. Forcible stretching of the cervix replaces the normal mechanism of safe dilatation.

c *Rupture of the Vagina and Perineum*. The presenting part being forced through the birth canal in too short a time to allow for its proper stretching.

d *Shock, Haemorrhage and Sepsis:* Owing to the above complications, these are more liable to arise than in a normal labour.

2 *Foetal*

a The main foetal complication is *Cerebral Haemorrhage*. This is usually due to forcible distortion of the head and the enclosed brain from the excessively rapid delivery.

b The fact that delivery often occurs with extreme suddenness can mean that the foetus falls to the floor. Alternatively, it is deposited in a lavatory bowl, the patient being under the impression that she was about to have a violent bowel action.

c A further foetal hazard is that birth often occurs in a place and among people where no obstetric care is immediately available. In consequence, resuscitation may be impossible.

Management

Owing to the rapidity with which labour is completed in these cases, little in the way of obstetric management can ever be provided.

a Where the patient gives a past history of precipitate labour, arrangements should be made for her admission to hospital during the last weeks of pregnancy to avoid the possibility of delivery occurring in an unsuitable place.

b A doctor should be called as soon as labour starts since what management as is possible will consist of reducing the strength of the contractions by strong sedation or with a general anaesthetic.

c A generous episiotomy may reduce the risk both of severe trauma to the lower genital tract and of cerebral haemorrhage.

d A prophylactic injection of Synkavit or Konakion should be given to the baby at birth.

It need hardly be stressed that in no circumstances whatsoever should the patient be left alone during labour.

If outside hospital, the midwife should, in an emergency, proceed as follows:

a Arrange either for a doctor and an ambulance or for the Emergency Obstetric Unit to be called

b Deliver the patient as safely as the facilities permit

c Arrange for the mother's transfer to hospital after delivery so that any trauma may be properly treated.

Transfer to hospital *during* labour should be avoided unless it is clear that the foetus will not be born until the patient's arrival in the labour ward. An ambulance is one of the worst places in which to conduct a delivery.

Summary

General Considerations

Normal uterine contractions are strong, regular and frequent. Starting at the fundus they spread downwards to the lower segment. Each contraction is followed by a period of relaxation. Such uterine action is spoken of as being well-co-ordinated.

Abnormal Uterine Action is of three main types:

a Where the contractions are well-co-ordinated but weak and infrequent. This is known as Hypotonic Uterine Inertia.

b Where the contractions are poorly-co-ordinated. This is called Hypertonic Uterine Inertia.

c Where the contractions are abnormally strong and frequent. This is Precipitate Uterine Action.

Hypotonic uterine inertia is characterised by slow cervical dilatation and prolonged labour. The maternal and foetal conditions remain good. As a rule cervical dilatation eventually occurs and labour ends with a vaginal delivery, either spontaneous or operative.

Hypertonic uterine inertia consists of uncoordinated and painful contractions. Cervical dilatation is slow and irregular. The maternal and foetal conditions soon deteriorate and dehydration and ketosis are common. In severe cases it is rarely possible to allow labour to last for more than a few hours. In milder instances a vaginal delivery may eventually become possible.

Precipitate uterine action results in dangerously rapid labour. Rupture of the uterus and extensive lacerations of the lower genital tract are common maternal dangers. Cerebral haemorrhage is a frequent foetal complication.

The causes of abnormal uterine action are not known. Some cases of hypotonic and hypertonic inertia appear to be associated with a badly-fitting presenting part.

Prolonged Labour

Prolonged labour is labour lasting over twenty-four hours. It is always associated with some degree of uterine inertia.

The maternal dangers of prolonged labour are dehydration and ketosis. These predispose in their turn to maternal distress. Post-partum haemorrhage is another complication. The foetal hazards are anoxia and trauma.

The investigations necessary in such cases may be subdivided into three groups:

a Those concerned with the nature of the contractions

b Those concerned with the progress of labour

c Those concerned with the development of maternal or foetal complications.

The nursing care of such cases includes consideration of the patient's general well-being, comfort and morale. Attention must also be paid to the state of the bladder.

Dehydration requires the intravenous infusion of saline, dextrose saline or glucose solution. Ketosis is treated by giving glucose intravenously.

Cases of hypotonic inertia usually need sedation rather than analgesia. Where hypertonic inertia is present, analgesics rather than sedatives are called for.

In hypotonic inertia the uterine contractions may be stimulated by intravenous Syntocinon or by Buccal Pitocin. Such measures are generally contra-indicated in hypertonic inertia. Less sophisticated and safer means of increasing the power of the uterine contractions are an enema and digital dilatation of the cervix.

Premature Labour: Precipitate Labour

Labour is premature when it starts before the thirty-seventh week of pregnancy. This definition is preferable to one based upon the weight of the baby – 2·5 kg or less.

Premature labour is particularly likely to occur in multiple pregnancies, elderly primigravidae, grand multiparae, women of poor social class and unmarried mothers.

There are no purely maternal dangers associated with premature labour. The foetal dangers are related in part to the delivery and in part to the subsequent care of the delicate premature infant.

Since the premature infant requires special neo-natal care and supervision, it should always be delivered in a hospital equipped with a Special Care Unit.

The conduct of labour differs from normal in that sedatives and analgesics must be given with caution and that a routine episiotomy should be performed to reduce the risk of trauma to the soft foetal head. Synkavit or Konakion should be given to the baby after birth.

Precipitate labour is characterised by unduly strong contractions, only a few of which are needed to complete all stages of labour.

Rupture of the uterus, extensive lacerations of the cervix, vagina and perineum, together with shock and haemorrhage are common maternal complications.

Foetal dangers include cerebral haemorrhage and trauma with anoxia from delivery in an unsuitable place lacking nursing and medical facilities.

Management consists of controlling the strength of the uterine contractions with heavy sedation or a general anaesthetic, together with a wide episiotomy to reduce trauma to the lower genital tract and to the foetal head.

In an emergency situation, the midwife should deliver her patient as well as circumstances allow and then arrange for her transfer to hospital.

CHAPTER TWELVE

Other Abnormalities of Labour

Multiple Pregnancy

Although not as frequently encountered as either an occipito-posterior position or a breech presentation, a multiple pregnancy is still one of the more common abnormalities of pregnancy and labour, occurring in about 1·2 per cent of cases. Much of its importance from the midwife's point of view lies in the fact that since a correct diagnosis is often not made until late in labour, the actual delivery is often her direct responsibility.

Definition

A Multiple Pregnancy is one in which two or more foetuses are present, twins, triplets or quadruplets. A twin pregnancy is one in which there are only two foetuses present. However, since triplet and, especially, quadruplet pregnancies are extremely rare, the two terms are to a large extent interchangeable.

Types of Twins

Twins may be 'Like' – Uniovular – or 'Unlike' – Binovular. The former are due to the early separation of a single ovum into two equal halves, the foetuses then being of the same sex and similar in every respect. The more common binovular twins develop from the simultaneous fertilisation of two different ova and thus resemble each other no more than would any two children born to the same parents. Uniovular twins appear to be at greater risk during pregnancy and labour than binovular, but since the type of twins cannot be recognised until after delivery, this fact is of no practical importance.

Maternal and Foetal Hazards

Although almost every known obstetric complication has been attributed at one time or another to a multiple pregnancy, the dangers may be simplified and more easily understood if considered along the following lines:

1   The main risk to the foetus is that of Prematurity, both by dates and by weight, nearly half of all twins weighing less than 2·5 kg at birth. The fact that the majority of these prematures are comparatively large accounts for the relatively low perinatal mortality rate of about twelve per cent in this group. That this is still a high figure is shown by the finding that the perinatal loss among mature twins is only about two per cent. It follows that if the high prematurity rate in multiple pregnancies could be reduced the perinatal mortality would be considerably lower.

2   The other foetal risks of twin pregnancies are associated in part with certain of the maternal complications and in part with difficulties encountered at delivery. The latter are largely due to the high incidence of abnormal presentations in these cases.

3   The maternal hazards can be divided into three groups, depending upon whether they arise in pregnancy, labour or the puerperium. They may be summarised as follows:

a   *In Pregnancy*
Premature rupture of the membranes
Premature onset of labour

Pre-eclampsia – usually mild and of late onset

Ante-Partum Haemorrhage – both accidental and unavoidable

Hydramnios – especially with uniovular twins

Anaemia – both iron deficiency and megaloblastic.

b *In Labour*
Prolonged labour
Operative delivery
Post-Partum Haemorrhage.

c *In the Puerperium*
Anaemia
Infection
Phlebothrombosis.

Despite the length and sinister appearance of this list, it should be emphasised that the very great majority of patients succeed in passing through pregnancy and labour without developing any of the conditions mentioned above and that the maternal morbidity associated with a twin pregnancy is only slightly greater than normal.

Diagnosis

Since the outcome for the patient as well as for the foetuses depends upon proper management during pregnancy as well as in labour, it is important to reach a correct diagnosis not later than the thirtieth or thirty-second week. This diagnosis is based upon the following features:

1 There is often a *family history* of twins, involving either the parents, the grandparents or other siblings.

2 The uterus is larger than the dates would suggest. Alternative conditions related to this finding are discussed on page 144.

3 More than two foetal poles – head or breech – may be felt. If only two poles are palpable, these may be too close together to belong to a single foetus.

4   If only one head is felt, it may seem to be unduly small in relation to the apparent size of the foetus.

5   In many cases a mass of apparently unrelated and unrecognisable foetal parts is all that can be made out. This is a valuable sign since it is rarely encountered in singleton pregnancies.

6   At times two foetal hearts may be heard, but in order to distinguish these from one heart heard in two separate places, two observers must listen simultaneously and record a difference in rates of at least fifteen beats a minute.

7   When in doubt, an X-ray examination will settle the question. This of course can be ordered only by a doctor, who in any event must be informed whenever a multiple pregnancy is suspected.

Management in Pregnancy

The principles of management during pregnancy are:

1   To reduce the incidence of prematurity

2   To prevent the development of maternal complications.

1   It is often said that the prematurity rate of twins may be reduced by resting the mother in hospital from the thirty-second week to the thirty-sixth week. The arguments upon which this idea is based are not, however, entirely sound and its real value has never been proved. Moreover the social difficulties arising from such a course of action are often considerable. For these reasons, many obstetricians now advise admission only for those patients in whom a genuine obstetric indication for hospital treatment has arisen.

2   While the development of maternal abnormalities cannot always be prevented, careful and frequent ante-natal supervision

will usually reduce their extent. For that reason, all twin pregnancies should be seen weekly after the thirty-second week, a careful watch being kept for the development of pre-eclampsia and hydramnios and the patient being closely questioned at each visit about any vaginal bleeding, however slight.

Lastly, since there is evidence that the perinatal mortality starts to rise after the thirty-eighth week, no twin pregnancy should be allowed to go beyond term.

The Presentation of the Foetuses

Although the most common way in which twins present is as two vertices, this particular combination is only met with in about forty per cent of cases. This implies that either the first or the second or both foetuses will present abnormally in a majority of instances. The frequency with which the various presentations are seen is as follows:

Twin 1	Twin 2	Per cent
Vertex	Vertex	44
Vertex	Breech	30
Breech	Vertex	10
Breech	Breech	9
Other Combinations		7

Management in Labour: General Remarks

It goes without saying that all twin labours should be conducted in hospital, where medical aid can, if necessary, be secured at once. Moreover, the second stage should never be completed without the presence in the labour ward of an experienced obstetrician, an anaesthetist and a paediatrician. The reason for these precautions is the high incidence of prematurity, of malpresentations and of post-partum haemorrhage seen in these cases.

The First Stage

The management of the first stage of a twin labour does not differ greatly from that of a normal labour. Particular care should be taken to guard against an unsuspected prolapse of the cord, particularly when the membranes rupture, while oral feeding should be severely restricted in view of the likelihood of a general anaesthetic being needed for delivery.

The Second Stage

As soon as the cervix is fully dilated the patient must be transferred to the labour ward and a consultant or registrar obstetrician and the duty anaesthetist and paediatrician informed. Preparations for an operative delivery and for a general anaesthetic should, of course, have already been made.

In the event of no doctor being available, due either to misdiagnosis or to the unduly rapid advance of labour, the midwife should proceed as follows:

1   The method of delivery of the first twin should be similar to that adopted for a singleton foetus, whether presenting by the head or by the breech.

2   An episiotomy should always be performed, partly in case of difficulty arising over the birth of the second twin and partly because of the probable prematurity of the foetuses.

3   After the birth of the first twin the cord is divided between clamps and the baby passed to an assistant for resuscitation.

4   The patient's abdomen is now palpated to determine the lie and presentation of the second foetus. A vaginal examination should be made to confirm these findings.

5   If the lie is transverse, version is carried out, either the head or, preferably, the breech, being made to present.

6   The foetal heart should then be auscultated.

7   If uterine contractions do not start again within ten minutes, the forewaters should be ruptured.

8   Little difficulty is usually experienced over the delivery of the second twin, since by now the maternal soft parts have been widely stretched.

9   An oxytocic, preferably Syntometrine – 1 ml – should be given either intravenously or intramuscularly with the crowning of the head or the birth of the anterior shoulder of the second twin.

10   Owing to the high incidence of post-partum haemorrhage in these cases, special care is needed in the management of the third stage of labour.

Disproportion

Disproportion is present when there is not enough room for the foetal head to pass safely through the maternal pelvis. In the not too distant past it was one of the most common abnormalities of labour. Today, owing to improvements in nutrition during childhood and adolescence, together with the recent reduction in the incidence of bony disease, it is seldom seen.

Causes

Disproportion may be of either maternal or foetal origin.

1   *Maternal.* Here the shape and size of the pelvis are inadequate for the passage of a foetal head of normal size presenting in a normal manner. Examples of this are:

a   Alterations in the pelvis from hereditary, environmental or nutritional causes

b   Diseases of the pelvis such as tuberculosis

c   Deformities of the pelvis such as those caused by serious fractures *d* Deformities in the spine or lower limbs. These lead to compensatory alteration in the shape of the pelvis and could result from poliomyelitis, congenital dislocation of the hip or Perthé's disease.

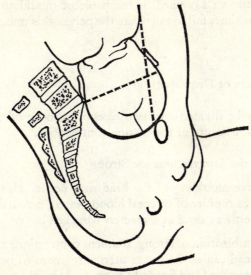

Fig. 43 Disproportion: lateral view of pelvis and head

It is often said that disproportion is common in women under 150 cm in height. If those cases where such short stature is due to disease or malnutrition are excluded, this statement is probably untrue. Although the pelvis may be small in such women, they usually have small babies.

2 *Foetal.* Here the head is too large to pass safely through a pelvis of normal size and shape.

a In theory, a foetus may have an abnormally large head for purely genetic reasons. In practice this is rarely seen.

b The size of the foetus, including that of its head, may be increased in pre-diabetes and diabetes mellitus.

c Congenital malformations such as hydrocephalus result in a greatly enlarged head.

d Abnormally large diameters of engagement are encountered in deflexed occipito-posterior positions, brow and incompletely extended face presentations. These may result in disproportion.

Although it is taught that the skull of the 'postmature' foetus, being unduly well ossified, is incapable of moulding and will therefore at times fail to negotiate the pelvis, this must be a rare event.

The Dangers of Disproportion

These may be divided into two categories, both of which are related to the nature of the uterine contractions.

1 Where the Contractions are Strong

a Excessive moulding of the head may occur. This can lead ultimately to rupture of cerebral blood vessels, cerebral haemorrhage and either a dead or a severely damaged baby.

b The combination of strong, frequent contractions and a non-engaged head causes the lower uterine segment to become abnormally stretched and finally to rupture. As might be expected, this accident carries a high maternal and foetal mortality.

c By reducing the placental blood-flow, the uterine contractions cause foetal anoxia to develop. If untreated, this may lead to intra-uterine death of the foetus.

2 Where the Contractions are Weak
Here the large head, remaining above the pelvic brim, constitutes a badly fitting presenting part. As such it predisposes to premature rupture of the membranes, weak uterine contractions, prolonged labour and prolapse of the cord.

Diagnosis

In view of its associated dangers, disproportion should be confirmed or excluded at the thirty-sixth-week examination so that time may be available for deciding upon the best method of delivery. If at this examination the foetal head is either engaged or can be made to engage by applying supra-pubic pressure, disproportion is absent, since it is practically never confined to the pelvic outlet.

If, however, the head is not engaged and cannot be made to enter the pelvic brim, disproportion *may* be present. In such a case a vaginal examination is necessary to determine the size and the shape of the lower cavity and of the outlet of the pelvis. If these are normal, it is unlikely that the brim will be significantly abnormal. If the opposite is the case, it is *possible* that the brim will also be smaller than normal.

It should be unnecessary to add that the responsibility for such a decision rests entirely in the hands of the doctor in charge of the case.

Subsequent Management

1 *X-ray Pelvimetry.* Although it might be supposed that an X-ray of the pelvis would be necessary whenever disproportion was suspected, such an examination is of little value before the onset of labour. The reason for this is that if disproportion is severe it will be easily recognised clinically while if it is only slight an X-ray will not tell whether it could be safely overcome by head moulding during labour. X-ray pelvimetry is thus of greater value during labour in cases where clinical examination yields equivocal results.

2 *Elective Caesarean Section.* An elective Caesarean section is usually carried out at or shortly after the thirty-eighth week if there is no prospect of a safe vaginal delivery.

Management in Labour

a Where it is thought that vaginal delivery may be possible pregnancy is usually allowed to proceed until term, induction being then carried out to avoid the risk of placental insufficiency which so often arises when pregnancy is prolonged.

b Since disproportion is an entirely medical responsibility, a doctor must be informed when labour has started.

c Close supervision during labour is essential. The dangers of foetal and maternal distress for reasons such as prolapse of the cord, excessive head moulding and undue distension of the lower segment, characterised by supra-pubic pain and tenderness, must be borne in mind. This applies particularly to those cases where the contractions are strong and engagement of the head delayed.

d Vaginal examinations to assess the degree of engagement and descent of the foetal head and the extent of cervical dilatation are usually carried out by a doctor. Where delegated to a midwife, careful note must be made of the level, the position and the degree of flexion of the head, the amount of caput formation and the state of the cervix.

e If the foetal head engages and foetal and maternal distress do not supervene, a spontaneous vertex delivery may be expected. If, despite engagement of the head and full cervical dilatation, distress develops, an operative vaginal delivery will be called for. If foetal or maternal distress arises before engagement or full cervical dilatation, Caesarean section is usually the treatment of choice.

Trial of Labour

In the past, cases of disproportion were often subjected to what was known as a Trial of Labour. This term implied that labour was allowed to take place under special conditions of supervision and management with the object of determining whether the foetal head would engage or not. Nowadays, such Trials of Labour in their strictest sense are regarded as out-of-date and unnecessary and are rarely if ever carried out. The phrase, however, is still sometimes used to denote the method of managing disproportion as outlined in this chapter.

Foetal Distress: Maternal Distress: Obstructed Labour

These three complications may arise either during the first or the second stage of labour. The hazards they present to the patient and to the foetus are such that they must be regarded as serious obstetric emergencies.

Foetal Distress

Foetal distress is a sign that the foetus is suffering from anoxia which, if not rapidly relieved, may cause its death. Although some hospitals now possess sophisticated monitoring apparatus for the early detection of foetal distress, this is not generally available and conventional means of diagnosis must therefore still be studied.

The Signs of Foetal Distress

1   Alteration in the Foetal Heart Rate
The following alterations in the rate of the foetal heart are indicative of foetal distress:

a   A drop to below 100 or a rise to over 160 beats a minute.

b   Temporary slowing *between* contractions

c   Although of lesser importance, variations in rate of a lesser degree than those indicated above or temporary slowing *during* contractions still suggest that foetal oxygenation may be deficient.

2   Alterations in the Rhythm of the Foetal Heart Rate
Here the actual *rate* may be within normal limits but the *rhythm* is irregular.

3   The Passage of Meconium
This is a less reliable sign than those involving the foetal heart rate. The reason for this is that meconium may be passed but not

revealed, either because the membranes are intact or because of the close fit of the presenting part in the pelvis.

4 Tumultuous Foetal Movements
These usually indicate that the foetus is on the point of death.

It is sometimes said that an alteration in the *intensity* of the foetal heart sounds is suggestive of distress. This is untrue and no attention need be paid to this particular sign.

Conditions Often Associated with Foetal Distress

Although foetal distress may develop during any labour, no matter how normally it may seem to be progressing, it is more likely to complicate the following conditions:

1 Placental Insufficiency

a Where pregnancy has been prolonged beyond term, especially past forty-two weeks

b Where the foetus is small-for-dates

c Where there is a history of ante-partum haemorrhage or of bleeding in early pregnancy

d Where pregnancy has been complicated by pre-eclampsia, eclampsia, essential hypertension or unexplained albuminuria

e Where the patient is an elderly primigravida – over 35 years of age.

2 Abnormal Labour

a Where the first or second stages are abnormally prolonged

b Where hypertonic uterine inertia is present

c Where the presenting part fails to engage despite strong contractions

d Where the cord prolapses.

Maternal Distress

Maternal distress is less common than foetal distress. It is also less common than might be supposed from the behaviour of some women in labour. It should be diagnosed only when one or both of the following signs are present:

1 A pulse rate of over 100 beats a minute

2 A temperature of over 37·2°C.

Although maternal distress is often accompanied by dehydration and ketosis, and indeed is exacerbated by these conditions, it can exist in their absence. In the same way, dehydration and ketosis are often seen in the absence of true maternal distress.

It is sometimes said that a rise in the maternal blood pressure is a sign of distress. This is not so.

Conditions Often Associated with Maternal Distress

1 Where the Resistance of the Patient is Lowered

a In older patients, especially Elderly Primigravidae

b Where the patient is suffering from some serious systemic disease such as cardiac or pulmonary disease, or where there is a severe degree of anaemia

c Where dehydration and ketosis are present.

2 Where Labour has Become Abnormal

a Where the first or second stage is abnormally prolonged

b Where hypertonic uterine inertia is present

c Where labour has become obstructed.

Obstructed Labour

Labour is said to be obstructed when no advance occurs despite strong uterine contractions. This may occur either during the first stage or, more usually, during the second, when it is more serious and requires more urgent treatment.

Diagnosis

In the first stage, an obstructed labour may be diagnosed if the presenting part fails to engage or if the cervix fails to dilate. In the second stage it must be taken to be present if the presenting part fails to advance. The time which may be allowed to elapse before reaching a diagnosis depends upon the maternal condition and the strength and frequency of the uterine contractions. As a rule this should not be more than one to two hours in the first stage and twenty to thirty minutes in the second.

Dangers

The dangers of an obstructed labour are:

1 The rapid development of foetal distress from placental ischaemia

2 Cerebral damage from over-moulding of the foetal head

3 Severe maternal distress, often leading to shock and collapse

4 Rupture of the uterus.

The Management of Foetal and Maternal Distress

1 As soon as either of these conditions arises, an immediate examination, both abdominal and vaginal, must be carried out.

This will serve to determine, if possible, the cause of the distress and to exclude prolapse of the cord.

2　Medical help must now be sent for urgently.

3　The doctor in charge of the case will consider the degree of distress and the point to which labour has advanced. He must then decide whether:

a　To deliver the patient at once, or

b　To treat the distress conservatively in the hope that full cervical dilatation will occur rapidly enough to allow a vaginal delivery.

If immediate delivery is indicated, this will either be by Caesarean section or with the forceps, depending upon the nature, position and engagement of the presenting part and the state of the cervix. Owing to the time needed for its application, the ventouse is seldom of use in these cases.

If it is decided to allow labour to proceed, the following steps must be taken:

1　Careful and frequent monitoring of the maternal and foetal conditions is necessary, the pulse being recorded half-hourly and the foetal heart rate quarter- to half-hourly.

2　Dehydration and ketosis must be corrected.

3　Strong sedatives and analgesics are contra-indicated owing to the possibility of having to deliver the foetus at short notice.

4　An attempt may be made to improve the supply of oxygen to the foetus by giving oxygen to the patient by means of a face-mask. Alternatively, the placental blood flow may be improved by the intravenous infusion of a plasma expander such as Rheomacrodex.

Summary

Multiple Pregnancy

A twin pregnancy, although not so common as an occipito-posterior position or a breech presentation, is still fairly frequently encountered.

Twins may be either uniovular – derived from the same ovum – or binovular – arising from separate ova. Uniovular twins are similar in all respects. Binovular twins resemble one another no more closely than other members of the same family.

The main foetal hazard of a twin pregnancy is prematurity. Nearly half of all twins weigh 2·5 kg or less at birth. The perinatal mortality in this group is several times larger than that associated with mature twins.

Other foetal risks are associated in part with the various maternal hazards and in part with difficulties encountered at delivery.

A variety of maternal hazards may arise either in pregnancy, labour or the puerperium. The great majority of patients, however, succeed in passing unscathed through pregnancy and labour.

Diagnosis is reached on the basis of the family history, abdominal palpation, auscultation of two foetal hearts and X-ray examination.

The principles of management during pregnancy are to reduce the incidence of prematurity and to prevent, by careful antenatal supervision, the development of maternal complications.

All twin labours must be conducted in hospital. An experienced obstetrician, an anaesthetist and a paediatrician should be present for the delivery of the foetuses.

In the management of the first stage of labour, special care should be taken to detect prolapse of the cord, while oral feeding should be drastically reduced in view of the possibility of a general anaesthetic being later required.

In the event of a midwife having to conduct the delivery unaided, particular attention should be paid to the need for an episiotomy, the correction of the lie and presentation of the second twin, early rupture of the forewaters of the second sac, the administration of an oxytocic at the delivery of the second twin and the careful management of the third stage in view of the frequency of post-partum haemorrhage in such cases.

Disproportion

Although in the past disproportion was one of the most common abnormalities of labour, it is now far less frequently encountered owing to improved standards of health and nutrition.

Disproportion may be of either maternal or foetal origin. Maternal causes include alterations in the size and shape of the pelvis from hereditary factors as well as from diseases or deformities involving either the pelvis itself, the lower limbs or the spine.

Disproportion of foetal origin may be due to an abnormally large head or to a normally sized head presenting by abnormally large diameters.

If the uterine contractions are strong, the dangers of disproportion are cerebral haemorrhage, foetal anoxia and rupture of the uterus. If the contractions are weak, premature rupture of the membranes, prolonged labour and prolapse of the cord are likely complications.

Disproportion should either be confirmed or excluded at the thirty-sixth-week examination. If, at this time, the foetal head is engaged, it is absent. If the head cannot be made to engage it may be present. In such a case clinical assessment of the pelvis may allow a correct diagnosis to be reached.

Where there is no prospect of a safe vaginal delivery, elective Caesarean section is the best treatment. If vaginal delivery appears possible, labour may be induced at the fortieth week to avoid the risk of placental insufficiency.

If the head engages and dilatation of the cervix proceeds normally, a vaginal delivery may be expected. If foetal or maternal distress develops before engagement or full dilatation, section is usually the treatment of choice.

Foetal Distress: Maternal Distress: Obstructed Labour

Foetal distress is a sign that the foetus is suffering from anoxia. This, if not speedily corrected, may cause its death.

The signs of foetal distress consist of alterations in the rate and rhythm of the foetal heart, the passage of meconium and, as a terminal event, tumultuous foetal movements.

Conditions associated with foetal distress are related to placental insufficiency, prolonged labour, disproportion and prolapse of the cord.

Maternal distress is characterised by a rise in pulse rate and in body temperature, often accompanied by dehydration and ketosis. A rise in blood pressure is *not* a sign of maternal distress.

Conditions particularly associated with maternal distress are age, serious systemic diseases, prolonged labour, hypertonic uterine inertia and obstructed labour.

Labour is obstructed when no advance takes place despite good contractions.

In the first stage, such a complication is revealed by failure of the presenting part to engage or of the cervix to dilate. In the second stage it is present if the presenting part fails to advance.

The dangers of obstructed labour are foetal distress, cerebral haemorrhage, maternal distress and rupture of the uterus.

The management of either foetal or maternal distress consists of a full abdominal and vaginal examination to determine, if possible, the cause of the distress. Medical aid must be called immediately.

The doctor in charge of the case will decide whether to deliver the patient at once or to treat the distress conservatively.

If the latter course is adopted, careful and frequent checking of the maternal and foetal conditions is necessary. Any dehydration or ketosis present must be corrected. In view of the possibility of early delivery, strong sedatives or analgesics should be withheld.

CHAPTER THIRTEEN

Abnormalities of the Third Stage

Post-partum Haemorrhage from the Placental Site

For a midwife, the importance of the various abnormalities of the third stage of labour is related to the following features:

1 They are relatively common, even in otherwise normal labours

2 They tend to arise suddenly and unexpectedly

3 The hazards they present to the patient are often serious and may even at times result in her death

4 They are frequently avoidable. Hospital reports show that about half of all fatalities attributable to post-partum haemorrhage might have been prevented had reasonable precautions been taken.

It follows that abnormalities of the third stage may arise in labours conducted by midwives and that treatment may have to be started while awaiting the arrival of a doctor. For that reason, an understanding of the causes and of the management of these abnormalities is necessary if serious accidents are to be avoided.

The three complications to be considered in this chapter are Post-partum Haemorrhage, Retention of the Placenta and Inversion of the Uterus. Of these, the first is by far the most important owing to the frequency with which it is still encountered and because of the dangers it presents to the patient.

Post-partum Haemorrhage

Post-partum haemorrhage may be either primary or secondary. Primary post-partum haemorrhage is bleeding from the birth canal of 500 ml or more, occurring after the birth of the baby until twenty-four hours after the delivery of the placenta. Secondary post-partum haemorrhage is abnormal bleeding from the genital tract occurring during the puerperium after the first twenty-four hours. Since this is a complication of the puerperium rather than of labour, it is considered on page 367.

Primary Post-partum Haemorrhage

1   Dangers
The most immediate dangers of post-partum haemorrhage are shock and collapse from excessive blood loss. More remote hazards include sepsis, anaemia, chronic ill-health and impaired lactation.

2   The Source of the Bleeding
Post-partum haemorrhage may arise either from the placental site or, less commonly, from extra-placental sources such as uterine, cervical, vaginal or perineal lacerations. In the present section only the first of these will be considered.

3   Incidence
The incidence of post-partum haemorrhage depends both upon the management of the third stage and upon the accuracy with which blood loss is measured. Its reported frequency thus varies widely from centre to centre. In general, a post-partum haemorrhage complicates about three per cent of all deliveries in which

an oxytocic is given either at the end of the second stage or at the start of the third. When no such drug is given, abnormally heavy bleeding occurs in between five and ten per cent of all labours.

4 Management

Most cases of post-partum haemorrhage result from some disturbance of the normal process of placental separation and expulsion. They thus depend for their treatment on the correction of such disturbances. For this reason, the consideration of the causes and management of these haemorrhages should start with a review of the normal physiology of the third stage of labour.

Review of the Physiology of the Third Stage of Labour

The third stage of labour consists of two main events:

1 The separation and expulsion of the placenta

2 The control of bleeding from the placental site.

1 *The separation and expulsion of the placenta* is brought about by:

a Contraction and retraction of the uterine muscle. This reduces the area of the placental site and forces the placenta off the uterine wall.

b This process of separation is assisted by pressure from the retro-placental haematoma.

c The detached placenta acts as a foreign body, stimulating the uterus to contract and to expel it.

    Separation of the placenta is normally completed within a few minutes of the birth of the foetus.

2 *Haemorrhage is controlled* by:

a Contraction of the myometrial bundles around the vessels running to the placental site. This reduces the blood flow through them.

b The increased thickness of the uterine wall stretches these vessels and reduces their lumen.

c The formation of a firm clot in the mouths of these vessels.

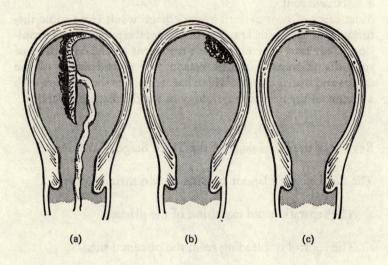

(a)   (b)   (c)

Fig. 44   The causes of post-partum haemorrhage

The Causes of Post-partum Haemorrhage

Since a post-partum haemorrhage usually results from some disturbance of the above process, it follows that the basic reasons for such haemorrhage could be:

1   Faulty and incomplete separation of the placenta

2   Retention of part of the placenta

3   Atony of the uterus following separation and expulsion of the placenta

4   Clotting defects in the maternal blood.

1 Faulty and Incomplete Separation of the Placenta
This is usually due to weak and inefficient uterine contraction
and retraction, as a result of which the placenta is incompletely
severed from its attachments. Even where the placenta is
separated and lying free in the cavity of the uterus, the contractions may not be strong enough to expel it into the vagina.
The placental site cannot, therefore, contract down in the usual
way; the mouths of the vessels running to it are kept open and
bleeding results.

2 Retention of Part of the Placenta
At times a part of the placenta may be detached from the main
mass and either fail to separate or, having separated, remain
within the uterine cavity. In either event the result is the same as
when the entire placenta is retained, save that the bleeding is as a
rule less severe.

3 Atony of the Uterus following Separation and Expulsion of
the Placenta
Here the main factor responsible for closing the vessels running
to the placental site, namely contraction of the myometrial
bundles, is absent. Bleeding therefore occurs.

4 Clotting Defects in the Maternal Blood
The most common clotting defect is Afibrinogenaemia – a reduction in the amount of Fibrinogen in the circulating blood. If
this complication is present bleeding will start whenever the
uterus relaxes, no matter how slightly.

Predisposing Factors to Post-partum Haemorrhage

It is often taught that uterine exhaustion predisposes to faulty
action during the third stage of labour. Exhaustion of this sort is
usually attributed to a number of widely differing conditions
such as grand multiparity, chronic medical diseases, long labour,
precipitate labour, ante-partum haemorrhage and drugs given
during labour. In practice, however, there are only four important predisposing factors to post-partum haemorrhage, none
of which is obviously related to the above states.

L

1   General Anaesthesia
This presumably acts by interfering with normal uterine action.

2   Multiple Pregnancy
Although the precise reasons for the high incidence of post-partum haemorrhage in multiple pregnancies is not known, several factors are probably involved. Among these are the greatly increased area of the placental site and the frequency with which a general anaesthetic is needed for the delivery of one or other of the foetuses.

3   Faulty Retraction of the Placental Site
Bleeding from this cause is seen if the placenta is implanted in a relatively inactive part of the uterus, such as the lower segment – Placenta Praevia.

4   Mismanagement of the Third Stage
Repeated and unnecessary manipulation of the uterus immediately after the birth of the foetus encourages faulty uterine action and hence post-partum haemorrhage.

The Prevention of Post-partum Haemorrhage

Although not all post-partum haemorrhages can be avoided, much may be done to reduce the incidence and severity of this complication if the following principles are observed:

1   All women likely to have a post-partum haemorrhage must be delivered in hospital, a doctor being present for the whole of the second and third stages of labour. This rule applies particularly to patients with a past history of this complication, since the factors responsible for the original haemorrhage are likely to recur.

2   Maternal distress, dehydration and ketosis arising during labour must be detected and treated promptly.

3   Wherever possible, pudendal block or local infiltration analgesia are preferable to general anaesthesia.

4 The most important requirement of all, however, is the correct management of the third stage. Unnecessary manipulation of the fundus and forceful efforts at placental expression must be avoided and the placenta delivered by controlled cord traction after the administration of an oxytocic at the end of the second stage.

The Management of a Post-partum Haemorrhage

The main difficulty in treating a case of post-partum haemorrhage is that so much has apparently to be done in so short a time. For this reason it is best to act in accordance with a few fundamental principles rather than to drift from one expedient to the next. The first thing to remember is that AN EMPTY AND FIRMLY CONTRACTED UTERUS WILL NOT BLEED and that, in consequence, treatment must aim first at *emptying the uterus* and then at securing its *firm contraction*. It may be argued that this will not control bleeding due to a clotting defect, but as a loss due to this cause can only occur when the uterus relaxes, so long as a firm contraction is maintained, and this is usually possible until help arrives, serious bleeding will not occur.

1 Emptying the Uterus
Here it is essential to act early so as to prevent the patient's condition deteriorating to a point where resuscitation will be impossible. The midwife should therefore:

a Give an oxytocic, preferably Syntometrine (1 ml) if this has not already been done. In cases of this sort the intravenous route is by far the best.

b Pass a catheter if there is time and if the bladder has not been recently emptied.

c Once the uterus contracts an attempt should be made to deliver the placenta by the method referred to on page 199. The so-called Crede expression must *never* be attempted, as it is likely to cause severe shock.

d Even if the placenta cannot be delivered, the contraction produced by the oxytocic will almost always control the bleeding sufficiently to justify waiting for the doctor's arrival. Where, however, the blood loss continues the placenta must be removed manually. This operation is carried out as follows:

i   A gloved hand is passed into the vagina, through the cervix and into the cavity of the uterus

ii   The placenta is identified

iii   The fingers are inserted between the placenta and the uterine wall and by a gentle sawing motion gradually separate it from its remaining attachments

iv   During this process the opposite hand is placed on the patient's abdomen and exerts counter-pressure on the fundus

v   When the placenta has been completely separated it is grasped by the fingers and carefully withdrawn

vi   The placenta is inspected to check that it is complete

vii   Should bleeding continue, it may be controlled by compressing the uterus bimanually, as described below.

It should be emphasised that since the heavy loss that has already occurred is a sign that the placenta has already largely separated, this operation is unlikely to prove difficult. Moreover, if carried out so soon after the birth of the foetus it will cause little pain or discomfort.

2   Causing the Uterus to Contract
Bleeding after the delivery of the placenta may be due either to retention of a portion of the placenta or to atony of the uterus. Since it is not easy to be sure that the placenta is, in fact, complete, an exact diagnosis of the cause for this type of haemorrhage is not always possible. Atony of the uterus, however, is usually associated with heavier bleeding than is seen where a cotyledon or a succenturiate lobe are retained. In addition, the uterus may be obviously relaxed. In such a case, if the bleeding is to be brought under control, it is essential to stimulate the uterus to contract. This may be achieved as follows:

a   A further injection of Syntometrine may be given

b External compression of the uterus should be attempted as described on page 199.

c Should both these measures fail, bimanual compression must be carried out. To do this, one hand is inserted into the vagina, made into a fist and placed in the anterior fornix. The opposite hand, on the lower abdomen, anteflexes the uterus which can then be compressed between the two hands. Firm pressure must be kept up for at least two minutes. This manoeuvre will almost always succeed in persuading the uterus to contract.

d Other measures which are occasionally necessary to control bleeding are hot intra-uterine douches and packing the uterus under general anaesthesia. These procedures, however, are a doctor's responsibility.

Retention of a Cotyledon

When it is thought that a post-partum haemorrhage is due to the retention of a cotyledon or of a succenturiate lobe a vaginal examination must be carried out. This may reveal the cotyledon to be lodged in the partly reformed cervix, in which case it may easily be removed merely by hooking it out with the fingers. Otherwise the bleeding may usually be arrested, at least temporarily, by means of a further injection of Syntometrine.

The treatment of the shock so often associated with the various conditions described above is naturally a doctor's responsibility. The midwife, however, should always make the necessary preparations for blood or plasma transfusion or for glucose-saline infusion.

Medical Management

This usually consists of manual removal of the placenta or the evacuation of a placental polyp or a succenturiate lobe under general anaesthesia, together with the resuscitation of the patient along the lines indicated above.

Coagulation Defects: Afibrinogenaemia

The clotting mechanism of blood may be summarised as follows:

1 Platelets + Thromboplastinogen = Thromboplastin

2 Thromboplastin + Prothrombin = Thrombin

3 Thrombin + Fibrinogen = Fibrin

It is Fibrin which Provides the Basis for the Clot

Although clotting failures may at times arise from a deficiency of platelets, thromboplastin or prothrombin, they are usually due to lack of Fibrinogen. This may arise either from rapid depletion of the body stores from massive intravascular clotting or from the destruction of existing clots by abnormal Fibrinolysins. Both these mechanisms usually exist side by side.

Predisposing States

Afibrinogenaemia is encountered in cases of severe accidental ante-partum haemorrhage, especially if this is mainly concealed, where intra-uterine death of the foetus has occurred and the foetus has been retained for some weeks and after the intravenous administration of substances such as Dextran.

The Recognition of a Coagulation Defect

Since it is inevitable that after the delivery of the placenta some degree of uterine relaxation must sooner or later occur, the presence of firm clots in the mouths of the vessels running to the placental site is necessary to control further bleeding. A clotting defect is thus associated with a post-partum haemorrhage which occurs in the presence of normal uterine action. In cases of this sort, which fortunately are rare, examination of the patient often reveals multiple small bleeding points on the cervix, steadily oozing perineal lacerations and abnormal loss from any puncture wounds caused by intramuscular or intravenous injections. Moreover, the blood accumulated in containers or on the towels and leggings fails to clot.

Management

In the management of this serious condition it is vital to remember two points:

1 With proper treatment prompt recovery is the rule; without it death may easily result

2 The sheet anchor of treatment is the replacement of fibrinogen.

Fibrinogen is available in the following forms:

1 As pure fibrinogen for intravenous infusion. This is in short supply and may therefore not be readily available.

2 As fresh whole blood. This presents difficulties in collection and for that reason is seldom given.

3 As reconstituted plasma. One pint of this contains 1·5 grammes of fibrinogen. This is always obtainable. It is usually given in triple strength to provide the maximum amount of fibrinogen in the minimal volume of fluid. One or two pints of this mixture are usually all that is necessary to produce firm clotting, after which blood loss can safely be made good in the usual way.

It should be emphasised that the potential dangers of afibrinogenaemia are so great that treatment should always be started on suspicion without awaiting laboratory confirmation of the diagnosis. If first suspicions turn out to have been ill-founded, no harm will have been done. If they prove correct, the patient's safety will have been assured while serious and possibly fatal blood loss will have been prevented.

Haemorrhage of Extra-Placental Origin:
Retention of the Placenta:
Inversion of the Uterus

1 Haemorrhage of Extra-Placental Origin

Although bleeding from the placental site accounts for the vast majority of post-partum haemorrhages, serious losses sometimes arise from other sources, notably the cervix and the vaginal walls. While haemorrhage of this sort usually occurs after an operative delivery, it is occasionally encountered after an apparently normal labour.

a Cervical Lacerations

Small cervical tears which do not cause any appreciable bleeding are extremely common and require no immediate treatment. At times, however, these lacerations extend upwards, involve the cervical vessels and cause severe bleeding. Since this is at first controlled by pressure from the foetus it is noticed only after delivery and thus constitutes one variety of post-partum haemorrhage. It may be distinguished from bleeding from the placental site in that it is continuous irrespective of the state of the uterus and that it is not controlled by oxytocics. It may be diagnosed from Afibrinogenaemia by the fact that the extravasated blood clots in the normal manner. Treatment consists in suturing the laceration under general anaesthesia. Since it is useless to attempt to control the loss by insertion of a vaginal pack, owing to the distensibility of the vagina, a doctor must be called at once.

b Vaginal and Perineal Lacerations

Lacerations of the vaginal walls and of the perineum always result in a certain amount of bleeding. This is rarely enough to constitute a post-partum haemorrhage. At times, however, such as when a large vessel or a varicosity is torn, the haemorrhage is much more severe. Diagnosis is usually obvious, although difficulties may arise when the bleeding vessel is situated high up in the vaginal vault. Treatment consists of suturing the laceration under either general or local anaesthesia. As a first-aid measure, if the bleeding point is readily accessible, it may be secured with an artery forceps.

2   Retention of the Placenta

Retention of the placenta without haemorrhage is uncommon. It is due either to complete failure of the normal mechanism of separation, since once this has occurred some bleeding always results, or to abnormal adherence of the placenta – Placenta Accreta. As a general rule, failure of the placenta to separate is not associated with any other abnormality although occasionally maternal shock may develop. While it is usually claimed that such shock is due solely to the presence of the placenta in the uterus, it is more likely that it is related to repeated and ill-advised attempts at its delivery.

Abnormal retention of the placenta must be assumed to have occurred if the cardinal sign of separation, namely vaginal bleeding, is not seen within twenty minutes of the birth of the baby. In such circumstances a doctor must be called and preparations made for manual removal of the placenta.

3   Inversion of the Uterus

In this rare accident the uterus, to a greater or lesser degree, turns inside out, the inverted fundus either projecting into the vagina or, in extreme cases, hanging outside the vulva. Since this involves the adnexa being drawn into the inversion from above, shock is usually severe. On the other hand, haemorrhage is often surprisingly slight, presumably owing to kinking and distortion of the uterine vessels.

If the inverted uterus appears at the vulva the diagnosis is obvious. In less pronounced cases the reason for the sudden development of shock may not be apparent unless a careful examination, both abdominal and vaginal, is carried out at once. This should reveal the fundus to be abnormally low – it may not even be palpable per abdomen – while the upper vagina will be occupied by the inverted uterus. Management consists in the first-aid treatment of shock while awaiting the arrival of a doctor. Reposition of the inverted uterus is usually carried out under general anaesthesia, following which the patient should be resuscitated by the usual methods. It is doubtful whether it is worth while attempting fully to restore the patient's condition before undertaking operation, since so long as the uterus remains inverted, the shock will, to a large extent, persist.

Summary

Post-Partum Haemorrhage from the Placental Site

The importance of the abnormalities of the third stage of labour is due to the frequency with which they occur and the dangers they present to the patient. Furthermore, a large proportion of these abnormalities are avoidable.

One of the chief complications of the third stage is Post-Partum Haemorrhage. This may be either primary or secondary, of which the former is the more common and the more serious. Haemorrhage of this sort can arise from a variety of sources, of which the most usual is the placental site.

The immediate dangers of Primary Post-Partum Haemorrhage are shock and collapse from excessive blood loss. More remote risks are sepsis, anaemia and impaired lactation.

The correct management of a post-partum haemorrhage depends on an understanding of the normal process of the third stage of labour.

The chief causes of post-partum haemorrhage are:

a Faulty and incomplete separation of the placenta

b Retention of part of the placenta

c Atony of the uterus following delivery of the placenta

d Clotting defects in the patient's blood.

Predisposing factors to such haemorrhage are:

a General Anaesthetics

b Multiple Pregnancy

c Placenta Praevia

d Mismanagement of the Third Stage.

The incidence and severity of post-partum haemorrhage may be reduced:

a By arranging for the hospital delivery of all women likely to present this complication *b* By the prompt treatment of maternal distress, dehydration and ketosis

c By the avoidance, wherever possible, of a general anaesthetic in favour of infiltration analgesia

d By the correct management of the third stage of labour.

The management of a post-partum haemorrhage is governed by the concept that AN EMPTY AND FIRMLY CONTRACTED UTERUS WILL NOT BLEED. It is therefore necessary first to EMPTY the uterus and then to secure its CONTRACTION.

As a general rule, this may be achieved by the injection of a suitable oxytocic followed by the delivery of the placenta by controlled cord traction. Only rarely will a manual removal or bimanual compression be required. Any associated shock must be managed in the usual manner.

Coagulation defects are usually due to lack of Fibrinogen in the blood – Afibrinogenaemia. Such a defect can be recognised by persistent oozing from the genital tract despite firm uterine contraction and by failure of extravasated blood to clot.

Immediate treatment consists of the replacement of Fibrinogen, usually in the form of triple strength reconstituted plasma. Only after this should blood loss be made good.

Due to the grave dangers presented by this abnormality, treatment should be started on suspicion without awaiting laboratory confirmation.

Post-Partum Haemorrhage of Extra-Placental Origin:
Retention of the Placenta: Inversion of the Uterus

Although blood loss from the placental site accounts for most instances of post-partum haemorrhage, at times heavy bleeding can come from cervical or vaginal lacerations.

Bleeding from cervical lacerations is due to their upward extension to involve the cervical vessels. Treatment consists of suturing the laceration under a general anaesthetic. It is useless to attempt to control the haemorrhage with a vaginal pack.

Heavy bleeding from a vaginal or perineal laceration is occasionally seen. Such a tear should be sutured under general or local anaesthesia.

Retention of the placenta in the absence of haemorrhage sometimes occurs. It may be assumed to have happened if the cardinal sign of separation, vaginal bleeding, is not seen within twenty minutes of the birth of the baby. In such a case the placenta must be removed manually.

Inversion of the uterus is a rare accident. While complete inversion is obvious, partial inversion cannot be diagnosed without a full abdominal and vaginal examination. Treatment consists of first-aid measures to combat shock followed by reposition of the uterus under general anaesthesia.

PART FIVE

The Puerperium

CHAPTER FOURTEEN

The Normal Puerperium

Introduction

Pregnancy, labour and the puerperium are always said to be of equal importance and to deserve the same degree of attention. Despite the truth of this statement, a tendency nevertheless exists to regard the puerperium, coming as it does after the stresses and dangers of labour, as a period of lesser moment in which, thanks mainly to the passage of time, the patient makes a gradual return to normal life.

Yet although such an unaided transition can and does occur in a large proportion of instances, this is not always so, nor is it desirable that it should ever be allowed. Pregnancy and labour impose many demands on a woman, both mental as well as physical. If a return to a normal life is to be rapidly and smoothly attained, a woman requires a period of readjustment during which help and understanding must be provided by her medical and nursing attendants. Such a period is represented by the first days of the puerperium, whether they are spent in hospital or at home. Their importance in shaping a woman's future outlook on life and its problems, both old and new, cannot be too strongly emphasised.

Since, from a purely medical viewpoint, the vast majority of puerperal women are normal, the amount of care they require from a doctor is strictly limited. This does not apply to nursing care, which consists not so much in ensuring that all proceeds uneventfully from a physical standpoint as in encouraging the mother in the readjustment necessary to her altered environment and in helping her to overcome the problems with which she may be presented.

It is with the consideration of these two basic principles that the nursing management of the puerperal woman is concerned.

General Considerations

The puerperium may be defined as the time taken for the uterus to involute, arbitrarily accepted as six weeks. In uncomplicated cases, however, medical and nursing care are provided only for the first few days of this period. After this it is generally assumed that the mother has, to all intents and purposes, returned to normal and that she may safely resume her everyday activities. This is far from being the case, the full resumption of the non-pregnant state, mental as well as physical, occupying well over a month. This must be explained not only to the patient herself but also to her husband and relatives. Meanwhile, in the limited time set aside for nursing care, everything possible must be done to prepare the mother for her return to her home and to her responsibilities. With this in mind, the objects of obstetric care during the first days of the puerperium should be:

1   To give the anatomical and physiological changes in the genital tract and the breasts an opportunity to develop normally

2   To prevent the onset of complications such as infections and thrombosis

3   To provide adequate rest after the physical and mental stresses of pregnancy and labour

4   To assist in the psychological readjustment of the mother to her baby and to the rest of her family.

1   Anatomical and Physiological Changes

In order to allow the various anatomical and physiological changes which characterise the puerperium an opportunity to take place under the most suitable conditions, it is necessary to understand the nature of these changes. This may be considered under the following headings:

a   The general physiology of the puerperium

b   The involution of the genital tract

c   The re-establishment of menstrual function

d   Breast changes in relation to breast feeding.

a   The General Physiology of the Puerperium

Provided that the patient's health has been good during pregnancy, that her heart and lungs are normal and that she is not anaemic, the stress imposed by a normal labour should be little more than that of very strenuous physical exercise. No cardiac or respiratory distress is therefore normally apparent, although at the end of labour both the pulse rate and the temperature may be slightly raised. In some women a sudden rise in blood pressure occurs at the end of labour. This is more marked where hypertension has been present during pregnancy or if Ergometrine is given as an oxytocic. Normally this rise is of only short duration, the patient becoming normotensive again within a few hours. From then onwards, temperature, pulse and blood pressure remain within normal limits.

Since most of the fluid retained during pregnancy is eliminated in the first days of the puerperium, a moderate diuresis is common at this time. Care must be taken not to confuse this with the frequency which often characterises a urinary tract infection (page 92).

Psychological Changes

A woman's reaction to the birth of her child is unusually variable. To the great majority the event brings a sense of pleasure and of relief, together with some apprehension concerning both the baby's well-being and the mother's own re-entry into normal family, social and professional life. Such emotions, which to some extent are conflicting, tend to produce a rather typical unstable reaction, the patient's moods alternating rapidly between elation and depression. It is therefore necessary, while observing all puerperal women for any evidence of a developing psychosis, to realise that the alterations in emotional behaviours outlined above are normal and that readjustment will almost always be both rapid and complete.

b The Involution of the Genital Tract

The organ most closely concerned with the process of involution is the uterus. An idea of the changes taking place in it after delivery may be gained from the fact that at the end of the third stage it measures about $25 \times 18 \times 10$ cm and weighs about 900 grammes, while when fully involuted it measures only some $7\cdot5 \times 5 \times 2\cdot5$ cm and weighs only 60 grammes, a 16-fold decrease. Most of this decrease occurs during the early days of the puerperium, about 450 grammes being lost in the first week and a further 225 grammes in the second. Thereafter its reduction in weight becomes progressively slower until the end-point of 60 grammes is reached. Uterine involution is brought about by gradual diminution in both the size and the number of individual fibres of the myometrium, the reverse of what happens during pregnancy.

It should, perhaps, be stressed that a complete return to the size of the nulliparous uterus is rarely if ever achieved. This is due to a permanent deposition of hyaline tissue in the myometrium and in the blood vessels. These are later recanalised to provide a second set of vessels literally within the first.

The Regrowth of the Endometrium

Although most of the decidual lining of the uterus is shed either at the end of labour or in the early days of the puerperium, islands of endometrial tissue are still to be found in the deepest portions of the uterine glands and in the layer of tissue adjacent to the myometrium. It is from these remnants that the endometrium is regenerated, the process being completed comparatively rapidly save in the region of the placental site. Several weeks are needed for this area to be completely covered.

The outward sign of involution is a progressive reduction of the height of the fundus, so that by the twelfth or fourteenth day it is no longer palpable above the symphysis pubis. It must be emphasised that this is a very rough guide to the size of the uterus, since many variable factors such as the thickness of the abdominal wall, the position of the uterus and the state of the bladder and of the bowel influence either the height of the fundus or the ease with which it can be felt. For that reason, in many centres, assessment of uterine involution is not considered to be of any practical value and is no longer carried out as a routine procedure.

The Cervix reforms in an extremely short space of time. It is recognisable as a short, patulous and ill-formed structure within an hour of delivery, and is largely reconstituted in three days. The process involved is the reverse of that which characterises its 'taking up' into the lower segment during the last days of pregnancy and in early labour. Full cervical dilatation is usually accompanied by minor lacerations and these lacerations rarely heal completely. Because of this the involuted cervix presents a different appearance from that of a nulliparous woman and instead of being conical in shape with a small, circular external os, tends to be flatter and bulkier with a slit-like or patulous os.

After-Pains

The uterus, being a muscular organ, continues to contract during the puerperium and these contractions, especially in multiparae, are often painful. Since they are reflexly stimulated by the act of suckling, they tend to be particularly severe in women who are breast feeding (page 343). These 'after-pains' soon become less and disappear completely within a few days.

The Lochia

After the delivery of the placenta and the immediate control of haemorrhage, a certain amount of blood loss continues to occur from the genital tract, particularly from the placental site. This loss develops into a typical bloody discharge known as the Lochia.

The lochia consists of red blood cells, degenerated decidual cells and bacteria resulting from the invasion of the uterine cavity by the normal flora of the lower genital tract. As healing and regeneration take place, the lochia becomes scantier and changes its colour, becoming first brown – from the presence of altered blood – and later pale. The total duration of the lochial discharge is usually about four weeks, during the first two of which it is either bloody or blood-stained. It is not uncommon, however, for such red loss to recur for no very obvious reason later in the puerperium, when it may be mistaken for a menstrual period.

The Lower Genital Tract

Even where there is no gross trauma to the lower genital tract, multiple small tears and extensive bruising invariably accompany labour, however normal this may have been. These lesions heal remarkably rapidly and within a few days the vagina and perineum have largely regained their original appearance, although the vaginal walls may for some time seem more congested than normal.

c   The Re-Establishment of Menstruation and Ovulation

While many women maintain that their periods return four weeks after delivery, this is seldom true and in fact less than a quarter of mothers start to menstruate within six weeks of confinement. Earlier losses are thus more likely to be due either to a renewal of the lochial discharge, as mentioned above, or to some variety of secondary post-partum haemorrhage (page 367). As a rule, menstruation is re-established later in nursing mothers than in those who are not breast feeding. When the periods do return, they may not at first be either regular or related to ovulation.

Ovulation itself does not apparently occur within six weeks of delivery, a point of some importance in relation to contraception (page 336) and indeed may be delayed until much later. Once fully re-established, however, both menstruation and ovulation continue in a normal and regular manner.

d   Breast Changes in Relation to Breast Feeding
This subject is considered on page 342.

2   The Prevention of Complications

a   General Nursing Principles
Nowadays, normal puerperal women require little skilled attention, early rising having made them largely independent of nursing care. The temperature and pulse rate should be recorded twice daily for three days and then daily until discharge from hospital, the lochia inspected daily for undue blood loss or offensive smell – possible evidence of infection – and care taken to ensure that bowel function is regular and painless and that no frequency, dysuria or urinary retention is present. Where the repair of a laceration or of an episiotomy has been necessary, the suture line should be inspected daily for the first five days to check that healing is proceeding satisfactorily and that the stitches themselves are not causing any undue discomfort. Where non-absorbable suture material has been used, the stitches should be removed on the sixth or seventh day of the puerperium. A haemoglobin estimation is usually carried out on the fourth day and iron therapy started should the result suggest that this is needed.

b   The Prevention of Infection
In the past, puerperal infection of the genital tract was one of the gravest accidents that could befall a woman. Such infections were associated with an extremely high mortality, and even if the sufferer were fortunate enough to survive, the various sequelae often resulted in serious and lasting disability. More recently, however, both the severity and the incidence of puerperal infections have sharply declined and the risk they present is thus far less (page 353). It has also become apparent that this decline is not entirely due to the various precautions against infection which at one time were thought to be essential. Partly as a result of this realisation, and partly owing to lack of nursing facilities, these precautions have gradually been modified and relaxed

without adverse effects. At present it is not thought necessary to do more than to keep the perineum clean and dry, the methods adopted to achieve this depending on the standard of equipment available to the hospital or the midwife concerned.

Early Rising

During the puerperium, the blood develops an increased tendency to clot. This peculiarity is associated with a greater liability to Thrombo-embolic disease (page 360). Since this clotting tendency is encouraged by any slowing of the blood flow through the legs, one of the main sites for the formation of a thrombus, and since such slowing is in turn encouraged by immobility, it follows that if ambulation is allowed from an early date the incidence of thrombosis should be reduced. Mainly for this reason, early rising in the puerperium has become an accepted practice, its other advantage being that it allows an earlier return to normal life and activities than would be possible had the patient been confined to bed for ten days, as was the practice in the past.

At present, therefore, the puerperal woman is allowed to sit out of bed on the first day post-partum, activities being rapidly increased to full ambulation by the end of the third day.

3 The Provision of Adequate Rest

One of the problems of puerperal care is to arrange for adequate rest while the patient is in hospital, since this requirement conflicts with the demands of washing, feeding, exercise, rehabilitation, caring for the baby, entertaining visitors and the often unnecessary rounds of senior medical and nursing staff. Yet rest is necessary if a woman is to be returned to her family in a fit state, both mentally and physically, and if a chance is to be provided for satisfactory involution of the uterus and for the repair of damage to the lower genital tract.

It is therefore necessary to arrange for all mothers while in hospital to have the chance of securing sufficient rest and sleep both at night and during the day. This involves not only providing enough time, e.g., early 'lights out', relatively late awakening to the duties of the morning, setting aside a period of two hours during the afternoon, but also ensuring that rest and in particular sleep is possible at these times. This in its turn requires the avoidance of all unnecessary disturbance during these rest periods, babies being removed to a separate nursery and visitors to the wards discouraged, as well as prescribing an efficient hypnotic in cases where sleep is slow to come. There can be few reasons for withholding such a drug which, if given in moderation for a few nights only, will neither affect the baby nor encourage habit formation.

The Restoration of Tone to Damaged and Stretched Muscles

Two groups of muscles are liable to be damaged as a result of pregnancy and labour:

1 Those of the abdominal wall, particularly the rectus abdominis

2 Those of the pelvic floor, particularly the levator ani.

Restoration of tone in these muscles is necessary if the support they normally provide is to be regained and if utero-vaginal prolapse is to be avoided. Tone is best restored by means of exercises, during which the weakened muscles are made to undertake progressively more work and thus recover their original strength and elasticity. For this reason, post-natal exercises, initially taught and supervised by a physiotherapist and later practised at home, are an important feature of present-day puerperal management. A midwife can do much to impress on her patients the long-term value of this course and the extent to which these exercises are practised after discharge from hospital is an index of her ability in this particular direction.

4 The Psychological Readjustment of the Patient
The majority of recently delivered women, despite some initial emotional instability, referred to earlier in this section, adjust

rapidly and satisfactorily to their altered circumstances. This process of readjustment can be greatly assisted by visitors, the visiting hours being made as flexible as possible and not confined to a particular time during the late afternoon or early evening. The value of visitors, however, lies in what they bring to the patient in the way of news of her home and of her family, always provided that this is not disturbing. Nothing is worse for a woman in hospital to hear stories of family crises, often grossly exaggerated by the narrator. Visitors should also remember that it is their function to entertain the patient, not hers to amuse them, and that if she is compelled to adopt this active role, much of the value of their visit will be lost. Lastly, efforts should be made to avoid large numbers of visitors at any one time, since this often proves both tiring and upsetting to the mother.

Where the midwife feels that a woman's problems, social, domestic or professional, are becoming too great, she should arrange a visit from the medical social worker, who can often be of great help in such cases.

The Post-Natal Examination

A post-natal examination is usually carried out by a doctor on the day prior to discharge. Although in some centres this examination is still extremely thorough, this probably represents misdirected effort, unless the patient presents symptoms and signs suggestive of some abnormality. Where all has been straightforward throughout the patient's stay in hospital, all that is required is to record the blood pressure, test the urine for abnormal constituents, make sure that the uterus is involuting normally and exclude any pathological masses or undue tenderness. If the perineum has been sutured, a vaginal examination should be carried out to check that healing is proceeding satisfactorily and that no swab has been left in the vagina. Where the perineum is intact it is best to avoid such an examination at this stage.

The Forty-eight-hour Discharge

Where a woman has arranged to return to her home within forty-eight hours of delivery, the puerperal nursing care provided during her brief stay in hospital should follow the usual pattern. She should also be examined by a doctor on the second day to exclude the presence of any complication which might require further hospital treatment. Where no contra-indication to early discharge is discovered, arrangements should be made for suitable transport and the District Midwife and the patient's general practitioner notified of her departure from hospital.

The Post-natal Clinic

Unless alternative arrangements have been made, all puerperal women should attend the post-natal clinic six weeks after their confinement. The objects of this visit are to ensure that post-natal progress has been normal, that no complications have arisen since delivery and that nothing now stands in the way of the woman's full return to her everyday life. At the same time the opportunity should be taken to enquire, if necessary, into the patient's social circumstances and to check on the baby's progress. Lastly, it is widely accepted nowadays that the question of contraception should be raised at this time.

Although the original reason for selecting the end of the sixth post-partum week as the best time for this examination is not clear, it happens, by chance, to be a most suitable moment. The reason for this is that, as already pointed out, ovulation, while never occurring before this time, will probably take place shortly afterwards and this event, more than any other, marks the physiological return to normal.

While details of the procedures adopted in a post-natal clinic vary from one centre to another, the following points should always be considered:

1 The history of any complaints noted since leaving hospital

2 The general physical examination

3 The vaginal examination

4 Advice regarding further treatment

5 Advice on social and economic problems

6 Advice on coitus and contraception

7 Advice on the baby's management and feeding.

1 The History
In taking the patient's history, attention should be paid to the following features:

a *General Health.* Has she felt unduly tired and, if so, can she offer an explanation for this? Does she get sufficient sleep? Does the baby waken her repeatedly at night? Has she any headaches? Is her appetite good?

b *Vaginal Bleeding.* Since leaving hospital has there been any abnormal vaginal bleeding? Was this loss light, or heavy and associated with the passage of clots? Was it painful? Is it still continuing or has it now stopped?

c *Vaginal Discharge.* Has she had any discharge? What is its colour? Is it profuse enough to need a pad? Does it cause irritation or soreness?

d *Abdominal Pain.* Has she had attacks of abdominal pain? Were they associated with nausea or vomiting? Were they related to food, bowel action or micturition?

e *Backache.* Has she had any backache? Is it incapacitating? Is it worse on standing, or walking, or at the end of the day? Is it relieved by rest? Does it ever waken her at night? Is it associated with pain radiating down either leg?

f *The Breasts.* Is there any pain or discomfort in the breasts? Have any lumps been noticed?

g *Micturition.* Is micturition painful? Is there any frequency by day or by night? Does the urine ever escape involuntarily on coughing? Or on sneezing or straining?

h   The Bowels. Are the bowels regular? Is there any pain or bleeding associated with defaecation?

i   Other Symptoms. Are there any other symptoms which are causing worry, pain or discomfort?

While it is obviously not possible to consider all the possibilities raised by this list, two general principles should be mentioned:

a   The doctor, when carrying out the physical examination of the patient, should pay particular attention to any symptom possibly responsible for any complaint.

b   For that reason, should any symptom seem more than trivial, or should a straightforward explanation for it not be forthcoming, the clinic doctor must be informed.

2   The General Physical Examination
This is always carried out by a doctor, usually along the following lines:

a   The blood pressure is recorded

b   A sample of urine is tested for the presence of albumen and sugar.

These two investigations are usually the responsibility of the midwife.

c   The mucous membranes are inspected to exclude clinically evident anaemia

d   The breasts are examined for any abnormal masses, any nodularity or any undue tenderness

e   The abdomen is palpated to exclude any masses or tenderness. The tone and strength of the abdominal muscles are tested by asking the patient to lift her head forwards or to raise one or both legs while keeping the knees straight.

3   The Vaginal Examination
As in the ante-natal clinic, this consists of a speculum and a bimanual examination.

The Speculum Examination

Before a speculum is passed, the vulva and perineum are inspected to ensure that any lacerations have healed satisfactorily. The patient is then asked to strain down and any tendency to *prolapse* of the vaginal walls is noted. She is then asked to cough to determine whether any *stress incontinence* is present.

Although the type of speculum used depends on the wishes of the doctor, a bivalve or Cusco model is, as a rule, the most popular. The patient will be either in the left lateral or in the dorsal position. Attention is first paid to the state of the vaginal walls; these are usually redder than normal. The amount and appearance of any discharge is then noted, a high vaginal swab being taken if it seems likely that a trichomonas or monilial infection is present.

The Cervix is now inspected. Characteristically this is somewhat congested, an erosion often being present on one or both lips. The external os will almost certainly be torn laterally and some degree of ectropion may also be present. At this stage a cervical smear should be taken – if this has not already been done during pregnancy – to exclude a carcinoma-*in-situ*.

The Bimanual Examination

The state of the pelvic floor is first checked by palpating the perineal muscles between two fingers in the vagina and the thumb placed externally. The cervix is then felt, its position and size being noted as well as the presence of any lacerations and the nature of the external os – whether patulous or closed. The size, shape, position and mobility of the uterus is now assessed and any undue tenderness noted. Lastly, the adnexa are examined for any abnormal masses or tenderness.

Rectal Examination

While a rectal examination is not usually carried out at the postnatal clinic, if there is a history of pain or bleeding on defaecation, the anal margin must be inspected for the presence of a *fissure*. This fairly common complication, which is responsible for a disproportionate amount of pain and misery, is readily amenable to simple surgical treatment.

4   Advice Regarding Further Treatment

Should the physical examination have revealed any abnormality requiring further treatment, arrangements will now be made for this to be carried out. Once this question has been decided, the midwife should make certain that the patient understands the practical details involved and knows, in addition, when she is to return to the Clinic for further investigation.

5   Advice on Social and Economic Problems

In the course of a woman's visit to the post-natal clinic, it often becomes clear that certain social or economic problems, relating to her home and family life or to her professional employment, are causing her concern. Further enquiry may sometimes point to a relatively straightforward solution which the midwife herself may feel qualified to suggest. Where the situation is more complex, the advice of a medical social worker is often invaluable and can be of the greatest help in solving what, at times, may first appear to be intractable problems.

6   Advice Regarding Coitus and Contraception

Many women resume intercourse considerably before the sixth post-partum week. Others postpone such activities until after their post-natal examination. This side of life should always be enquired into, if only to reassure the patient that coitus may once again be practised. At the same time she should be warned that unless adequate contraceptive measures are taken she may well become pregnant again within a few weeks. It follows that contraceptive advice should always be made available at the post-natal clinic, a question which is more fully considered on page 336. It need only be mentioned here that a midwife is never expected to *give* such advice, but merely to indicate to the patient where, if she so wishes, she may obtain it and to see that she understands how to proceed in this matter.

Family Planning

A detailed knowledge of the various contraceptive methods available today and of their application to the individual woman is outside the province of the midwife. On the other hand, responsible as she is for the physical and mental well-being of her patients, it is necessary for her to understand their problems and wishes in respect of family limitation and to be able to inform them of where they may obtain expert advice on this important aspect of their lives.

It may be argued that a midwife should not provide such information if either her own or her patient's religious beliefs are such as to render contraception morally unacceptable. This is never the case and where a midwife herself feels unable to help her patient in this matter, she is morally obliged to refer her to someone else who is willing to do so. Again, if the patient, despite her religious upbringing, asks for such advice, the midwife should never refuse her.

It follows that all those who practise midwifery should, in the present day and age, have a general knowledge of contraception and, more specifically, of where reliable advice on Family Planning may be obtained by their patients.

1   Contraceptive Methods Available
The contraceptive methods in common use today are:

a   The Sheath or Condom
The rubber sheath or condom is an appliance placed over the penis during intercourse, thus preventing spermatozoa from reaching the female genital tract. It is a purely male method of contraception over which the woman can obviously have little direct control.

b   The Vaginal Diaphragm or Dutch Cap
This is a circular metal spring covered by a thin rubber dia phragm. Prior to intercourse it is placed in the vaginal vault, covering the cervix and preventing spermatozoa from entering the uterine cavity. It is usually used in conjunction with some form of spermicidal jelly or cream which provides an additional safety margin. Since the diameter of the vault varies considerably

from woman to woman, it is important that the correct size of diaphragm be selected. For this reason it should be fitted by an expert in this field if the maximum degree of protection – about 98 per cent – is to be obtained.

c   The Pill

Most contraceptive pills contain a mixture of two hormones, oestrogens and progestagens, the action of which suppress ovarian function and, in particular, the maturation of the ovum (page 6). Such pills, therefore, act mainly by inhibiting ovulation, although a secondary action on the receptivity of the cervical mucus to spermatozoa is also present. The pill is usually taken daily for twenty-one days at a time, starting on the fifth day after the onset of a period. About three days after the end of such a course, another period will begin. A further course of pills should be started seven days after stopping the previous one.

If taken regularly, the pill gives almost complete protection against pregnancy, but in some women side-effects such as nausea, headaches, depression, irritability, loss of libido and weight gain may be troublesome. These, however, are usually short-lived and disappear after a few months. Apart from a slightly increased tendency to thrombo-embolic disease (page 360), the dangers of this method of contraception have been much exaggerated. In the interests of complete safety the pill should not be given to women with hypertension or varicose veins or to those with a history of liver disease, carcinoma or venous thrombosis.

d   The Loop, Coil or Intra-uterine Contraceptive Device – I.U.C.D.

Although the Loop has recently gained the reputation for being the simplest, most efficient and safest contraceptive, this is an overstatement. Of various designs, these plastic Loops or Coils are intended to be inserted into the uterine cavity and left there for periods of up to five years. The reason why they prevent pregnancy from occurring is not clear; what is certain is that their efficiency is lower than is generally claimed and that the longer they are left in the uterus, the more probable is pregnancy. Further disadvantages of these appliances are that they are usually suitable only for multiparae and that they often cause menorrhagia, intermenstrual bleeding and pelvic sepsis. Their main advantage is that they make no demands upon a woman's time, memory or will-power. For these reasons they are best suited to those of low intelligence and poor motivation. It should be added that, for legal reasons, the signed consent of both wife and husband should be obtained before the loop is fitted.

2 The Places where Contraceptive Advice may be Obtained
As yet, few contraceptive clinics are attached to regional hospitals and under the control of doctors on the medical staff. The places and the people able to provide advice on birth control are therefore generally outside the hospital service.

a The Family Planning Association – F.P.A. – Clinics
These clinics, organised on a voluntary basis by the Family Planning Association, are to be found in most towns in this country. Staffed by doctors who have received a special training in this aspect of preventive medicine, they have a deservedly high reputation. Being unattached to the Health Service, any woman attending for advice is expected to contribute towards the expenses of the clinic, the sum required varying in accordance with her means.

b Local Authority Clinics
Contraceptive clinics run by the Local Health Authority have recently been developed in some boroughs. The cases seen at these clinics are usually those presenting some urgent medical or psychological reason for avoiding further pregnancy. In certain areas, where any such women are for some reason unable to attend the clinic, a domiciliary service is provided.

c The Catholic Advisory Clinics
Although all hormonal, chemical or mechanical barriers to conception are unacceptable to practising Catholics, the use of the safe period – that time at the beginning and end of the menstrual cycle when fertilisation of the ovum is less likely to occur – is allowed. Advice on the exact duration of the safe period is given at Catholic Advisory Clinics. This rhythm method, as it is sometimes called, while making great demands on the intelligence and self-control of both partners, is associated with a very

high incidence of unwanted pregnancies even in ideal circumstances.

d Consultant Obstetricians
Many consultant obstetricians are prepared to give contraceptive advice either privately or in hospital outpatient clinics. The quality of this advice naturally varies with the experience of the consultant dispensing it.

e General Practitioners
While the above remarks apply equally to most General Practitioners, an increasingly large number of such doctors have now received formal training in Family Planning methods and are thus well qualified to give advice on this matter.

In conclusion, a midwife's responsibilities towards those of her patients who enquire about the means of limiting their families is to outline to them the various contraceptive methods currently available, to inform them where adequate advice may be obtained and to ensure that no difficulties arise regarding appointments to the places or people chosen to provide this advice.

The Breasts in Pregnancy and the Puerperium

At present only a small proportion of mothers choose to breast feed their babies. Despite this, the midwife should still have a knowledge of the anatomy of the breasts, of the physiological changes that take place in them during pregnancy and the puerperium, and of some of the more common pathological conditions that may affect them at these times.

Anatomy

The breasts are paired hemispherical structures of a sort known as compound racemose glands. They are situated on the chest wall between the second and the sixth ribs. Medially they reach to the edge of the sternum, laterally they extend to the mid-axillary line. At this point an upward extension of breast tissue, the axillary tail of Spence, passes towards the axilla. At the centre

M

of each breast is the nipple, surrounded by the Areola. The skin of the breast is as a rule more elastic than elsewhere on the chest wall, while that covering the nipple and the areola is particularly thin and sensitive. On the surface of the areola are some eighteen to twenty small swellings known as Montgomery's tubercles. These represent modified sebaceous glands and produce a secretion which keeps the nipple soft and supple.

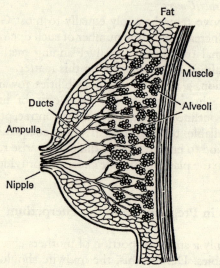

Fig. 45   General structure of breast

The interior of the breast is made up of both glandular and fatty tissue. As the proportions of these two elements vary from woman to woman, the breast's capacity for milk production bears little relation to its size. The glandular tissue is split up into between eighteen and twenty lobes by fibrous septa which radiate outwards from the nipple like the spokes of a wheel. As a result, each lobe is a separate secretory entity and is not connected with those on either side.

The glandular tissue may be divided into two parts, the Alveoli and the Ducts.

The *Alveoli* are the actual secretory elements of the breast. They consist of numerous clusters of cuboidal cells arranged around small ducts and surrounded themselves by specialised contractile cells, the myoepithelial or basket cells.

The *Ducts* appear as a many-branched system of collecting tubules which eventually unite to form the main lactiferous tubules. These pass towards the nipple where they open on to the surface. Immediately before reaching the nipple each duct expands into a small reservoir, the ampulla, in which milk is stored during lactation. As in the case of the alveoli, the ducts, lactiferous tubules and ampullae are all surrounded by myoepithelial cells.

The Development of the Breasts

The breasts are derived from the upper part of a line of specialised cells, the Milk Line, which extends along the ventral aspect of the embryo from the axilla to the groin. While only two breasts develop fully, accessory nodules of breast tissue are frequently present. These may at times be mistaken by the patient for papillomata, pigmented naevi or even malignant growths.

Between birth and puberty, little change occurs in the breast. Once ovarian activity develops, however, growth of both ducts and alveoli proceeds rapidly under the influence of oestrogens and progesterone. During early pregnancy, renewed stimulation from these two hormones, which are produced initially by the corpus luteum and later by the placenta, causes further breast growth to take place. At this time the alveoli are affected to a greater extent than the ducts. The outward and visible effect of this is a marked increase in the size of the breasts, occurring mainly between the sixth and the twenty-fourth week, while their consistency, previously soft and uniform, becomes nodular and irregular. Simultaneously, symptoms such as tingling, pain and tenderness are usually noted to a greater or lesser degree by the patient herself. In addition, pigmentation changes occur, involving the skin of the nipples and of the areolae. As already mentioned on page 17, these are more marked in dark-skinned women than in blondes and may be altogether absent in redheads. To allow for these growth changes, the blood supply of the breasts is greatly increased. This is shown by the engorgement of the superficial veins, referred to on page 16 and which is such an important diagnostic sign of pregnancy.

Alveolar secretory activity starts early in pregnancy with the production of colostrum. The main purpose of this is to clear the ducts of cellular debris and thus to simplify the later process of lactation. Unlike milk, colostrum is a clear, watery fluid containing leucocytes, fat globules and desquamated cells from the walls of the alveoli and the ducts.

Lactation

The production of milk as distinct from that of colostrum is under the control of prolactin, a hormone secreted by the anterior part of the pituitary body. Since the production of prolactin is inhibited by oestrogens, it follows that lactation cannot start until after delivery when the oestrogens from the placenta have been eliminated from the body. The onset of lactation is recognised by a sudden engorgement of the breasts which usually occurs three or four days after delivery and which is often associated with considerable pain and discomfort as well as with some degree of constitutional upset. Although milk is produced by the same cells as is colostrum, it differs from this substance both in its appearance and in its make-up, containing a far higher proportion of fat, protein and sugar. The average amounts of these components is as follows:

	Per cent
Fat	3·5
Protein	1·5
Sugar (Lactose)	7·0
Salts	0·2
Water	87·8

The Sucking Reflex

Stimulation of the nipple by suckling causes sensory nerve impulses to pass upwards to a part of the brain – the hypothalamus – which lies immediately above the pituitary body. Under this

stimulus, the hypothalamus produces releasing factors which act
directly upon the anterior and the posterior parts of the pituitary
causing the release into the circulation of prolactin and oxytocin.
The former hormone, as already stated, acts upon the secretory

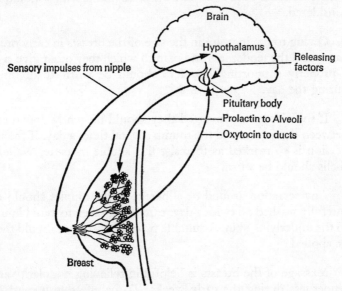

Fig. 46 Suckling reflex

cells of the alveoli, increasing the production of milk while the
latter causes the myoepithelial cells to contract. Milk is thus
driven along the ducts, through the lactiferous tubules and out
of the nipple.

In addition to the need for prolactin and oxytocin, one of the
chief factors in ensuring a good and steady supply of milk is the
regular and complete emptying of the breasts, preferably at each
feed. Failing this, the amount of milk produced will rapidly
decline.

It should be mentioned that in addition to its action on the
myoepithelial cells, oxytocin also causes the uterus to contract.
These after-pains are noted by many mothers who feed their
babies, especially during the first days of the puerperium. Apart
from assisting in the process of involution, they are of no significance.

The Care of the Breasts in Pregnancy

Maternity Units vary so much in the type of advice they give to patients regarding the care of the breasts that it is probably unwise to do more than to outline the main points which should be considered.

1   Owing to the increase in the size of the breasts in early pregnancy and the tenderness and pain to which they often give rise, a properly supporting brassiere should be worn at all times during the day.

2   If the nipples are inverted they should be gently drawn out between the fingers and the thumb several times a day. If the inversion is so marked as to resist this simple measure, Waller's shells should be worn.

3   Any secretion around or adherent to the nipples should be carefully washed off twice a day, care being taken to avoid injury to the underlying skin. A suitable proprietary cream should then be applied.

4   Massage of the breasts is helpful in relieving nodularity and tenderness during the early weeks. To be effective it must be carried out firmly but gently, working from the periphery towards the centre. Care should be taken to include the axillary tail in this manoeuvre.

5   The expression of colostrum during pregnancy probably helps to establish good lactation by removing any accumulated cellular debris from the ducts. Preferably expression should be carried out after massage, the thumb and forefinger being placed on the areola immediately behind the nipple and gentle pressure then exerted.

Breast Feeding

Here again, maternity units tend to evolve their particular systems for the education of mothers in the technique of breast feeding. For this reason it is only necessary here to remind the midwife of certain general principles:

1 No mother should ever be persuaded against her will to breast feed her child. Such an attempt will succeed in doing more harm than good and will weaken rather than reinforce the developing relationship between her and her baby.

2 If a mother who wishes to breast feed fails to do so for one reason or another, she must never be allowed to imagine that she is in any way abnormal or inadequate and that as a result of her 'failure' her relationship with her baby will be damaged.

3 A mother may need to be reassured that several days are normally required for the proper establishment of lactation and that for this reason immediate success in breast feeding should not be expected.

4 For successful breast feeding the following are required:

a The breasts should not be unduly tender or tense

b The nipples should be well formed and everted

c The baby should be encouraged to feed with equal frequency and with equal ease from either breast

d The breasts should be emptied at each feed, if necessary by manual expression

e The mother's diet and fluid intake should be sufficient to meet the added demands of lactation

f There should be no past history of acute mastitis or of breast abscess.

Some Common Pathological Conditions

1 *Engorgement of the Breasts*. As already mentioned, this commonly occurs at the third or fourth day of the puerperium. Although Stilboestrol was used in the past in the management of this condition, this is no longer acceptable owing to

the risk of provoking thrombo-embolic disease. At present, therefore, all that should be done is to ensure that the breasts are well-supported and to relieve discomfort with mild analgesics such as Aspirin, Panodol or Codeine, two tablets of any one of these drugs being given twice or three times a day.

2 *Cracked Nipples.* The soft, thin skin of the nipples can readily become cracked by the baby's attempts at feeding. This will rarely happen if breast feeding is properly taught and the child persuaded to take the whole nipple well into its mouth. The management of cracked nipples is thus initially preventive. Once established, the condition is best treated by the application of a suitable proprietary cream. While healing is in progress the baby should be removed from the affected breast and its feeds made up, if need be, with expressed breast milk – E.B.M. – given by spoon or bottle. Manual expression of the milk from the damaged breast must be persevered with if it is wished that lactation should continue.

3 *Acute Mastitis: Breast Abscess.* Acute inflammation of the breast is nowadays uncommon. The infection usually gains entry through a crack in the nipple. Since milk is an excellent culture medium, multiplication of the invading organisms is favoured by any degree of engorgement. Acute mastitis is characterised by the general signs of an infection – pyrexia, tachycardia, headache and malaise – as well as by local signs such as swelling, redness and tenderness of the affected breast. Treatment is with antibiotics such as Ampicillin and analgesics. Should the condition progress to pus formation, incision or aspiration of the abscess is usually necessary.

The Suppression of Lactation

In the past, lactation was almost always suppressed by giving large doses of Stilboestrol spread over several days. Such a measure is nowadays indefensible and it has come to be realised that it is also unnecessary. All that would seem to be needed in the great majority of cases are measures identical to those advised for the management of breast engorgement. It may, however, be an advantage to apply a firm binding to the breasts if a supporting brassiere seems to be inadequate. Restriction of fluids and purgation are both unnecessary and inhumane. In the occasional patient in whom engorgement persists despite the treatment outlined above, the intramuscular injection of 1 ml of Hexoestrol – 15 mg – repeated if need be in forty-eight hours, will be found to be of value.

Summary

General Considerations

The puerperium represents the period taken for the uterus to involute. It is arbitrarily accepted to occupy six weeks. Medical and nursing care are, however, needed only for the first few days of this time.

The objects of obstetric care during the puerperium are to allow involution to proceed normally, to prevent the development of complications, to provide adequate mental and physical rest and to help in the physical and psychological readjustment of the mother.

Apart from a slight rise in pulse and temperature, the maternal condition after a normal labour is little altered. In some cases a transient rise in blood pressure may occur, more marked where Ergometrine has been given.

From a psychological aspect, a puerperal woman is emotionally labile, her mood varying between elation and depression. Readjustment is usually rapid and complete.

The involution of the uterus is mainly completed during the first two weeks of the puerperium. A full return to the nulliparous size is rare. Menstruation is seldom resumed within six weeks of delivery while ovulation never occurs before this time.

Normally the puerperal woman requires little nursing care. The temperature and pulse rate should be recorded twice daily for three days and daily thereafter. The perineum should be inspected daily if sutures are present. Stitches should be removed on the sixth or seventh day. Precautions against genital infections have recently been considerably relaxed and now consist merely of keeping the perineum clean and dry.

Early rising should be encouraged in view of its effect in reducing the incidence of thrombo-embolic disease and its influence upon the rehabilitation of the mother.

Adequate rest periods must be provided both at night and during the afternoon. Unnecessary noise must be avoided at these times, babies being removed to a separate nursery. At night, a hypnotic may be given if needed.

Post-natal exercises, designed to improve the tone of the muscles of the abdominal wall and of the perineum, should be practised both in hospital and after the patient's return home.

A post-natal examination is usually carried out by a doctor before the patient's discharge from hospital. This need not include a vaginal examination unless the perineum has been sutured.

Where a forty-eight-hour discharge has been arranged, the District Midwife and the patient's General Practitioner must be notified of her departure from hospital.

The Post-Natal Clinic

A woman should attend the post-natal clinic about six weeks after her confinement. The objects of this visit are to ensure that her progress as well as that of her child have been normal and that no complications have arisen since delivery.

In questioning the patient, attention should be paid to her general health, the presence of abnormal vaginal bleeding or discharge or of abdominal pain or backache. Micturition and bowel action should be normal and painless. There should be no pain or discomfort in the breasts.

The physical examination covers such points as blood pressure, urinalysis – usually carried out by a midwife – and palpation of the breasts and abdomen.

Pelvic examination includes both a speculum and a bimanual examination. Before passing a speculum any tendency to prolapse or stress incontinence is noted. The state of the vaginal walls and of the cervix is then checked. If there is any undue discharge a swab should be taken to exclude a trichomonas or monilial infection. A cervical smear is also taken.

On bimanual examination the thickness and tone of the pelvic floor is estimated. The cervix and uterine body are then palpated. Finally the adnexa are examined for any abnormal masses.

Advice on any social or economic problems may be given either by the midwife herself or, should she feel it desirable, by the medical social worker.

If all is normal, the patient should be told that coitus may be resumed but that if precautions are not taken pregnancy may soon ensue. For that reason she should be offered contraceptive advice.

Family Planning

Since she is responsible for the physical and mental well-being of her patients, a midwife should be in a position to inform them, if asked, about the various contraceptive methods currently available and to advise them where advice on such methods may be obtained.

Reliable contraceptive methods at present in use are the sheath or condom, the vaginal diaphragm or Dutch cap, the pill and the intra-uterine contraceptive device – the loop or coil.

Contraceptive advice may be obtained from:

a Family Planning Association Clinics. These are voluntary organisations staffed by doctors specially trained in this branch of medicine.

b Local Health Authority clinics, which have been set up in a few boroughs for the purpose of assisting cases in special need of such advice.

c Catholic Advisory Clinics, where advice on the safe period or rhythm method is available to those unable, owing to their religious convictions, to make use of more reliable techniques.

d Consultant obstetricians and general practitioners, some of whom have received formal training in Family Planning methods.

The Breasts in Pregnancy and the Puerperium

The breasts are situated on the chest wall between the second and sixth ribs. They are hemispherical in shape with an extension, the axillary tail, passing upwards from their lateral aspect. The skin over the breast is thin and supple, especially in the region of the nipple and the areola.

The interior of the breast is divided by fibrous septa into about twenty lobes. In addition to fat, each lobe contains many secretory alveoli and collecting ducts. These unite to form the main lactiferous ducts which open on to the nipple. Both alveoli and ducts are surrounded by myoepithelial cells.

The growth of the breasts in pregnancy takes place between the sixth and twenty-fourth weeks under the control of oestrogens and progesterone. It is marked by pigmentation of the areola and nipple, increased vascularity, the secretion of colostrum and by certain subjective symptoms.

Lactation depends on the secretion of prolactin from the pituitary body. Its onset, usually on the fourth day of the puerperium, is characterised by sudden engorgement of the breasts with some constitutional upset.

Pain and tenderness of the breasts during pregnancy is best managed by providing proper support. The nipples should be kept clean of dried secretion. Inversion of the nipples may require the use of Waller's shells. Massage and expression of colostrum are of use in preparing the breast for lactation.

For satisfactory lactation the breasts should be soft and painless, the nipples everted and the sucking reflex well-established. Diet and fluid intake must be adequate. There should be no history of breast abscess.

Cracked nipples may be avoided if breast feeding is properly carried out. Once a crack has formed, the child must be taken from the affected breast until healing is complete. The crack should be dressed with a proprietary cream and the breast expressed to avoid engorgement.

Acute mastitis presents the signs, both general and local, of any acute infection. Treatment is with antibiotics and mild analgesics. If pus formation occurs, the abscess should be incised or aspirated.

Lactation is suppressed by binding the breasts firmly and providing mild analgesics. If these measures fail, Hexoestrol is of value. Purgation and fluid restriction are never necessary.

CHAPTER FIFTEEN

The Abnormal Puerperium

Introduction

In the past, complications of the puerperium, especially haemolytic streptococcal infections of the genital tract, were extremely common and accounted for a very high proportion of the maternal deaths encountered at that time. It is probably for this reason that many obstetricians and midwives are still apt to accord to puerperal infections an importance which cannot in fact be related to their present-day incidence or severity and to consider them in terms more suited to the past than to the present.

In the following pages an attempt will be made to alter this traditional attitude and to present a picture more in keeping with observed facts.

The complications to be considered may be divided into four groups:

1 Infections involving the genital tract

2 Infections involving the urinary tract and the breasts

3 Thrombo-embolic disease

4 Secondary post-partum haemorrhage.

Of these, infections of the genital tract, which at one time took pride of place among puerperal complications, are now uncommon and rarely present the clinical picture traditionally associated with them. On the other hand, infections involving extra-genital structures such as the urinary tract and the breasts are today relatively more significant while the dangers of thrombo-embolic disease are becoming increasingly evident.

The balance has thus greatly changed and the attitude of those who practise and teach midwifery must also change if the status and significance of present-day puerperal abnormalities is to be properly appreciated and if the best use is to be made of the various means available for reducing still further the hazards and long-term effects of these complications.

Infections of the Genital Tract

In addition to the variable amount of trauma inevitably inflicted by the passage of the foetus upon the cervix, vagina and perineum, the genital tract at the end of labour contains one of the largest wounds ever likely to be sustained, namely the placental site. Furthermore, the proximity of the vulva to the perianal area and the fact that the vagina itself normally harbours large numbers of potentially dangerous bacteria, makes it surprising that genital infections occur so relatively infrequently and that when they do they usually assume a mild form. This pattern, however, has only recently become apparent; previously these infections were both common and severe. The reasons for this important change are as follows:

1 Puerperal genital infections are usually caused by bacteria belonging to one of three main groups:

a Haemolytic streptococci

b Anaerobic streptococci

c Staphylococci and B. Coli.

Of these, haemolytic streptococci were responsible in the past for the great majority of severe infections and contributed almost exclusively to the high maternal mortality associated with puerperal sepsis.

2 The availability of sulphonamides and penicillin, drugs to which the haemolytic streptococcus is particularly sensitive, together with a diminution in the virulence of the organism, have together resulted in such infections being less serious and more easily controlled.

3 The change from difficult and hazardous vaginal deliveries to Caesarean section and the more careful repair of vaginal and perineal trauma have greatly decreased the number of infections due to anaerobic streptococci, as these organisms flourish mainly in dead or damaged tissues.

4 The continued production of new, wide-spectrum antibiotics has allowed most infections caused by staphylococci and coliforms to be brought under effective control.

Puerperal Pyrexia

Most infections, regardless of their site of origin, evoke a pyrexia. Pyrexia developing during the puerperium suggests the following possibilities:

1 A genital tract infection

2 A urinary tract infection

3 A breast infection

4 An infection in some structure unrelated to childbirth

5 A deep vein thrombosis.

Pyrexia alone is thus of no value in determining the site and nature of an infection. Moreover, the recent decrease in the number and severity of puerperal complications renders its clinical significance far smaller than in the past. This is the reason for the recent decision to abandon the compulsory notification of puerperal pyrexia, which used to be such an important feature of public health obstetrics.

The Sources of Genital Infections

A puerperal infection of the genital tract may be derived from one of three sources:

a *The Patient's Own Vagina.* The normal vagina harbours a variety of organisms. Many of these, although usually harmless, are capable under certain conditions of causing an infection. Infections from such a source are known as *Endogenous*.

b *From Other Sources on the Patient.* Examples of this are the upper respiratory tract, the bacteria spreading from here to the genital tract. An infection of this type is called *Autogenous*.

c *From Outside Sources*, such as nurses, doctors, lay staff or visitors to the ward, or from inanimate objects such as dust, bed-clothes, books, magazines or eating utensils. This sort of infection is called *Exogenous*.

Although all human beings are under constant attack from pathogenic bacteria, these rarely succeed in causing an infection. For this to happen, three requirements must be met:

i The *dose* of bacteria must be sufficiently large

ii A suitable *site* for infection must be present

iii The body's *immunity* must be lowered.

These conditions are often fulfilled during the puerperium, because:

i A post-natal ward provides an opportunity for the spread of a sufficient number of bacteria from one patient to another

ii A woman's natural resistance is often lowered by the stresses of labour, especially if this has been prolonged and associated with exhaustion, trauma, haemorrhage or shock

iii Damage to the perineum, vagina or cervix, together with the large open placental wound itself, provide satisfactory sites for the start of an infection.

d The lochia forms an excellent culture medium.

Types of Infection

The structures most likely to be involved in a puerperal genital infection are the perineum, the vagina and the cervix. The placental site, despite its size and the blood clots and decidual remnants adherent to it, is less accessible to invading organisms and is less frequently involved. As with most other infections, the symptoms and signs are in part general and in part local.

1 Infections of the Perineum and Vagina

These usually consist of infected lacerations or episiotomy incisions. The general constitutional upset is small and the patient seldom feels acutely ill. The temperature and pulse are thus only slightly raised. The local signs of infection consist of reddening and swelling around the suture line or laceration, together with some pain and tenderness.

2 Cervical Infections

The small lacerations which almost invariably accompany cervical dilatation during labour often become infected. These infections are usually mild and cause few symptoms other than vague lower abdominal pain and slight backache together with an increased amount of purulent vaginal discharge.

3 Infections of the Placental Site

Infections of the placental site, although uncommon, are potentially serious since unless they are brought under early and effective control, outward spread may occur involving the myometrium, the parametrium, the adnexa and the peritoneal cavity.

Fortunately, the infection usually remains well localised and causes only slight constitutional upset and such local signs as a bulky, tender uterus which involutes more slowly than normal.

Faced with the possibility that her patient has developed a puerperal infection, a midwife should proceed as follows:

a Medical aid must be called at once

b The doctor will examine the patient to determine the site of the infection, particular attention being paid to the state of the vagina, the perineum, the cervix, the uterine body and the adnexa

c A high vaginal swab, a throat swab and a mid-stream specimen of urine must now be sent for microscopy, culture and sensitivity tests. While awaiting the laboratory reports on these specimens an initial course of a wide-spectrum antibiotic will probably be prescribed. If necessary, this can later be changed to one to which the organisms discovered show greater sensitivity.

General Nursing Measures

Due to the need to limit the spread of a puerperal infection, the patient should be transferred to a ward specially adapted for the management of such cases. Once transferred, general measures include the provision of free fluids, a light diet, adequate amounts of analgesics, sedatives and, if necessary, hypnotics, and local applications of heat to the perineum – if this is infected – in the form of hot baths and radiant heat. Unless the temperature is high or the constitutional upset severe, complete bed-rest is not necessary. Under such management the symptoms and signs of infection will usually rapidly subside.

Should culture of the swabs originally taken from the throat or vagina reveal pathogenic organisms, swabbing must be repeated with negative result before the patient can be regarded as cured and discharged home.

The Prevention of Infection

In many respects, obstetrics is a branch of preventive medicine. It is therefore only reasonable for obstetricians and midwives to try to prevent rather than to treat a puerperal infection. While the detailed management of each case must naturally be in accordance with its particular needs, there are certain general principles which should always be followed:

1 All predisposing causes of infection must be eliminated. These include:

a The efficient management of anaemia during pregnancy

b The effective replacement of blood loss occurring during or after labour

c The avoidance of all unnecessary trauma during delivery

d The careful and thorough repair of all damage sustained at delivery

2 All patients should, if possible, be treated in a special ward

3 All reasonable precautions must be taken to avoid exogenous infections

a Since dust is a common carrier of bacteria, it must be kept to a minimum. Energetic sweeping, which spreads dust particles, must be avoided

b Since bacteria are often harboured in the cracks to be found in old crockery, any chipped or cracked cups or plates must be rejected. For the same reason, knives should be of all-metal construction rather than having bone or plastic handles

c Where practicable, exchange of books and magazines should be forbidden, since these allow the transfer of bacteria from one person to another

d Lastly, any nurse, doctor, lay administrator or visitor suffering from an upper respiratory infection should avoid entering the post-natal wards or, in the event of having to do so, wear an efficient face-mask.

General Principles Governing the Management of an Established
Outbreak of Puerperal Infection

Although a detailed description of the management of an outbreak of puerperal infection in a post-natal ward is beyond the
scope of this book, the general principles involved may conveniently be considered here. These are:

1   Treatment of the infected cases themselves

2   Detection of the source of the infection

3   Protection of the other patients in the ward

4   Protection of patients in the rest of the unit

5   Disinfection of the ward at the end of the outbreak.

1   The Treatment of the Infected Cases
The medical and nursing care of puerperal genital infections has
already been considered, as has the principle that such cases
should be transferred to a ward where they may be nursed with
greater safety both to themselves and to the rest of the com-
munity. In such a ward, as an added precaution, the system of
Barrier Nursing may be adopted to reduce still further the possibility of spreading infection to other patients.

2   The Detection of the Source of the Infection
Here the services of a pathologist are essential. Should the nature
of the infection warrant such a course, all contacts must be
screened to exclude the presence of carriers. This screening procedure involves:

a   The taking of throat, nasal and high vaginal swabs from all
patients in the ward in which the outbreak has occurred

b   The taking of throat and nasal swabs from all nurses and
doctors who have been in contact with infected patients

c   The transference of any carriers among the patients to an
isolation ward

d The suspension from duty and the adequate treatment of any carriers discovered among the hospital staff

e A search must be carried out for a source of infection in such places as sluices, lavatories and bathrooms.

3 The Protection of the Other Patients in the Ward
This may be ensured by:

a Removing from the ward all carriers of infection

b Returning the remaining patients to their homes as soon as their obstetric condition allows.

N.B.: The Medical Officer of Health must be notified of the discharge to their homes of any potentially infected patients so that the necessary arrangements may be made for their care.

4 The Protection of the Patients in the Rest of the Unit
This may be achieved by:

a Restricting all movement of equipment or of patients, medical staff, or nursing staff in or out of the affected ward

b Refusing admission to the ward to administrators or laymen unless this is absolutely necessary.

5 The Disinfection of the Ward at the End of the Outbreak
Once the ward has been emptied of patients, the walls, floor, furniture and beds must be washed down with disinfectant. This removes, in theory if not in practice, any remaining bacteria.

In conclusion it should be emphasised that the extensive measures outlined above apply only where a number of women are affected by a relatively virulent organism. They are not needed where the outbreak is merely sporadic and mild, provided that, in such cases, all reasonable precautions are taken to treat the affected patients energetically and to isolate them from their fellows.

Thrombo-Embolic Disease

During the puerperium, due to various complex changes, the clotting power of the blood is increased and a tendency to venous thrombosis develops. Since thrombosis is naturally more likely to occur where the blood flow is sluggish, the veins chiefly affected are those of the legs and, to a lesser extent, of the pelvis.

The usual sequence of events is for a clot to form in one of the deep veins of the calf and for it then to extent into progressively larger vessels. Being poorly attached at its point of origin and floating freely in the wider veins into which it has spread, the upper part of the clot is liable to break off and to find its way up the vascular tree into the heart. From there it passes into the lungs where, depending upon its size, it occludes a greater or lesser amount of the pulmonary arterial system and gives rise to signs and symptoms of variable severity.

The clinical evidence of such a pattern of events depends in part upon the effects produced locally by a deep vein thrombosis and in part upon those caused by a pulmonary embolus, in the unlikely event of this serious abnormality developing.

1   The Symptoms and Signs of Deep Vein Thrombosis
These are general and local. General signs consist of a mild and transient constitutional upset, the temperature being rarely higher than 38°C and often sustained for less than twenty-four hours, while the pulse rate is only slightly raised. Local signs are pain and tenderness in the affected leg, which, on examination, may appear swollen, pitting oedema being occasionally demonstrable over the malleoli and the dorsum of the foot. In addition, the muscles of the calf present a peculiar brawny sensation on gentle palpation. It may also, at times, be possible to outline a tender, thrombosed vein in the popliteal fossa or along the adductor aspect of the thigh. Lastly, pain is experienced on stretching the muscles of the leg by dorsiflexion of the foot.

2   Pulmonary Manifestations
Here the symptomatology is directly related to the size of the embolus.

a   A small embolus will pass into a lesser branch of the pulmonary artery and produce only a slight and transient disturbance. There may be momentary faintness and pain in the chest with the production, some hours later, of a small amount of rusty sputum. It is essential to recognise this train of events for what it is as it may be the sole warning of a future massive embolus and thus present the sole opportunity for starting effective treatment.

b A larger embolus, as would be expected, causes a greater and more prolonged disturbance with:

i Pain in the chest, respiratory distress and cyanosis

ii Tachycardia and engorgement of the veins of the neck

iii Blood-stained sputum due to infarction of the lung.

An X-ray reveals a variable amount of pulmonary consolidation. This later resolves and the circulatory defect is to a great extent made good.

c A massive embolus obstructs the pulmonary circulation at or just beyond the bifurcation of the pulmonary artery. It results in:

i Pain, suffocation and collapse, often followed within seconds by death from vagal inhibition.

ii If this initial onslaught is survived, the patient develops the symptoms and signs of pulmonary occlusion, such as extreme breathlessness, cyanosis, severe pain in the chest and evidence of right-sided heart failure with gross engorgement of the veins of the neck and acute enlargement of the heart and liver.

3 Treatment

a Deep Vein Thrombosis
In view of its potential dangers, a doctor must be called if ever a deep vein thrombosis is suspected. Treatment is primarily medical, the principles being to prevent extension of the clot and to reduce the chance of its becoming detached.

i *Preventing the Extension of the Clot*
Anti-coagulants are used for this purpose, Phenindione – Dindevan – being the drug usually selected. Since this takes time to act, initial treatment usually consists of Heparin, given by intravenous infusion at a rate of 25,000 units every twenty-four hours for two days. At the same time, 200 mg of Phenindione are given orally, followed by 100 mg twelve hours later. The dose is then adjusted to suit the Prothrombin Time, which must be estimated

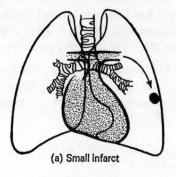

(a) Small infarct

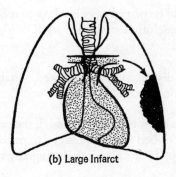

(b) Large Infarct

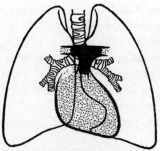

(c) Embolus occluding
pulmonary vessels

Fig. 47   Degrees of pulmonary infarction

daily by the Laboratory. About 50 mg twice daily are usually needed once control has been established. This regime is continued for between ten and fourteen days, depending on the extent of the thrombosis and its response to treatment.

ii   *Preventing Clot Detachment and Reducing the Symptoms*
Although limiting extension of the clot, anticoagulants also help to prevent its detachment; the following general measures are also useful in this respect:

1   The patient should be confined to bed until the acute symptoms have subsided

2   A cradle should be placed over her legs to relieve them of the pressure of the bedclothes since this itself might predispose to further thrombosis

3   If pain and discomfort are marked, analgesics such as Codeine, A.P.C. or Aspirin should be given

4   Once the acute symptoms have passed, the patient should be allowed to be out of bed and encouraged to move about. At this stage physiotherapy is of value in reducing any residual oedema of the affected leg.

b   Pulmonary Embolus
When a small warning embolus has occurred full anti-coagulant therapy must be started immediately. This is the best insurance against further emboli. In the presence of a larger embolus, first-aid treatment is aimed at reducing dyspnoea and venous congestion by means of oxygen, morphia, aminophylline and, if need be, venesection. Should the patient survive the immediate crisis, anti-coagulants must then be started.

   In conclusion, two points should be emphasised:

1   Most cases of demonstrable Deep Vein Thrombosis do not develop a Pulmonary Embolus

2   In most cases of Pulmonary Embolus no demonstrable Deep Vein Thrombosis is present. This, however, does not mean that

full anti-coagulant therapy should not be started immediately in order to avoid further and possibly fatal emboli.

Superficial Thrombosis in a Varicose Vein

During the puerperium, superficial varicose veins are often the seat of a local thrombosis which, although at times painful, differs from deep vein thrombosis in that it is never followed by a pulmonary embolus.

Treatment is by local applications of Icthyol in Glycerine or Kaolin, supplemented by mild analgesics and, if the pain is unusually severe, by Butazolidine, 200 mg twice daily for five days.

In cases of this nature there is no need to confine the patient to bed and, in fact, early ambulation has much to commend it. Since the thrombus has occluded a vein which was dilated and incompetent, the long-term result is often the cure of the affected varicosity.

Other Abnormalities of the Puerperium

I Urinary Tract Complications

1 Retention of Urine

Retention of urine due to bruising of or trauma to the urethra, vagina or perineum sometimes occurs immediately after labour. Treatment in the first instance consists of allowing the patient to go to the lavatory, since many women find it impossible to use a bed-pan. Should this measure fail, Carbachol – 1 ml intramuscularly – is sometimes effective, otherwise catheterisation will be necessary. It is important that this measure be not too long delayed, since over-distension of the bladder may result in the development of retention with overflow or residual urine.

2 Retention with Overflow

In this uncommon complication the bladder remains permanently over-distended, only small amounts of urine escaping at frequent intervals. Treatment is essentially the same as for Residual Urine.

3   Residual Urine

Residual urine in the bladder after micturition is occasionally encountered during the puerperium. It is due to an inability of the bladder to empty itself completely. As this may lead to an infection of the urinary tract if left untreated, the recognition of this condition is important. This may at times be difficult. Diagnostic points of value are frequency of micturition without pain or urgency, the passage of relatively small amounts of urine and a sensation on the part of the patient that even after micturition the bladder still feels full. When doubt exists a catheter should be passed immediately *after* micturition and the volume of residual urine thus obtained measured. Any amount exceeding 60 ml is of significance.

Management

It is important to ensure that the bladder is regularly emptied and for this reason, despite the risks involved, catheterisation as described above should be carried out in every suspected case. Where this confirms the diagnosis it must be continued twice daily until the volume of residual urine falls to and remains below two ounces.

4   Ascending Urinary Tract Infections

Ascending urinary tract infections are not uncommon during the puerperium for two reasons:

a   Infection may be introduced by catheterisation during labour

b   Infection may result from such abnormalities as retention of urine, retention with overflow or residual urine.

Whatever the cause, the symptoms and signs of this complication are similar to those outlined on page 92. They need not, therefore, be considered here.

5   Stress Incontinence

Stress Incontinence implies the involuntary passing of a small amount of urine whenever the intra-abdominal pressure is suddenly raised, such as on coughing, sneezing or straining. This distressing symptom is occasionally seen after childbirth.

Treatment consists of an extended course of physiotherapy. Operative correction is contra-indicated in these cases and should never be contemplated within one year of childbirth.

II   Breast Infections

These are considered on page 345.

III   Secondary Post-partum Haemorrhage

Secondary post-partum haemorrhage may be defined as abnormal vaginal bleeding during the puerperium, apart from the first twenty-four hours of this period. It is of less importance than primary post-partum haemorrhage for the following reasons:

1   It is far less frequently encountered

2   The loss, as a rule, is not so heavy

3   There is usually more time in which to call for assistance.

Causes

Secondary post-partum haemorrhage may come either from the placental site or from some extra-placental source. If from the former, it is usually due either to a placental polyp – a cotyledon which has failed to separate and be expelled and which produces its effects in precisely the same manner as a retained placenta in primary post-partum bleeding – or from the separation of a thrombus from the mouth of one of the larger vessels running to the placental site.

Extra-placental sources include secondary haemorrhage from infected lacerations of the genital tract and, rarely, blood dyscrasias such as Purpura. Carcinoma of the cervix is a very infrequent cause.

Although widely regarded as causative factors, retained portions of the foetal membranes do not give rise to secondary post-partum haemorrhage.

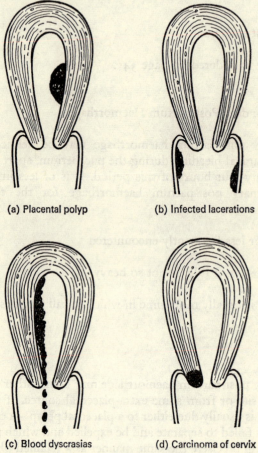

(a) Placental polyp   (b) Infected lacerations

(c) Blood dyscrasias   (d) Carcinoma of cervix

Fig. 48   Causes of secondary post-partum haemorrhage

Management

The management of a case of secondary post-partum haemorrhage should be along the following lines:

a   The patient must be put to bed and made to lie flat. The

Trendelenberg position should *not* be adopted as it allows blood to pool in the vaginal vault and thus escape notice

b A quarter-hourly pulse and blood pressure record must be started

c Medical aid must be called

d Preparations must be made for taking blood for grouping and cross-matching and for blood transfusion or plasma or saline infusion.

Other than this, no active treatment should be undertaken by the midwife.

Unless the source of the bleeding is both obvious and accessible, the doctor will probably decide to examine the patient under a general anaesthetic. If the bleeding is from an infected laceration, it can usually be controlled with further sutures; if from the uterine cavity, treatment consists of evacuating any placental tissue with a pair of sponge-holding forceps followed by gentle curettage.

After-care

On return to the ward, a watch should be kept for further bleeding or for the development of shock. Usually, however, recovery is rapid and complete.

IV Puerperal Psychosis

Although a description of puerperal psychosis is beyond the scope of this book, it may be of use to mention some of the early manifestations of this state since this may help to alert the midwife to the fact that her patient is in need of psychiatric assistance. These manifestations usually take the form of abnormal behaviour patterns and conform roughly to one of the following types:

1 The patient may complain of increasing insomnia for no obvious reason.

2   She may develop a violent aversion to someone for whom she has previously felt affection, such as her husband, a near relative or even her baby. In this last case, extreme care must be taken to ensure that she does not deliberately harm the child when it is within her reach.

3   She may become withdrawn and sullen, speak little and refuse to answer questions.

4   She may assume a more violent attitude, both in her actions and in her speech, threatening those around her.

5   She may complain of being persecuted by the other inmates of the ward, by the medical or nursing staff or by friends or relatives who visit her. Alternatively, she may declare that she is the object of some malign and improbable influence emanating from some distant source.

6   Rarely, she may suffer from frank hallucinations, seeing or hearing people, objects or voices which are not actually present.

Should a puerperal woman develop any of the above behaviour patterns, the midwife must inform a doctor immediately since the need for psychiatric treatment may be urgent if an early and complete return to a normal mental state is to be achieved.

Summary

Infections of the Genital Tract

The pattern of puerperal infections of the genital tract has altered in recent years. Such infections are now usually of a mild nature.

The reasons for this are the sensitivity of the haemolytic streptococcus to sulphonamides and penicillin, the lack of extensively traumatised tissues for the establishment of anaerobic streptococcal infections, and the efficacy of modern antibiotics against staphylococci and coliforms.

Pyrexia itself is of no value in indicating the site of an infection. This can be determined only from local symptoms and signs.

Genital infections may be endogenous, autogenous or exogenous. Of these, the last is the most important. For an infection to be established the *dose* of bacteria must be sufficiently great, the patient's *immunity* must be lowered and there must be a suitable *site* for invasion. These conditions are frequently fulfilled during the puerperium.

The more common genital infections are those of the perineum, vagina and cervix. These usually arise from infected lacerations or episiotomy incisions. In such infections both the general constitutional upset and the local symptomatology are usually mild. The potentially more dangerous infections of the placental site are uncommon. When they occur they usually remain well localised.

Any puerperal woman who develops a pyrexia must be examined by a doctor to determine the nature of her infection. If this is genital, a high vaginal swab, a throat swab and a midstream specimen of urine should be sent for microscopy and culture and a suitable antibiotic prescribed.

General nursing measures in these patients include their segregation to a ward adapted for their treatment, the provision of free fluids, a light diet, adequate analgesics, sedatives and hypnotics. Where the perineum is infected local applications of heat are often valuable.

The prevention of infection includes efficient correction of anaemia and blood loss and careful repair of damage sustained at delivery. Precautions must also be taken against the spread of bacteria by dust, crockery or droplet infection.

Where an outbreak of puerperal infection occurs in a postnatal ward, the principles of management include treatment of the infected cases, the detection of the source of infection and the protection of the other patients both in the ward itself and in the rest of the unit.

N

Thrombo-Embolic Disease

During the puerperium the clotting power of the blood is increased. As a result, venous thrombosis is liable to occur in the legs and in the pelvis, where the blood flow is relatively sluggish.

Once formed, a clot may spread into a larger vessel, break off and pass into the lungs, causing a pulmonary embolus.

Signs of deep vein thrombosis are low-grade pyrexia and slight tachycardia, tenderness and swelling of the affected leg and pain on stretching the muscles of the calf.

Signs of a pulmonary embolus depend upon its size and vary from transient and slight pleural pain with some productive cough to extreme respiratory and circulatory distress. In a few cases death is almost instantaneous.

The treatment of deep vein thrombosis consists of preventing extension of the clotting process with anti-coagulants, together with measures designed to relieve pain, tenderness and swelling. Once the acute phase has passed, physiotherapy is of value in reducing any residual oedema.

When a small warning pulmonary embolus has occurred, full anti-coagulant measures must be instituted immediately to limit the threat of further larger emboli. Where the initial embolus is large, first-aid treatment is aimed at overcoming dyspnoea and circulatory embarrassment.

The majority of demonstrable deep vein thromboses do not develop pulmonary emboli. Similarly, the majority of pulmonary emboli are not associated with demonstrable deep vein thrombosis.

Superficial thrombosis in a varicose vein does not carry the same risk as deep venous thrombosis. Treatment consists of early ambulation and, if pain and tenderness are marked, suitable analgesics.

Other Abnormalities of the Puerperium

Puerperal urinary tract complications consist of retention of urine, retention with overflow, residual urine, ascending urinary tract infection and stress incontinence.

Where any variety of urinary retention is present it is essential that the bladder be regularly emptied, if necessary by catheter, if infection of the urine is to be prevented.

Secondary post-partum haemorrhage is an occasional complication of the puerperium. Less important than the primary variety, its source may be either placental or extra-placental. In the former event the actual cause is usually a placental polyp, although at times the separation of a thrombus from the mouth of a large placental site vessel may result in bleeding. Extra-placental sources include infected lacerations, blood dyscrasias and, very rarely, carcinoma of the cervix.

Management depends on the cause. Bleeding from an infected laceration is usually controlled by suturing. Any loss from the placental site is dealt with by evacuation and curettage of the uterus under general anaesthesia.

Puerperal psychosis may assume a variety of forms. These usually appear as abnormal behaviour patterns, such as the development of a sudden aversion to a person for whom affection had previously been felt, sullen withdrawal from the every-day life of the ward, violent actions and speech or frank persecution mania and delusions. Insomnia is also a feature of many such cases.

Where the development of a puerperal psychosis is suspected from the patient's behaviour, medical assistance must be obtained at once since the need for psychiatric support is often urgent.

PART SIX

Neonatal Paediatrics

CHAPTER SIXTEEN

The Normal Newborn

The nursing care of the newborn differs from that of children of other age groups because a mother, being unfamiliar with her baby, may not realise that it is not perfectly well. Alternatively, the baby may become ill while its mother is still recovering from the effects of labour, before she has had an opportunity to see it. Although a baby may appear normal when examined by a doctor immediately after its birth, it can soon become seriously ill. For example, where there is a fistula between the oesophagus and the trachea, trouble will not develop until the baby is fed, when fluid will pass into the trachea and cause a severe and possibly fatal respiratory disturbance.

Again, if a newborn baby develops an infection such as gastro-enteritis, the dehydration and shock which may easily develop within a few hours will, if untreated, lead to permanent damage and even death. It should also be realised that, unlike an older child or an adult, a baby can often have a serious infection and yet show few signs of being unwell; even if gravely ill with meningitis it may merely go off its feeds.

For these reasons, the immediate responsibility for suspecting that a baby is unwell rests with the midwife. She, in turn, should at once tell a doctor of her suspicions so that a diagnosis may be reached and the appropriate treatment started without delay.

Only by so doing can the neonatal morbidity and mortality rates be reduced.

In order to be able to recognise that a newborn baby is abnormal or ill, the midwife must be familiar with its normal characteristics.

Weight. This varies considerably in full-time babies, being influenced by such factors as its own sex and the mother's race, height, parity, social class and smoking habits as well as by various maternal diseases and abnormalities of pregnancy. Although with early feeding the weight of some babies does not drop at all, as a rule the neonate loses about seven per cent of its birthweight during the first five days of life. This loss is usually made good by the eighth to twelfth day.

Subsequent Weight Gain. In general, a baby will double its birth weight in five months and triple it in one year, although this increase may be greater if its initial weight was low.

Length. The average Crown–Heel length of a baby at term is 51 cm – the normal range being from 46 to 56 cm. Accurate measurement of a baby's length provides an important standard from which to judge future growth.

The Skin. The skin is ruddy and often mottled. At birth it is usually covered in Vernix Caseosa – a white sebaceous secretion. Fine, downy hair – Lanugo – sometimes covers the shoulders and back. The following conditions may be observed on the skin of the newborn:

a   *Petechial Haemorrhages* are normally present on the face and neck but should not occur elsewhere.

b   *Mongolian Spots* are bluish, pigmented areas seen on the back and the buttocks of dark-skinned babies. They are of no significance.

c   *Milia* of the face are small papules which represent distended sebaceous glands.

d   *Superficial Naevi* occur as bluish-red patches on the eyelids, forehead and back of the head. Both these and Milia are normal findings.

e   *Toxic Erythema* is a blotchy, red rash, often associated with small pustular lesions. It needs no treatment.

f   A Midline Dimple is often present over the lower part of the sacrum. Provided that its base can be seen it is of no consequence, otherwise it must be investigated further as it may represent a sinus communicating with the spinal cord.

After about forty-eight hours the neonate may become jaundiced. This is due to immaturity of certain liver enzymes and clears after ten days. Jaundice which either develops *before* forty-eight hours or persists *after* ten days is abnormal.

The Head and the Face

The size of the head is large in relation to that of the body. Where the delivery was cephalic, moulding may be present (page 163). A Caput Succedaneum is often seen and may temporarily obscure the fontanelles. The *circumference* of the head should be carefully measured as it reflects the size of the intracranial contents. Normally 33 cm, it increases rapidly during early neonatal life due to the growth of the brain.

The Ears should be examined since deformities of the pinna are often associated with genito-urinary abnormalities. Accessory auricles, however, represented by small skin tags, are of no serious import.

The Eyes. At birth the irises are usually slate-grey while the sclera may be blue. Subconjunctival and scleral haemorrhages are common, of no significance and generally disappear within three weeks.

The Mouth and Jaws. The colour of the mucous membrane of the mouth is important. If pale, it suggests anaemia, if blue, cyanosis. *Epithelial Pearls* are small elevations at the gum margins and at the junction of the hard and the soft palate. They are not important. Occasionally the lower incisors have erupted at birth. Usually such teeth are soft and soon fall out. If they persist their removal may be necessary at some future date.

The Nose. Since a newborn baby breathes mainly through its nose, the patency of the nasal airway is of great importance. This can be checked by gently passing a small catheter up the nose.

The Baby's Cry. Much information can be gained from listening to a baby's cry. If high-pitched, it often denotes brain damage; if hoarse it suggests a naso-pharyngeal or respiratory obstruction.

The Abdomen

The abdomen of the newborn is normally somewhat protuberant. A slight prominence in the left hypochondrium may
develop immediately after a feed, sometimes accompanied by
visible peristalsis. This is normal. On the other hand a hollow or
scaphoid abdomen, associated with developing respiratory distress, points to the presence of a diaphragmatic hernia. *Abdominal Distension* is always abnormal and suggests intestinal
obstruction, an over-distended bladder or an intra-abdominal
tumour. An *Umbilical Hernia* which develops during the first four
weeks of life is very common and will always regress spontaneously. It therefore needs no treatment. A hernia either above
or below the umbilicus, however, is abnormal and calls for
operation.

The Umbilical Cord

The cord usually dries and sloughs off between the fifth and
tenth day. The slough may remain moist for a few days and a
small granuloma may form if the amount of Wharton's jelly was
excessive. Any umbilical discharge should be investigated
further as it may be due to a persistent urachus.

The Chest and Respiration

The newborn's breathing is abdominal in type and is commonly
shallow and irregular. Although the rate may vary momentarily
between 20 and 100 per minute, a rate persistently over 60 is
always abnormal. *Respiratory Distress* is of serious significance. It
is revealed by rapid, grunting respiration, flaring of the alae nasi,
rib recession and see-sawing of the sternum. *Stridor* – noisy
respiration – is associated with laryngeal obstruction due either
to pressure from without or to a congenital deformity.

The Breasts. Some degree of mammary engorgement occurs in
neonates of both sexes, the breasts being usually palpable and
sometimes very large. This enlargement persists for some weeks
but needs no treatment.

The Genitalia

In the male the prepuce is adherent to the glans penis and cannot be retracted without force. This should never be attempted. The *Testes* are usually palpable in the scrotum but sometimes may not have descended beyond the inguinal canal. In the female the labia minora and clitoris are relatively large and a hymeneal tag may protrude from the vulva. At times there may be a mucoid vaginal discharge or even a small amount of bleeding. None of these conditions requires treatment.

The Hips

In the newborn it is of great importance to exclude congenital dislocation of the hips. This can be done by placing the middle fingers on the greater trochanters, the thumbs over the region if the lesser trochanters and then abducting the hips. On applying pressure against the greater trochanters a click will be felt if the hips are dislocated. In such cases suitable treatment, if started in early life, will prevent any gross and permanent deformity of the hip joints.

Meconium and Stools

For the first three days of life the stools consist of Meconium, which is made up of mucus, desquamated epithelial cells, amniotic fluid and bilirubin. Thereafter they gradually assume a normal colour and consistency. The first stool is usually passed within twenty-four hours of birth although this may be delayed until the second or third day. Subsequently the daily number of stools varies considerably, although a breast fed baby will usually pass one at each feed. A *Meconium Plug*, which occasionally causes obstruction at the anus, can be removed with the tip of the finger or of a thermometer.

The Urine

A newborn baby should pass urine within twenty-four hours of delivery. Any delay beyond this time should arouse suspicions of a urinary obstruction and calls for a medical opinion.

Temperature

The neonate cannot easily tolerate changes in the temperature of his surroundings. As his surface area is relatively greater than that of an older child or of an adult he can lose heat very rapidly. For this reason care must be taken not to expose a baby to low environmental temperatures, especially when it is being bathed or changed. In warmer weather, or if excessive clothing is being used, a baby is liable to sweat and to develop a heat rash.

Behaviour and Response to Environment

While most babies sleep for the greater part of the time, waking up only for feeding, some stay awake for long periods. A baby born at term yawns and sneezes and frequently stretches its arms and legs. Hiccup is common. A number of reflexes are present at birth and provide an index of normal brain function. These reflexes are:

a   *The Grasp Reflex.* In response to pressure on the baby's palms or soles, the arms and legs exert counter pressure.

b   *The Moro Reflex.* This is elicited by supporting the baby in a supine position and then suddenly allowing the head to fall back a few inches when both arms will fly outwards with extension at all joints.

c   *The Rooting Reflex.* Here, stimulation of the upper lip causes the mouth to open and the head to move upwards.

Summary

The midwife must be familiar with the characteristics of the normal newborn baby so that she may be able to recognise the presence or development of any abnormality.

In the examination of the newborn, attention should be paid to the following points:

a The weight and weight changes

b The baby's length

c The condition of its skin

d The shape and circumference of its head and the condition of the ears, eyes, mouth and jaws, nose and throat

e The shape of the abdomen, the presence of any hernias and the condition of the cord

f The state of the breasts and of the external genitalia

g The presence or absence of congenital dislocation of the hips

h The temperature, pulse rate and respirations

i The nature of the stools, the frequency with which they are passed and the time when urine is first voided

j The baby's behaviour, reflexes, sleep pattern and movements.

Prematurity

The Premature Baby

As stated on page 276, a premature baby is often defined as one weighing 2500 grammes or less at birth. However, since many of such babies are small-for-dates rather than premature in the strictest sense, it is perhaps better to regard as premature a baby born before the end of the thirty-sixth week of pregnancy. Such babies usually, although not invariably, weigh less than 2500 grammes, have a crown–heel length of less than 37 cm and a head circumference of under 33 cm.

Conditions Associated with Prematurity

Although the precise cause or causes of prematurity are not known, in the majority of instances it is associated with certain conditions affecting the mother or the foetus.

a   *Maternal Conditions*. Prematurity is more common if the mother is under twenty or over forty years of age, if she is unmarried or if she is of high parity. It is also associated with smoking in pregnancy and with such features as hypertension, cardiac disease and urinary tract infection as well as pre-eclampsia and ante-partum haemorrhage. In addition, mothers who have a low standard of living are more likely to give birth to a premature baby than the well-to-do.

b *Foetal Conditions.* Prematurity is more common in twins, first-born babies and those possessing congenital malformations.

The Physical Characteristics of the Premature Baby

The premature baby differs in many respects from one born at term. Due to the fact that its muscles are poorly developed it is usually less vigorous, its cry is more feeble and its respirations more irregular. Its eyes, which are rather prominent, usually remain closed for long periods of time. Its head is larger in proportion to its overall size and its abdomen is more protuberant. Its skin is wrinkled and red with little or no vernix caseosa although lanugo hair is abundant. There is only scanty subcutaneous fat although this may be simulated by oedema to which it is very prone. Breast tissue is small in amount and breast engorgement absent, although in the female the labia are very prominent. The ears are flabby, lacking cartilage. Creases on the soles of the feet are absent.

The Assessment of Gestational Age. Where doubt exists about the duration of pregnancy or where the size of the uterus did not correspond to the period of amenorrhoea, it is important to assess the precise age of the newborn. This is because the management of the premature differs in many respects from that of the small-for-dates baby. Gestational age may be established both by testing for the presence of certain reflexes and by looking for certain clinical signs. These are set out in Tables 1 and 2.

The Hazards of Prematurity

Since the premature baby is less fully developed both anatomically and physiologically than the mature, it is subject to many hazards which do not affect the latter to the same extent.

a *The Body Temperature* varies greatly with changes in the temperature of the environment. This is partly because the baby is poorly insulated against heat loss due to lack of subcutaneous fat and partly because its surface area is very great

Table 1

Reflex	Stimulus	Positive Response	Gestation if Reflex is Absent	Present
Pupil reaction	Light	Pupil contraction	Under 31	29 or more
Traction	Pull up by wrists from supine	Flexion of neck or arms	Under 36	33 or more
Glabella Tap	Tap on Glabella	Blink	Under 34	32 or more
Neck righting	Rotation of head	Trunk follows	Under 37	34 or more
Head turning	Diffuse light from one side	Head turning to light	Doubtful	32 or more

Table 2

	To 36 weeks	37–38 weeks	39 weeks or more
Sole creases	Anterior Transverse Crease only	Occasional creases anterior 2/3rds	Sole covered with creases
Breast nodule diameter	2 mm	4 mm	7 mm
Scalp hair	Fine and fuzzy	Fine and fuzzy	Coarse and silky
Ear lobe	No cartilage	Some cartilage	Thick cartilage
Testes and scrotum	Testes in lower canal – small Few rugae	Intermediate	Testes pendulous Scrotum full Extensive rugae

in relation to its weight. Other reasons are that the baby, being inactive, does not shiver, that its temperature regulating mechanism is immature and that the blood supply to its skin and its sweating ability are both undeveloped.

b *Respiratory Hazards* are the poor cough and gag reflexes which allow aspiration to occur, the weak respiratory muscles and the soft, pliable thoracic cage which may not prevent retraction of the chest on respiration, the immature respiratory centre and the undeveloped alveoli.

c *Gastro-Intestinal Handicaps.* Apart from causing feeding difficulties, the poor swallowing reflex and the limited capacity of the stomach favour vomiting and aspiration of gastric contents.

d *The Immature Liver* of a premature baby is low in glycogen, resulting in a tendency to hypoglycaemia, while, owing to its undeveloped enzyme systems, jaundice is more common (page 399).

e *The Blood* is deficient in clotting factors, particularly Prothrombin. Haemorrhage is thus more common, particularly within the brain, owing to the weak vessel walls and the high incidence of anoxia (page 394).

f *Deficiency States.* The limited iron reserves of the premature favour the development of anaemia later in life. The immature Parathyroid glands cause a tendency to hypocalcaemia. Rickets may develop from the combination of low calcium and Vitamin D levels with a rapid rate of growth.

g *An Increased Susceptibility to Infection* is present due to a decreased rate of transfer across the placenta of antibodies from the mother (page 402).

The Management of the Premature Baby

A paediatrician, or some person trained in the resuscitation and care of the newborn should always be present at the delivery of a premature baby. After the pharynx has been sucked out, proper respiration established and 1 mg of Vitamin K given intramuscularly, the baby, kept well covered in order to prevent any drop in body temperature, should be placed in an incubator and transferred to the Special Care Baby Unit. Once there, it should be nursed unclothed in an incubator of a type which allows easy observation, the temperature of which should be high enough to maintain the baby's rectal temperature at 36–37°C or the skin temperature at 36°C. Handling should be kept to a minimum, especially if the baby weighs less than 1500 grammes, when the risk of apnoeic attacks is particularly high. No premature should be bathed during the first week of life unless it weighs over 2000 grammes.

Observations. The various observations necessary for the proper care of a premature baby should be carried out with the least possible disturbance, especially if it weighs less than 1500 grammes, when a No Touch technique should be used. Since opening the incubator allows a baby's temperature to drop, this must be avoided unless absolutely necessary.

a *The Heart Rate* should be recorded hourly for the first twenty-four hours. An oscilloscope or cardiorator makes this observation easier.

b *Respirations* should be checked at frequent intervals. An apnoea monitor is useful if the baby is very small. In addition, a ribbon should be attached to one of the baby's ankles and the end led out of the incubator. If apnoea occurs, breathing can usually be re-established by pulling on this ribbon. Should this fail, intubation will be needed. This has the disadvantage of entailing some handling of the baby. It may also allow the body temperature to fall as the incubator has to be opened.

c *Temperature*: This should be recorded frequently, preferably by means of a skin thermistor or a rectal probe, appliances which both permit of remote monitoring.

d *As Hypoglycaemia* is particularly common in premature babies, the blood sugar should be estimated routinely by means of a Dextrostix.

e *Weight.* The premature should be weighed regularly, incubator scales being used to avoid undue disturbance.

Protection from Infection (see also Chapter 18)

Premature babies are particularly prone to infection. For this reason, when in the Special Care Baby Unit, they should be well separated from one another, any obviously infected baby being isolated in another room. The number of people allowed to care for the babies should be strictly limited and all should wash their hands carefully both before and after handling them. In addition, the greatest care must be taken over the preparation of feeds and the disposal of soiled linen. It need scarcely be added that no known carrier of any infection should be allowed into the Unit.

Feeding

A premature baby should be fed within one hour of birth. If it weighs under 1500 grammes, a small feeding tube should be passed into its stomach, the other end being led out of the in-cubator and attached to a syringe. Although babies above this weight may be strong enough to suck a bottle or take the breast, if in doubt tube feeding should be started since it carries less risk of aspiration. The tube need not be changed for at least a week. Because of its limited stomach capacity, a premature baby needs frequent feeding, in some cases as often as every fifteen to thirty minutes. The amount of food needed during the first forty-eight hours is shown in Table 3.

Table 3   Feeding Regime for Premature Babies

Weight (g)	Age in Hours		
	1–3 (ml) hourly	4–22 (ml) every 2 hours	22–48 (ml) every 3 hours
750	2	4	9
1000	2·5	5	12
1250	3	6	15
1500	4	8	18
1750	4·5	9	21
2000	5	10	24
2250	6	12	27
2500	6·5	13	30

At the end of the first week all babies should be receiving at least 150 ml/kg body weight a day.

The Type of Feed. The first two feeds should consist of five per cent Dextrose in sterile water. Half strength milk feeds may then be given for twenty-four hours, after which full strength feeding can be started. The milk of choice is breast milk. Failing this, S.M.A. is preferable to other artificial feeds. *Supplements* in the form of Vitamins A, C and D should be given as Abidec, 0·3 ml increasing to 0·6 ml daily. Iron in the form of Ferrous Gluconate, 50 mg daily, should be started only after three weeks.

Complications Associated with Prematurity

Most 'At Risk' neonates are premature babies. These, as already pointed out in the previous section, are particularly likely to develop complications directly ascribable to their immature state.

a   *Respiratory Distress Syndrome.* This develops immediately after birth. It is characterised by cyanosis with rapid, grunting respirations, flaring of the alae nasi, intercostal recession and see-sawing of the sternum. In mildly affected cases it lasts for twenty-four to forty-eight hours before gradually subsiding. In more severe instances respiration may be embarrassed for two to three days before improvement sets in. Severely affected babies become increasingly distressed and die within forty-eight hours. The exact cause of this syndrome is not known. It is almost always restricted to premature babies, particularly to those of very low birth weight. It is also more common where the mother has had diabetes or an antepartum haemorrhage and where foetal distress has occurred during labour. No specific *treatment* exists. General measures include giving oxygen, avoiding heat loss and providing frequent small feeds, by tube if necessary. If acidosis is present, intravenous bicarbonate is needed. At times it may be advisable to put the baby on a ventilator.

b   *Intracranial Bleeding.* Even where labour has been uneventful the premature baby is liable to sudden and sometimes fatal intracranial bleeding.

c *Retrolental Fibroplasia.* This is usually seen in prematures of less than 1500 grammes birth weight and is particularly likely to arise if the baby is placed in a high concentration of oxygen. The disease affects the eyes and may cause blindness. For this reason, prematures should never be given oxygen unless this is really necessary, in which case its concentration should not exceed thirty per cent unless there are special reasons to the contrary.

d *Hypoglycaemia.* As already stated (page 387), hypoglycaemia is common in premature babies. It usually occurs within twenty-four hours of birth but may be delayed for some days. Although usually characterised by irritability, muscle jerking or convulsions, it may be symptomless. As hypoglycaemia can lead to permanent brain damage, the baby's blood sugar level must be frequently checked with Dextrostix. Once hypoglycaemia develops, treatment with oral or intravenous glucose must be started without delay.

e *Kernicterus.* This condition, described on page 400, can develop in prematures at lower levels of bilirubin than in babies born at term. For this reason, the serum bilirubin level in any jaundiced premature must be checked at frequent intervals, exchange transfusion being carried out if necessary.

f *Congenital Malformations.* These are also more likely to be found in babies of low birth weight.

The Prognosis for the Premature Baby

This is influenced by the degree of prematurity as well as by the baby's actual birth weight. Although approximately 50 per cent of all deaths among prematures occur during the first twenty-four hours of life, the precise mortality and morbidity rates associated with this group of babies vary widely between hospitals and depend largely upon the standard of medical and nursing care, the availability of mechanical and electronic aids to treatment and existing laboratory facilities. If prematurity can be anticipated before delivery, transfer to a hospital possessing a properly equipped and staffed Special Care Baby Unit will greatly increase the neonate's chances of survival, especially if it weighs under 1500 grammes. As a general rule, while babies weighing over 2000 grammes are unlikely to die, the mortality among those of under 1500 grammes birth weight is fifty per cent. Even if such a baby survives, it may suffer from mental retardation or cerebral palsy. Premature babies tend to remain shorter and lighter than babies born at term until about five years of age.

Summary

The Premature Baby

A premature baby is one whose gestational age is less than thirty-six weeks. This definition is preferable to one based on weight alone, since many babies of under 2500 grammes are born at or even after term.

Prematurity is often associated with certain well-defined maternal, foetal and social factors.

The physical characteristics of the premature differ in many important respects from those of the mature baby.

Where the duration of pregnancy is uncertain, the gestational age of a baby can be established by looking for certain reflexes and clinical signs. These do not depend upon the baby's weight.

The hazards of prematurity are:

a   Poor temperature control

b   Immaturity of the respiratory system, the gastro-intestinal tract and the liver

c   An increased tendency to haemorrhage, infection, feeding difficulties and hypoglycaemia.

The immediate management of the premature is aimed at preventing hypothermia. Once transferred to the Special Care Baby Unit, the baby should be placed in an incubator and handled as little as possible.

In all premature babies a careful record must be kept of the heart and respiration rates, the temperature, the blood glucose and the weight.

Particular attention must be paid to the avoidance of infection in the premature baby.

In small prematures tube feeding may be advisable. In all cases early and frequent feeding is necessary. The feeds of choice are breast milk or S.M.A. At the end of the first week a premature baby should be receiving 150 ml/kg body weight/day. Supplements of Vitamins A, C and D as well as of iron are also necessary.

Complications Associated with Prematurity

The anatomical and physiological immaturity of premature babies renders them particularly prone to complications such as the respiratory distress syndrome, cerebral haemorrhage, retrolental fibroplasia, hypoglycaemia and kernicterus. Congenital malformations are also more common in such babies.

The survival rate as well as the permanent health of premature babies depends upon the degree of medical and nursing care available as well as upon the laboratory and mechanical facilities that are to hand.

Fifty per cent of babies weighing under 1500 grammes at birth die. Of the survivors, many suffer from some type of cerebral damage.

For the first five years of life, premature babies remain smaller than those born at term.

CHAPTER EIGHTEEN

Complications of the Newborn

Anoxia

Anoxia can be defined as an inadequate supply of oxygen. Its greatest danger is that it can cause irreversible brain damage, characterised by cerebral palsy, mental retardation and, occasionally, death. Anoxia may arise before or after birth.

Anoxia before Birth can arise in several different ways:

a *Placental Insufficiency* may be present, as in cases of pre-eclampsia, prolonged pregnancy or ante-partum haemorrhage

b The placental circulation may be impaired, such as during a prolonged labour, as a result of a sudden drop in the maternal blood pressure

c The umbilical blood flow may be cut off by compression or a knot in the cord

d The oxygen concentration of the maternal blood may be too low, as in serious anaemia or during diseases such as pneumonia.

Anoxia after Birth is also due to a variety of causes.

a The baby may fail to breathe spontaneously, either because of cerebral damage or because its respiratory centre has been depressed by drugs given to the mother during labour

b The baby may be unable to oxygenate its blood owing to respiratory obstruction or because of pulmonary or cardiac abnormalities

c The baby may be severely anaemic

d Oxygenation of the baby's tissues may be impaired due to severe shock, blood loss, adrenal haemorrhage or infection.

The Clinical Signs of Anoxia

Before birth, these are alterations in the foetal heart rate, meconium staining of the liquor and a drop in the pH of the foetal scalp blood. After birth, the anoxic baby is characterised by absent or irregular respiration, cyanosis or pallor, bradycardia, poor muscle tone and a diminished response to stimuli.

The Apgar Score (Table 4)

This is a useful standard for evaluating the condition of the neonate. A score of 0, 1 or 2 may be recorded for each one of five clinical observations, making a maximum of 10.

Table 4

	Observation		Score	
		0	1	2
1	Heart rate	Absent	Slow: Under 100	Above 100
2	Respiratory effort	Absent	Occasional gasp	Regular
3	Colour	Blue or Pale	Trunk pink Extremities pale	Completely pink
4	Muscle tone	Limp	Some flexion of extremities	Active movements
5	Response to stimulation of nose or feet	Nil	Grimace Weak movement	Cough or sneeze Withdrawal

The Apgar Score should be recorded at 1 and 5 minutes after birth. A score of 8–10 shows that the baby's condition is good, one of 5, 6 or 7 that it is moderately depressed. A score of 4 or less will be recorded if the baby's state is very poor – limp, cyanosed, pale, apnoeic, with a slow or absent heart beat.

The Prevention of Anoxia

The following routine should be followed in every case:

a Gently remove any excess mucus from the mouth and the nostrils

b Record the Apgar Score at 1 and 5 minutes

c If the mother has been given either Morphine or Pethidine within four hours of delivery, give the baby Levallorphan (Lorfan) 0·25 mg either into the umbilical vein or intramuscularly. This will reverse any respiratory depression

d Give Vitamin K (Konakion) 1 mg intramuscularly to prevent any tendency to haemorrhage

e Always handle the baby gently and keep it warm and dry to prevent its temperature from falling

f Do not bath any baby weighing less than 2000 grammes or whose birth has been difficult or abnormal.

If the establishment of normal respiration is delayed the midwife must first call for medical aid and then proceed as follows:

a Place the baby on the 'Resuscitaire' and give oxygen by funnel

b Stimulate respiration by flicking the soles of the feet

c If breathing is still not established after one minute or if the baby's heart rate is below 100 per minute, an endotracheal tube must be passed and intermittent positive pressure ventilation carried out at a rate of 20 per minute, the manometer pressure being kept below 25 cm of water. It must be remembered that delayed respiration in the newborn is as serious as cardiac arrest in an adult.

Trauma

Trauma may be either minor or major. Minor varieties of trauma such as a caput succedaneum or a subconjunctival haemorrhage present no dangers to the baby although they may cause considerable anxiety to the mother who should be reassured by the hospital staff that her worries are groundless. Major trauma, on the other hand, such as cerebral haemorrhage, is of the greatest importance as it may lead to permanent impairment of function and thus severely affect a baby's subsequent development.

Varieties of Trauma

a *Caput Succedaneum*. This is an oedematous swelling affecting the presenting part of a baby's head. It occurs in the course of a normal labour, is of no pathological significance and disappears within fourteen days of birth. This should be explained to the mother who may otherwise worry unnecessarily, believing the caput to be a swelling of the underlying brain.

b *Cephalhaematoma*. This is a collection of blood beneath the periosteum of one of the bones of the cranial vault. It is thus limited by the suture lines. It is caused by pressure on the skull during labour and is therefore often associated with a forceps delivery. As in the case of a caput succedaneum, no treatment is needed although the swelling may take up to three months to resolve.

c *Skeletal Trauma*. Several types of damage to the skeleton may be seen. *Linear fractures of the skull* are sometimes associated with a cephalhaematoma. They are usually of no clinical significance. *Depressed fractures of the skull* are occasionally seen after a difficult forceps delivery. If they do not resolve spontaneously, surgical elevation of the depressed area of bone is necessary. *Fractures of the clavicle* are occasional complications of breech delivery or shoulder dystocia. Such fractures may not be immediately apparent and often are noticed only when a baby refuses to move the affected arm or cries when its shoulders are touched. No treatment is required and healing is always good. *Fractures of long bones* – the humerus or the femur – may occur in the course of a difficult delivery, especially when the breech presents. These fractures heal extremely well, even where reduction seems to have been poor.

d   *Trauma to Peripheral Nerves. Facial Palsy* is usually due to pressure by the forceps on the facial nerve. The muscles on the affected side droop, the naso-labial fold is obliterated and the eye cannot close. This sort of paralysis is almost always temporary. *Erb-Duchenne Palsy* is due to stretching or tearing of the upper part of the Brachial Plexus. It may complicate shoulder dystocia. The affected limb is held close to the chest, the arm hanging in a pronated position. The muscles of the wrist and hand are unaffected. The outlook depends on whether the nerves involved are merely stretched – when recovery is the rule – or whether they have been torn – in which case the outlook is poor despite operation. In all cases the arm should be tied above the cot in abduction with the elbow flexed and the forearm supinated. *Klumpke's Paralysis* results from damage to the lower part of the Brachial Plexus, usually in association with difficulty in the delivery of the after-coming head. As the muscles of the wrist and hand are affected both the grasp reflex and wrist movements are absent. In treating this condition, a flat splint is needed to support the hand and wrist to prevent wrist drop and flexion contractures. Although spontaneous recovery is usual, this type of paralysis may be permanent.

e   *Trauma to the Spinal Cord.* Excessive lateral flexion of the baby's trunk may cause the spinal cord to be torn across, resulting in sensory loss and flaccid paralysis below the level of the lesion. Bladder and bowel disturbances may also be present. The outlook is poor.

f   *Trauma to Abdominal Organs.* Rupture of a viscus such as the liver, kidneys, stomach or gut is rare, as it can occur only as a result of excessive abdominal pressure. As such, it is less uncommon in premature than in mature babies.

g *Brain Injury.* This may take the form of either haemorrhage or oedema. *Haemorrhage* is more likely to occur in premature babies, after a precipitate delivery, in association with disproportion or in any condition which predisposes to anoxia (page 394). Such haemorrhage may also result from tears of the Tentorium Cerebelli or Falx Cerebri or from laceration of a subdural vein. Haemorrhage into the ventricles of the brain is common in premature babies. The *clinical signs* of such an accident are either present at birth or develop within a few hours. As a rule the baby is irritable, with increased muscle tone and a high-pitched cry. The Moro reflex is either increased or absent. Twitching and convulsions can occur. Suckling is impaired. At times, however, the baby may be depressed and hard to rouse. Such a case may develop cyanotic attacks and respiratory difficulties.

Management. As there is no specific treatment for cerebral haemorrhage, its prevention is of the greatest importance. The nursing care of the affected baby should be conducted along the same lines as those suggested for prematures (page 387).

Prognosis. This is difficult. Some babies showing minimal signs of cerebral irritation may be mentally defective or develop cerebral palsy. Others, with apparently severe cerebral injury at birth may nevertheless progress normally.

Jaundice

Jaundice is an extremely valuable indication of disease in the neonate. Although the serum bilirubin of all babies rises above the normal level of 1 mg per cent during the first ten days of life, in only half of these does jaundice become apparent. In such a case the problem arises of distinguishing this so-called 'Physiological Jaundice' of the newborn from some pathological state which may need urgent treatment.

Bilirubin. This is a pigment formed when red blood cells are destroyed in the body. Although normally broken down in the liver, this process sometimes fails either because the amount of bilirubin is too great for the liver to deal with – too many red cells being destroyed – or because liver function is itself impaired. In either case the level of bilirubin in the plasma will rise, jaundice becoming clinically apparent when this exceeds 5 mg per cent.

Kernicterus. If, during the first weeks of life, the bilirubin concentration rises above 20 mg per cent, there is a risk that certain cells in the brain will absorb the pigment and be permanently damaged. This condition is known as Kernicterus. Since once it has developed no treatment is of any avail, it is important both to measure the level of bilirubin in the plasma and to know what conditions are likely to cause this level to rise. Early signs of kernicterus are diminished muscle tone, lethargy, poor suckling and feeding and upward deviation of the eyes. Later, spasticity and opisthotonus may supervene, with mental retardation and high-tone deafness. Sometimes the teeth may be stained yellow. The mortality is very high.

Causes of Jaundice in the Newborn

As has already been stated, the bilirubin level rises in all newborn babies. The reason for this is that the liver of the neonate is at first too immature to be able to deal with the amount of bilirubin resulting from the normal breakdown of its red cells, a function which in intra-uterine life is carried out by the mother. This immaturity of the neonate's liver is in no way abnormal and is analogous to the incomplete development at birth of such other functions as digestion and temperature regulation.

The clinical characteristics of physiological jaundice are that it becomes apparent within forty-eight hours of birth, is rarely severe and disappears by the tenth day. It follows that jaundice which starts *before* forty-eight hours, which is *severe* and which lasts *beyond* the tenth day is not physiological.

Factors aggravating *Physiological Jaundice* are:

a   *Prematurity*. The liver of the premature is even more immature than that of the baby born at or near term. It is therefore even less able to break down bilirubin. For this reason, jaundice in the premature may start earlier and last longer. Furthermore, kernicterus is likely to occur at lower bilirubin levels.

b *Drugs.* Drugs such as salicylates, sulphonamides, steroids and Chloramphenicol may, for various reasons, increase the depth of jaundice in the newborn

c *Dehydration and starvation* have the same effect

d *Breast Milk.* Some mothers excrete a steroid in their milk that exacerbates neonatal jaundice.

The Treatment of Physiological Jaundice. As a rule, physiological jaundice requires no treatment unless the level of bilirubin becomes abnormally high when an exchange transfusion should be carried out.

Haemolytic Jaundice (First Day Jaundice)
Excessive haemolysis – destruction of red cells – occurs either when the baby's blood group is incompatible with its mother's or when there is an abnormality of the baby's blood. In either case the immature liver is unable to deal with the excessive amount of bilirubin produced and a variable degree of jaundice results. *Blood Group Incompatibility* occurs in one of two ways:

a *Rhesus Incompatibility* is still the most usual cause of severe jaundice in the newborn. It has already been discussed on page 140.

b *ABO Incompatibility* arises when the mother's ABO group differs from that of her baby. In such an event haemolysis may take place although this is rarely severe enough to warrant an exchange transfusion.

Abnormalities of the Baby's Blood. Rarely certain enzymes normally present in the red corpuscles are absent. This allows excessive breakdown of these cells to take place with resultant jaundice.

Jaundice persisting beyond the tenth day is usually abnormal and should always be investigated. It may be due to:

a   *Biliary Atresia*. In this condition the bile ducts fail to canalise. Jaundice starts as usual on the third day but persists beyond the tenth. Unless corrected surgically – which is rarely possible – death occurs from biliary cirrhosis at nine to twelve months.

b   *Congenital Hypothyroidism*. Jaundice is often the earliest indication that a baby is hypothyroid. In such a case early diagnosis and treatment are necessary if brain damage is to be avoided.

c   *Certain Congenital Diseases* such as Galactosaemia and Fructosaemia may present as jaundice in the neonate. Treatment consists in altering the baby's sugar intake.

d   *Infection*. In the newborn jaundice, often of a dangerously high degree, may accompany an infection such as a generalised bacteraemia or a localised hepatitis.

The Management of Jaundice in the Newborn

Whatever the cause of the jaundice, the plasma bilirubin must not be allowed to rise above 24 mg per cent in the mature and 20 mg per cent in the premature neonate. The only effective way of preventing such a rise is by means of an exchange transfusion. For this reason, frequent estimations of the plasma bilirubin should be carried out in order to determine when such a transfusion is needed.

Infection

Bacterial infection is commonly seen both in the mature and, more particularly, in the premature neonate. This is because although some types of maternal antibodies are transferred across the placenta and provide the baby with a passive immunity to diseases such as measles, mumps and chicken-pox, antibodies which give protection against several common bacteria such as Staphylococci, Streptococci, Pneumococci and B. Coli, cannot reach the baby in this way. Moreover, since the newborn is unable to form these antibodies himself during the first two to three months of life, he is particularly susceptible to infection from such organisms.

In the newborn, a characteristic feature of infection, whether mild or severe, is that it may well produce few signs of illness. Thus the baby may merely go off its feeds, vomit occasionally or become lethargic. Pyrexia may be slight or absent, in some cases the temperature may even be subnormal.

Since all bacterial infections in the newborn are associated with an increased mortality and morbidity, it is important to reach a diagnosis as soon as possible so that effective treatment can be started without delay.

Infection usually reaches the baby by one of three routes:

a *Via the Placenta*, resulting in a congenital infection. Examples of this are syphilis, viral hepatitis and toxoplasmosis

b *From the liquor amnii* which has itself become infected following prolonged rupture of the membranes or in the course of labour

c *After Birth* from the mother, doctors, nurses, other babies or contaminated feeds.

The infection may enter the baby by way of the mouth, nose, ears, eyes, skin or umbilicus. The exact portal of entry may not always be obvious.

The following signs indicate that a newborn has an infection:

a Lethargy or reluctance to feed, especially if the baby has previously fed well

b Diarrhoea and vomiting, leading to dehydration and weight loss

c Ashen pallor, with or without cyanosis

d Hypoglycaemia.

As already stated, the temperature may be raised, normal or subnormal. Indications of the site of infection naturally vary with the site itself. Thus a skin infection is usually revealed by some visible lesion, a gastro-intestinal infection by loose stools

o

or vomiting and a urinary infection by white cells in the urine. A blood stream infection is associated with a positive blood culture, meningitis with convulsions, coma and a bulging fontanelle. Jaundice suggests a liver infection, a swelling at the end of a bone osteomyelitis and redness of the ear drum a middle ear infection.

Common Infections of the Newborn are:

a *Thrush* (*Moniliasis*). Although this is not a bacterial infection, being caused by the fungus *Candida albicans*, it can conveniently be considered here. It is characterised by white patches on the buccal mucosa which bleed if an attempt is made to remove them. Treatment consists of applying 10 drops of Nystatin – 10,000 units per ml – to the mouth four times daily after feeds, care being taken to cover each lesion. Since thrush is often transmitted to the baby from the mother she should be investigated and, if need be, treated.

b *Staphylococcal Skin Infections* take the form of small pustules, occurring either as isolated lesions or in crops. They carry a risk of abscess formation or septicaemia.

c *Paronychia* are small red lesions around the finger-nail beds. They are best treated by covering the affected finger and giving an antibiotic.

d *Ophthalmia Neonatorum.* Although in the past the commonest cause of ophthalmia neonatorum was infection by the gonococcus, this is no longer the case since the incidence of untreated gonorrhoea is now much lower than formerly. Today such eye infections are usually caused by the TRIC viruses, Staphylococci and Pneumococci. The eye becomes red and swollen and discharges copiously. If untreated, corneal ulceration may result with permanent damage to the eye. Treatment consists of the local application of an antibiotic. This condition must not be confused with 'sticky eyes' which need only irrigation with sterile water.

e *Umbilical Infection* is characterised by a serous or purulent umbilical discharge. The infection may remain confined to the umbilicus, extend to the surrounding skin which becomes red and indurated or spread by way of the umbilical vessels to distant organs. Unless the infection is limited to the umbilicus, antibiotics should be given.

f   Epidemic Gastroenteritis. The causative agent of this highly contagious disease is usually either the B. Coli or a staphylococcus. It may also be due to infection with one of a number of viruses. The infection is usually introduced into the nursery by an adult carrier. The affected baby goes off its feeds, vomits and passes frequent loose stools. Shock and dehydration soon develop. Treatment consists in rapidly replacing lost fluid and in correcting the electrolyte imbalance. Antibiotics are of doubtful value in this disease.

The Prevention of Infection

a   All nurses and doctors working in the Nursery or in the Special Care Baby Unit should be regularly swabbed to detect carriers, especially of staphylococci. No nurse or doctor with an infection should come into contact with any newborn child. Similarly, an infected mother must be separated from her baby until she has been successfully treated.

b   Medical and Nursing Staff in charge of neonates should wash their hands with Hexachlorophane soap before and after handling a baby

c   Feeds should be prepared with scrupulous care

d   Babies should be handled as little and by as few people as possible

e   After a baby has been bathed its skin should be dusted with Hexachlorophane powder

f   All instruments and equipment used in the nursery or Special Care Baby Unit should be regularly and frequently checked for infection. This applies in particular to incubators, Resuscitaires and ventilators

g   Overcrowding encourages cross infection and should be avoided in nurseries and Special Care Baby Units

b The prophylactic value of antibiotics in babies at special risk is still not established. These drugs are, however, given in certain cases where infection is particularly liable to arise.

The Effect on the Baby of Maternal Diseases

The effect on the baby of abnormalities of pregnancy or labour such as pre-eclampsia, essential hypertension, ante-partum haemorrhage, prolonged labour and prolapse of the cord has already been mentioned in earlier sections of this book. It should be emphasised that in all these conditions the chief danger to the baby is *anoxia* which if not fatal at the time may result in permanent damage. There are, however, certain diseases which, if present in the mother during pregnancy, may affect the neonate in a very different way. Thus, he may either develop the disease itself or reveal abnormalities directly related to it but departing widely from its symptomatology in the adult. For this reason, when assessing the state of a baby at birth, details of the mother's medical history during pregnancy should always be available.

The principal conditions which may be transmitted directly to the baby either during pregnancy or immediately after birth are:

a *Syphilis.* A syphilitic mother who has not received adequate treatment may transmit the disease to her child who will then be born with Congenital Syphilis. Since treatment given during pregnancy will prevent this, the Wassermann and Kahn Reactions of all mothers must be tested antenatally. Where this has not been possible, these tests should be carried out immediately after delivery since the sooner the baby can be treated, the less the chance that it will suffer irreversible damage.

b *Tuberculosis.* Although a tuberculous mother is very unlikely to infect her child during pregnancy, this is not so after delivery, neonates being particularly susceptible to this disease. Babies of such mothers should therefore be separated from their parent at birth and given B.C.G. on the seventh day. Careful screening of other members of the family is also desirable before allowing the baby home.

c   Thyrotoxicosis. Mothers with uncontrolled thyrotoxicosis give birth to similarly affected babies, since thyroxin can cross the placenta. In such a case the baby may be extremely ill and may even develop cardiac failure, although rapid recovery is the rule. Normally, however, thyrotoxic mothers are under treatment with antithyroid drugs which, by crossing the placenta, give rise to a temporary hypothyroidism in the neonate.

Diseases causing abnormalities in the baby which differ from the symptoms they produce in the adult are:

a   Rubella. If a mother contracts Rubella in pregnancy, especially during the first ten to twelve weeks, the baby may be born with a number of abnormalities including cataract, deafness, microcephaly, mental retardation and cardiac defects as well as hepatic and splenic enlargement. In addition, the rubella virus can be detected in the respiratory tract and the urine of the neonate for several weeks after birth. As such babies are very infectious, midwives in charge of their care should avoid all contact with pregnant mothers.

b   Cytomegalic Inclusion Disease is caused by a virus transmitted from the mother during pregnancy. Although in an adult the disease is almost always mild, in the newborn it can assume a serious form, jaundice, petechial haemorrhages, enlargement of the liver and spleen and cerebral haemorrhage being its principal features.

c   Toxoplasmosis. In the adult this again is a mild illness. If transmitted to the foetus during pregnancy, however, it can cause severe cerebral damage, microcephaly, hydrocephaly and, rarely, jaundice, purpura and enlargement of the liver and the spleen.

d   Diabetes. Perinatal mortality and morbidity rates among the babies of diabetic mothers are above average. The incidence of congenital malformations is also raised. The babies tend to be overweight and are frequently lethargic and hard to rear. They are liable to Respiratory Distress Syndrome and to hypoglycaemia. Early feeding and frequent monitoring of the blood sugar are essential in these babies which, despite their weight must be considered to be high risk cases.

The Effect of Maternal Age

The older the mother, the greater the likelihood that the baby will suffer from Mongolism (Down's Syndrome). The risk that this particular abnormality will be present in the baby of a woman over forty is as high as one in sixty. Other genetic disturbances are also related to maternal age but these are rarely seen in the course of general midwifery practice.

Summary

Anoxia

Anoxia can be defined as lack of oxygen. In the newborn it may cause irreversible brain damage. Such damage may occur before or after birth.

The clinical signs of anoxia before delivery are alterations in the foetal heart rate, meconium staining of the liquor and a fall in the pH of the foetal scalp blood. After delivery anoxia is characterised by irregular or absent respirations, pallor or cyanosis, bradycardia, deficient muscle tone and a poor response to stimuli.

The Apgar Score is a useful way of evaluating the clinical state of the newborn.

The development of anoxia after birth may be prevented by adopting the following routine:

a   Remove excess mucus from mouth and nostrils

b   Record the Apgar Score at 1 and 5 minutes

c   Give Levallorphan if indicated

d   Give Vitamin K

e   Prevent a fall in the baby's temperature.

If the onset of respiration is delayed or if the baby's heart rate remains low, intubation and intermittent positive pressure ventilation are needed.

Trauma

Trauma sustained at birth may be major or minor. The chief disadvantage of minor trauma is that it may cause the mother unnecessary anxiety. This should always be foreseen. Major trauma, on the other hand, may result in the baby being permanently disabled.

The main varieties of trauma affecting the newborn are:
Caput succedaneum
Cephalhaematoma
Damage to the bony skeleton
Damage to peripheral nerves
Damage to the spinal cord
Damage to abdominal viscera
Damage to the brain.

Of these, damage to the brain is the most common. It is often irreversible. As no specific treatment is available, it is important to do everything possible to prevent its occurring during labour.

Jaundice

Jaundice, due to a rise in the level of the plasma bilirubin produced by the breakdown of red blood cells, is a useful index of disease in the newborn.

Due to the immaturity of the liver, all neonates develop some degree of physiological jaundice although this is apparent in only 50 per cent of cases.

The danger of a high level of bilirubin is that it may lead to a type of irreversible brain damage known as Kernicterus.

Physiological jaundice is more marked in prematurity, dehydration and starvation and occasionally when certain drugs have been given.

Haemolytic jaundice starts on the first day of life. It has three main causes: blood group incompatibility between the baby and the mother, abnormalities of the baby's red cells and infection.

Jaundice persisting beyond the tenth day is almost always abnormal. It may be due to congenital atresia of the bile ducts, hypothyroidism, congenital diseases of the baby or infection.

Whatever the reason for the jaundice, if the plasma bilirubin rises to a dangerous level exchange transfusion is the only effective means of treatment.

Infection

Owing to lack of antibody protection the newborn is particularly liable to develop an infection.

A neonate may have a serious infection and yet show few signs of illness.

Infection is an important cause of preventable mortality and morbidity in the newborn. Delay in diagnosis and treatment is specially dangerous.

A baby may become infected via the placenta, the liquor amnii or after birth.

Signs of an infection are lethargy, reluctance to feed, diarrhoea, vomiting, dehydration, weight loss, pallor, cyanosis, alterations in body temperature and hypoglycaemia.

The primary sites of infection are the skin, the liver, the gastro-intestinal tract, the blood stream, the meninges, the bones and the ears.

Common infections of the newborn are thrush, staphylococcal skin infections, paronychia, ophthalmia neonatorum, umbilical sepsis and epidemic gastroenteritis.

Infection can be prevented by careful and restricted handling of the newborn, prompt detection and isolation of infected carriers, staff or mothers and of any infected baby, and by strict attention to asepsis and antisepsis. In some cases where the baby is at special risk antibiotics are given prophylactically.

The Effect on the Baby of Maternal Diseases

Since several maternal diseases may be transmitted to the baby during pregnancy or immediately after delivery, the health of the mother must always be taken into account when assessing the condition of the neonate.

In some cases the disease is passed on to the baby in its usual form. Examples of this are syphilis, tuberculosis and thyrotoxicosis.

In other instances the baby may present symptoms which differ widely from those seen in the adult. The principal conditions producing this effect are rubella, cytomegalic inclusion disease, toxoplasmosis and diabetes.

Increasing maternal age is associated with a rising incidence of chromosomal abnormalities in the baby. The most common of these is Mongolism (Down's Syndrome).

Appendix 1

Obstetrical Definitions

The following is a list of definitions of some of the more common terms in use in present-day obstetrics.

Abortion
The ending of pregnancy before the twenty-eighth week, the foetus being born dead
Antepartum Haemorrhage
Bleeding from the birth canal after the twenty-eighth week until the birth of the baby

a *Accidental Antepartum Haemorrhage* Antepartum haemorrhage resulting from the separation of a normally situated placenta

b *Unavoidable Antepartum Haemorrhage* Antepartum haemorrhage from a Placenta Praevia

c *Incidental Antepartum Haemorrhage* Antepartum haemorrhage from a source other than the placental site

Asphyxia Neonatorum
A condition in which a living foetus fails to breathe within thirty seconds of birth although its heart is beating
Attitude of the Foetus
The relation of the various parts of the foetus to one another
Breech Presentation
A foetus which presents by the breech

a   *Extended Breech*   A breech presentation in which the foetal legs are extended

b   *Flexed Breech*   A breech presentation in which the foetal legs are flexed

Cervix: Full Dilatation
Where the cervix is sufficiently dilated to allow the presenting part, whether the head or the breech, to pass through
Cord: Presentation
Where the cord is in advance of the presenting part and the forewaters are intact
Cord: Prolapse
Where the cord is in advance of the presenting part and the forewaters are ruptured
Engagement of the Head
The head is engaged when the biparietal diameter is below the level of the pelvic brim
Hydramnios
A demonstrable excess of liquor amnii
Involution of the Uterus
The decrease in size of the uterus following labour or abortion
Labour
The process whereby the foetus and the placenta are expelled from the uterus via the birth canal

a   *Onset of Labour*   When the external os begins to dilate

b   *Normal Labour*   Labour lasting between two and twenty-four hours in which a living mature foetus presenting by the vertex is delivered without complications other than an episiotomy or a first or second degree perineal tear

c   *Premature Labour*   Labour resulting in the birth of a premature baby *d*   *Precipitate Labour*   Labour lasting less than two hours

e   *Prolonged Labour*   Labour lasting more than twenty-four hours

Lie of the Foetus
The relation of the long axis of the foetus to the long axis of the mother
Live Birth
A baby which has breathed
Lower Uterine Segment
That part of the uterus immediately above the internal cervical os which does not retract during labour
Malpresentation
Any presentation other than vertex
Maternal Mortality Rate
The number of mothers dying as a result of childbirth or abortion per 1000 total births
Multigravida
A woman pregnant for the second or subsequent time
Multipara
A woman bearing or having borne two or more viable children
Neonatal Mortality Rate
The number of babies dying during the neonatal period per 1000 live births
Neonatal Period
The first twenty-eight days of life after birth
Oedema
A demonstrable excess of extracellular tissue fluid
Pelvic Diameters

a   *True Conjugate*   The shortest distance between the sacral promontory and the back of the symphysis pubis

b   *Diagonal Conjugate*   The distance between the sacral promontory and the lower border of the symphysis pubis

Perinatal Death
A baby which is either stillborn or which dies during the first week of neonatal life

Perinatal Mortality Rate
The number of perinatal deaths per 1000 total births
Placenta Praevia
A placenta situated wholly or partially in the lower uterine segment
Post-partum Haemorrhage
Abnormal bleeding from the genital tract after the birth of the baby until the end of the puerperium

a   *Primary Post-partum Haemorrhage*   Blood loss of or over 500 ml occurring after the birth of the baby until twenty-four hours after the delivery of the placenta

b   *Secondary Post-partum Haemorrhage*   Abnormal blood loss from the genital tract occurring during the puerperium after the first twenty-four hours

Pregnancy
The state in which a fertilised ovum is embedded and growing in the maternal tissues
Prematurity
A state in which a baby weighs 2500 grammes or less at birth
Presentation

a   *Presentation during Pregnancy*   That part of the foetus lying nearest to the external cervical os

b   *Presentation during Labour*   That part of the foetus lowest in the birth canal

Primigravida
A woman pregnant for the first time
Primipara
A woman bearing or having borne her first viable child
Promontory of the Sacrum
The upper, anterior, border of the sacrum
Puerperium
The time taken for the uterus to involute, arbitrarily occupying six weeks
Show
The discharge of blood and mucus which often heralds the start of labour

Still-birth
A baby born at or after the twenty-eighth week which never shows any sign of life
Version
Turning the foetus in the uterus in order to substitute one presentation for another
Vertex
A lozenge-shaped area on the top of the foetal skull, bounded posteriorly by the posterior fontanelle, anteriorly by the anterior fontanelle and laterally by the parietal eminences
Vertex Presentation
Where the vertex is the presenting part
Viable Foetus
A foetus that has existed in the uterus for twenty-eight weeks or more.

Appendix 2

Instruments Required for Vaginal Obstetric Operations

1 Basic Equipment Needed for all Vaginal Obstetric Operations
   a Sterile Equipment
   Towels and Leggings
   Gown
   Sterile disposable gloves
   Lotion bowl containing 1/10,000 Hycoline or Hibitane
   Bowl for gauze swabs, tampon and pads
   Small bowl for obstetric cream
   Kidney dish
   2 pairs of swab holding forceps

   b Non-sterile Equipment
   Mackintosh sheet
   Catheters – plastic disposable
   Ampoules of Syntometrine, Syntocinon, Ergometrine
   Bottle of 0·5 per cent Lignocaine.

2 Special Instruments for Particular Procedures
   Artificial Rupture of the Membranes
   1 pair of sponge holders
   1 pair Kocher forceps

1 pair Smythe forceps
1 Drew-Smythe cannula
1 Sims speculum
1 20-oz measure

Suture of Perineum
1 × 20 ml sterile disposable syringe
1 × 2 ml sterile disposable syringe
1 No. 1 gauge needle
1 No. 12 gauge needle
4 pairs of straight 6-inch Spencer-Wells forceps
1 needle holder
1 pair of 6-inch toothed dissecting forceps
1 pair of 6-inch non-toothed dissecting forceps
1 pair of straight scissors
1 pair of sponge holders
2 towel clips
2 × ½ circle round bodied needles: No. 12
2 × ½ circle cutting needles: No. 12
Ampoules of No. 2/0, 0 and 1 20 day catgut
1 bobbin of black thread for skin suture

Suture of Cervix
As for perineal suture with additional:
4 pairs of 8-inch Spencer-Wells forceps
6 pairs of 12-inch swab holding forceps – for grasping edge
   of cervix

Manual Removal of Placenta
As for Perineal Suture with additional:
4 pairs of 8-inch Spencer-Wells forceps
2 pairs of 9-inch blunt-ended scissors
1 large receiver for placenta

Forceps Delivery
As for perineal suture with additional:
1 pair of 9-inch blunt-ended scissors
Obstetric Forceps: Wrigleys
                   Simpsons
                   Neville-Barnes – with traction handle
                   Kiellands
                   Milne-Murray.

N.B. Always ask the obstetrician what type of forceps he normally uses if in doubt about this. *Always* have ready Simpsons and Kiellands forceps.

Vacuum Extraction
As for forceps with in addition the 3 cups for attachment to Extractor Bottle
N.B. *Always* check bottle and pump connections. These need *not* be sterile.

Breech Delivery
As for Forceps Delivery

Twin Delivery
As for Forceps Delivery with additional:
1 pair of Kocher forceps for rupturing membranes of second sac
Extra set of straight 6-inch Spencer-Wells forceps

Appendix 3

Drugs Used in Obstetrics

For many of the compounds included in this list the amounts which may safely be given vary widely from case to case. The doses indicated below must therefore be regarded as only approximate.

British Pharmacopoeia titles are given in small print, proprietary titles are given in capitals.

Ia   Analgesics and Antipyretics not normally prescribed in labour
A.P.C. – Aspirin, Phenacetin and Codeine tablets. 1–2 four times a day
Aspirin 300 mg tablets. 1–3 four times a day
Codeine Phosphate 30 mg tablets. 1–2 three times a day
PANADOL (Paracetamol) 500 mg tablets. 2 three times a day.

Ib   Analgesics Usually Prescribed in Labour
FORTRAL (Pentazocine) 25 mg tablets. 1–4 as required
Pethidine 50 mg in 1 ml. 1–2 ml by injection
PETHILORPHAN (Pethidine 50 mg/Levallorphan 0·625 mg). 1–2 ml by injection
Morphine Sulphate 10 mg per ml. 1 ml by injection
OMNOPON (Papaveretum) 10 mg per ml. 1 ml by injection.

II   *Antibiotics and Sulphonamides*

ACHROMYCIN (Tetracycline) 250 mg capsules. 1 six-hourly

AUREOMYCIN (Chlortetracycline) 250 mg capsules. 1 six-hourly

CRYSTAMYCIN (Penicillin/Streptomycin). 1 vial daily by injection

TERRAMYCIN (Oxytetracycline) 250 mg capsules. 1 six-hourly

PENBRITEN (Ampicillin) 250 mg capsules. 1 six-hourly

Penicillin V 250 mg tablets. 2–6 daily in divided doses

MIDICEL (Sulphamethoxypyridazine) 500 mg tablets. 2–4 initially, 1 daily

SULPHAMEZATHINE (Sulphadimidine) 500 mg tablets. 2 initially, 1 six-hourly

UROLUCOSIL (Sulphamethizole) 100 mg tablets. 2 five times a day.

III   *Anti-coagulants*

Heparin 5000–10,000 units by injection – intravenous or intramuscular

DINDEVAN (Phenindione) 10 mg tablets. 5–100 mg daily

Warfarin 3 mg tablets. 3–10 mg daily

IV   *Antiemetics*

DEBENDOX Tablets. 2 at night, 1 or 2 by day

Cyclizine 50 mg tablets. $\frac{1}{2}$–1 as required

FENTAZIN (Perphenazine) Ampoules, 5 mg in 1 ml. 1 ml six- to eight-hourly

NIDOXITAL Tablets. 1 three to four times a day

VIBAZINE (Buclizine) 25 mg tablets. 2 at night, 1 in the morning.

V   *Diuretics*

Bendrofluazide 2·5 mg tablets. 1–4 daily

LASIX (Frusemide) 40 mg tablets. 1–3 daily, usually as a single dose

SALURIC (Chlorothiazide) 500 mg tablets. 1–2 daily.

VI   *Hypotensive Agents*

ALDOMET (Methyldopa) 250 mg tablets. 1–2 six-hourly

APRESOLINE (Hydrallazine) 25 mg tablets. 2–8 daily

INDERAL (Propranolol) 10 mg tablets. 1–3 times a day

ISMELIN (Guanethidine) 10 mg tablets. 1–2 daily, increasing
as necessary
PUROVERINE (Protoveratrine) 0·25 mg tablets. 1–4 two- to
four-hourly
SERPASIL (Reserpine) 0·25 mg tablets. 1–2 daily.

VII   Hypnotics and Tranquillisers
AMYTAL (Amylobarbitone) 15 mg tablets. 1–3 three times a
day
Chloral Mixture 5–20 ml. Two- to six-hourly
GARDENAL (Phenobarbitone) 15 mg tablets. 1–2 three times
a day
LARGACTIL (Chlorpromazine) 25 mg tablets. 1 three times a
day
NEMBUTAL (Pentobarbitone) 30 mg tablets. 1–2 at night
OBLIVON (Methylpentynol) 250 mg capsules. 2–4 daily
SONERYL (Butobarbitone) 100 mg tablets. 1–2 at night
SPARINE (Promazine) 25 mg tablets. 2 six-hourly
TRICHLORYL (Triclofos) 500 mg tablets. 2 six-hourly
WELLDORM (Dichloralphenazone) 650 mg tablets. 2 six-
hourly.

VIII   Hormone Preparations
PRIMOLUT DEPOT (Hydroxyprogesterone Caproate) 250 mg
per ml. 1 ml weekly
PRIMODOS (Norethisterone Acetate/Ethinyloestradiol). 1 tab-
let for two days
ORASECRON (Ethisterone/Ethinyloestradiol). 1 tablet five
times a day for two days
Hexoestrol 15 mg per ml. 1 ml by injection as required.

IX   Iron Preparations
Ferrous Gluconate. 300 mg tablets. 1 three times a day
Ferrous Sulphate. 200 mg tablets. 1 three times a day
FERSOLATE (Ferrous Sulphate with Copper and Manganese
added). 1 tablet three times a day
JECTOFER (Iron Sorbitol/Citric Acid) 1 ampoule daily by deep
injection.

X   Oxytocics
Ergometrine 0·5 mg per ml. 1 ml by injection

SYNTOCINON (Oxytocin) 5 units per ½ ml. ½ ml by injection
SYNTOMETRINE (Ergometrine 0·5 mg/Syntocinon 5 units).
1 ml by injection.

XI Vitamin Preparations
KONAKION (Vitamin K 10 mg per ml). 1 ml by injection
MULTIVITE (Mixture of Vitamins A, B, C and D). 2 tablets
three times a day
PREGNAVITE FORTE (Mixture of Vitamins A, B, C and D
with Iron and Calcium). 1 tablet three times a day
SYNKAVIT (Vitamin K, 10 mg per ml). 1 ml by injection.

XII Miscellaneous Preparations
BUTAZOLIDIN (Phenylbutazone) 100 mg tablets. 2 once or
twice daily
Carbachol 0·25 mg per ml. 1 ml by injection
Kaolin poultice
Ichthyol and Glycerine poultice.

Index

Index

Index